"This book is a testament to how powerful food can be in transforming your health. The combination of quick, delicious recipes and the latest nutritional science offers an invaluable resource for anyone looking to make positive changes to their diet."

— **Jenné Claiborne**, author of *Sweet Potato Soul*

"*Powered by Plants* contains quick, easy, and scrumptious recipes, combined with the latest nutritional science, to offer a road map to a healthier, happier you and a healthier, happier planet."

— **Joel Fuhrman, M.D.**, 7-time *New York Times* best-selling author and president of the Nutritional Research Foundation

"One of the greatest tools a woman has for balancing hormones is to eat more plants. I'm massively grateful for Ocean's and Nichole's dedication to providing us with unique, delicious recipes that make it effortless to incorporate plants into every meal."

— **Mindy Pelz, M.D.**, author of *Fast Like a Girl*

"In a world where fast food is the easy option, this book is a lifesaver. It shows you how to whip up nutritious, plant-based meals quickly, proving that healthy eating can fit into even the busiest of lifestyles. A must-read for anyone serious about boosting their energy and health."

— **Kris Carr**, *New York Times* best-selling author, wellness activist, and cancer thriver

"Ocean Robbins masterfully bridges science and our food choices in this brilliant cookbook. The easy-to-follow, delicious recipes, backed by the latest scientific evidence, empower us to nourish our bodies and prevent chronic diseases. We wholeheartedly recommend this essential guide for anyone committed to vibrant living and sustaining a healthy future for our planet."

— **Drs. Dean and Ayesha Sherzai**, neuroscientists and best-selling authors of *The Alzheimer's Solution*

"An essential guide for anyone looking to improve their health through diet. The scientific credibility of the nutritional advice, combined with delicious and easy recipes, makes this book a must-have for my patients—and anyone interested in a plant-based lifestyle."

— **Joel Kahn, M.D., FACC**, founder of the Kahn Center for Cardiac Longevity

"*Powered by Plants* isn't just a cookbook; it's a prescription for vitality. As a physician, I prescribe its nutrient-loaded 30-minute meals to patients seeking delicious ways to achieve better health. With each dish, you'll not only be enjoying tasty, satisfying food, you'll be powering up your body's natural defenses. So, eat well, live well, and thrive with this great plant-powered guide!"

— **Michael Klaper, M.D.**, author of *Vegan Nutrition: Pure and Simple*

POWERED BY PLANTS

POWERED BY PLANTS

NUTRIENT-LOADED 30-MINUTE MEALS TO HELP YOU THRIVE

OCEAN ROBBINS
CO-FOUNDER AND CEO OF FOOD REVOLUTION NETWORK

AND NICHOLE DANDREA-RUSSERT, MS, RDN

HAY HOUSE

HAY HOUSE LLC
Carlsbad, California • New York City
London • Sydney • New Delhi

Published in the United States by: Hay House LLC: www.hayhouse.com®
Published in Australia by: Hay House Australia Publishing Pty Ltd: www.hayhouse.com.au
Published in the United Kingdom by: Hay House UK Ltd: www.hayhouse.co.uk
Published in India by: Hay House Publishers (India) Pvt Ltd: www.hayhouse.co.in

Indexer: J S Editorial, LLC
Cover design and interior: Julie Davison
Recipe photos: Angela MacNeil Photography
Photos on pages vii–84: Images used under license from Shutterstock.com

Cataloging-in-Publication Datais on file at the Library of Congress

Hardcover ISBN: 978-1-4019-7856-3
E-book ISBN: 978-1-4019-7857-0
Audiobook ISBN: 978-1-4019-7858-7

10 9 8 7 6 5 4 3 2 1
1st edition, October 2024

Printed in China

To your health!

And to the joy of being part of the solution on planet Earth.

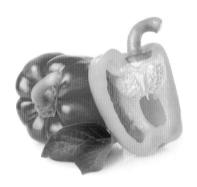

CONTENTS

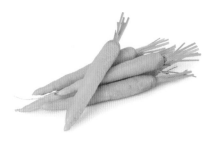

Introduction xiii

PART I: NOTABLE NUTRIENTS

CHAPTER 1   Protein 3

CHAPTER 2   Fiber 15

CHAPTER 3   Omega-3 Fatty Acids 23

CHAPTER 4   Selenium 31

CHAPTER 5   Zinc 37

CHAPTER 6   Iron 43

CHAPTER 7   Magnesium 51

CHAPTER 8   Calcium 59

CHAPTER 9   Supplements and
Other Key Nutrients 65

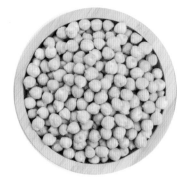

PART II: RECIPES

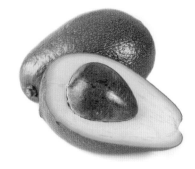

BREAKFASTS

Three-Grain Peaches and Cream
Breakfast Bowl 90

Berrylicious Poppy Seed Pancakes 92

Banana Bliss Chocolate Chip
Millet Muffins 94

Simply Savory Polenta and Greens
Breakfast Bowl 96

Rise 'n' Shine Breakfast Hash 98

Wrapped in Wellness Tofu Scramble 100

Morning Zen Buckwheat Muesli 102

SALADS

Bright and Lively Citrus Salad 106

Delightfully Creamy Avocado Salad
with Maple Tahini Dressing 108

Under the Italian Sun-Dried Tomato,
Cannellini, and Spinach Salad 110

Super Greens and Beans
Detox Salad 112

Perfectly Balanced 15-Minute
Pasta Salad 114

Creamy Almond Meets
Crunchy Slaw 116

Lettuce Go to the Farmers
Market Salad 118

Crunchy Southwest Salad with Zingy
Lime Dressing 120

Pea-Nuts about You
Thai Millet Salad 122

Yummy Tabbouleh Salad 124

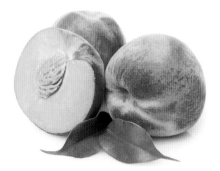

SOUPS AND STEWS

Simple and Savory Buckwheat Soup 128

A Bowl of Goodness Tortilla Soup 130

Creamy and Cozy Veggie Ramen 132

Nourish and Thrive Immune
     Support Soup 134

Creamy Dreamy Mushrooms, Greens,
     and Beans Soup 136

Buttery Vegan Corn Chowder 138

Sip and Shine Asparagus Soup 140

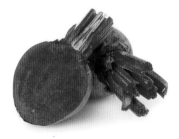

BOWLS

Purple Paradise Power Bowl 144

The Ultimate Loaded Mashed
     Potato Bowl 146

Bountiful Bulgur Bowl with Savory
     Orange Vinaigrette 148

Zesty Fiesta Mushroom Lentil Chorizo
     Taco Bowl 150

Deconstructed Sushi Bowl 152

Fantastically Fermented Natto
     Black Rice Bowl 154

Sweet On You Chili Broccoli and
     Tofu Bowl 156

Sweet Potato Lentil Bowl with Silky
     Green Tahini Sauce 158

SANDWICHES, WRAPS, AND PIZZA

Meet Me in the Mediterranean Tortilla
     Pizza with Tofu Ricotta 162

Smothered in Tzatziki Tempeh Gyro 164

Turn Up the Beet Burger with Smashed
     Avocado and Pickled Onions 166

Seoul-ful TLT with Pickled Veggies and
     Spicy Mayo 168

It's Slice to Meet You Plant-Powered
     Pesto Pizza 170

Sweet 'n' Smoky BBQ Tempeh
     Collard Wrap 172

Smashed Avocado
     Chickpea Salad Wrap 174

Pile 'Em High Pad Thai Tofu Burgers 176

Rolled Up with Love Vegetable Temaki
     Hand Roll 178

Garden of Goodness Sandwich 180

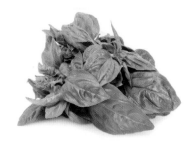

TACOS AND TOSTADAS

Banh Mi Oh My
   Vietnamese-Inspired Tacos 184

Clean Out the Pantry Everyday Tacos 186

Asparagus and Black Bean
   Tasty Tostadas 188

Air Fryer Crunchy Chickpea and
   Cauliflower Tacos 190

Warm and Smoky White Bean and
   Spinach Flautas 192

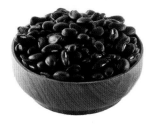

NOODLES

Veggielicious Mac 'n' Cheese 196

YUM-ami Cacio e Pepe 198

Miso Zen Spicy Noodle Bowl 200

Living and Thriving Zucchini Noodles
   with Raw Marinara Sauce 202

Presto Pesto Pasta 204

Zesty Ginger Soba Noodle Salad 206

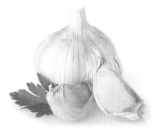

ONE-POT MEALS

A Taste of Africa Fonio Pilaf 210

All-In-One Mexicali Quinoa 212

Pot-to-Plate Tempeh Sausage Pasta 214

Wholesome 'n' Hearty One-Pot
   Farro Roma 216

Give Me 10 Minutes to Prep Chili 218

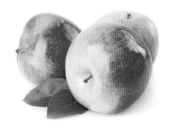

BLENDED MEALS

Apple Pie for Breakfast Smoothie 222

Island Time Kiwi Cooler 224

Wrap Me in Comfort Cold
   Brew Smoothie 226

Golden Sunrise Smoothie 228

Beets 'n' Berries Smoothie Bowl 230

Morning Motivator Spiced Shake 232

Sweet Pumpkin Spice and Everything
   Nice Smoothie Bowl 234

Appendix 237

Endnotes 247

Index 265

Acknowledgments 275

About the Authors 277

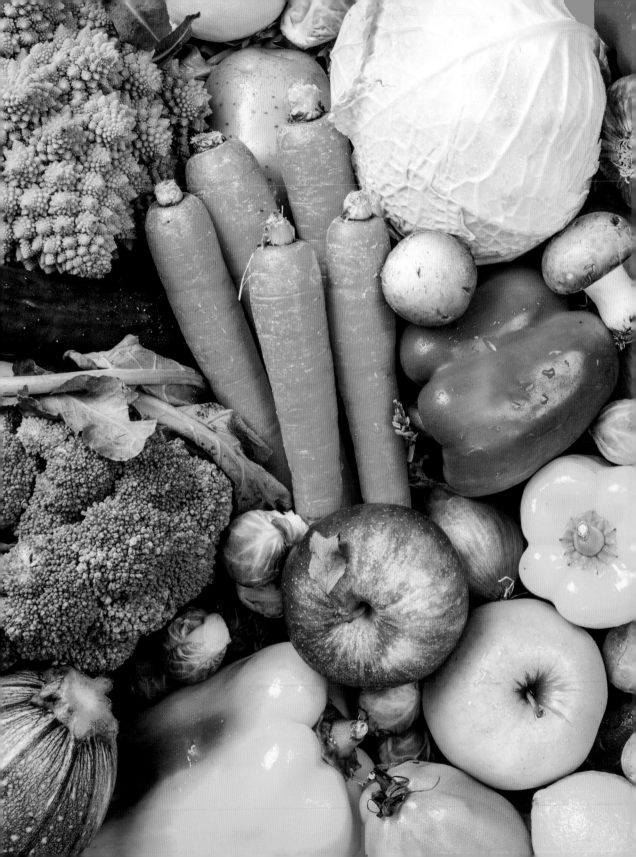

INTRODUCTION

My great-uncle Burt should have been the world's happiest man. He was an incredibly successful entrepreneur who had amassed something of a fortune. He had a family he loved and work that lit him up. And boy, did he love food—especially the modern American diet of burgers, pizzas, fries, sodas, and a double scoop of ice cream for dessert. Sadly, he died of a heart attack at the young age of 54, leaving his wife a widow and his kids fatherless.

His business partner and brother-in-law (and my grandfather), Irv, appeared to be heading down the same road. He also adored the modern American diet and by his early 70s suffered from diabetes, heart disease, and weight problems. His cardiologist told him that his days were numbered and that only radically changing what he ate could possibly relieve his suffering and avert a premature death.

Irv decided to live. He reduced his consumption of processed foods and cut back on meat. He put a lot more fruits and veggies on his plate. And most amazing of all, he gave up sugar, and with it his beloved ice cream. The results came quickly; Irv lost 30 pounds, got off his diabetes and hypertension meds, and felt a renewed surge of energy. He started walking, and soon was up to several miles a day. His golf game improved. He lived for 19 more years and got to meet my children (his great-grandchildren). And by all accounts, he had a heck of a good time.

Burt and Irv's contrasting stories illustrate the old saying: A person with their health has a thousand dreams. But a person without it has just one dream—to get it back.

According to the United Nations, preventable, chronic illness prematurely takes the lives of more than 41 million people every year.[1] And I want to emphasize the word *preventable* here. Because the wonderful truth is that most of the chronic diseases that are threatening our lives and taking our loved ones don't have to happen. They may look inevitable, like Uncle Burt's early demise, but Grandpa Irv's experience shows that we have a lot more power over our health destiny than we've been led to believe.

The evidence shows that the number one factor that can bend the odds in our favor is the food on our plates.[2] Credible researchers tell us that with a healthy diet and lifestyle, we can prevent at least 80 percent of cardiovascular disease[3] and 90 percent of type 2 diabetes.[4]

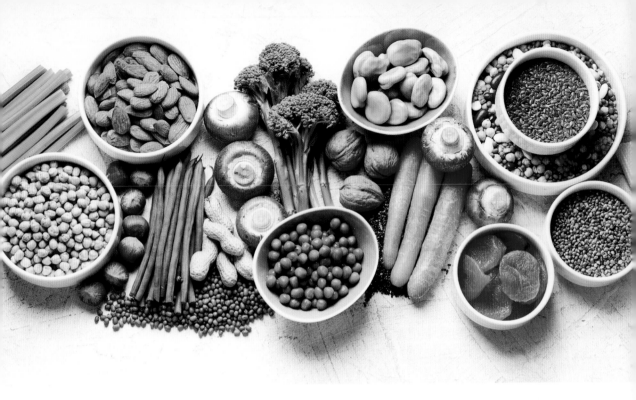

And dietary changes alone have been shown to reduce risk of Alzheimer's by 53 percent.[5]

When I think about a joyful life, I think about both the quality and quantity of years. Thousands of studies published in peer-reviewed medical journals make it abundantly clear that when you move away from a diet based around factory-farmed animal products, ultraprocessed foods, added sugars, and chemical additives, and instead base your diet on real, whole, plant foods, you can radically extend your life span, and perhaps even more importantly, your health span.

The good news is, it's never too late to make a shift and start reaping benefits. In fact, a recent meta-analysis found that shifting from a typical diet to an optimized diet (which happens to be plant-rich) and incorporating more legumes, nuts, and whole grains—even as late as age 60—can still add eight healthy years of life. And if you start earlier, you add even more.[6]

Why Eat More Plants?

There are many dietary patterns that can be significant improvements over the modern industrialized diet. You don't have to go "vegan" to get some big benefits to your health. But there are some compelling reasons to move in a solidly if not exclusively plant-based direction.

For one, most of the longest-lived people on the planet eat largely plant-based diets. Residents of the "Blue Zones," regions of the world with the highest concentrations of centenarians (those who live to 100 or more), all consume large quantities of whole plant foods, including vegetables, grains, and legumes.[7]

One big reason for the impact a healthy plant-based diet has on life expectancy has to do with the harmful effects of dietary saturated fat—which is found almost exclusively in meat, dairy, and eggs. Consuming saturated fats has been linked to increased risk of high LDL ("bad") cholesterol, cardiovascular disease, chronic inflammation (which itself is a contributing factor to pretty much every other chronic disease), weight gain and obesity, Alzheimer's disease, and multiple sclerosis.[8] Only two common plant-based ingredients, coconut oil and palm oil, deliver any meaningful quantities of saturated fats.[9]

Another key factor that partly explains the positive health effects of a whole-food, plant-based diet is fiber. Animal-derived foods do not contain this vital nutrient (which we'll meet in detail in Chapter 2), and the number of people who are chronically fiber-deficient is staggering; the most recent statistics published by the U.S. Department of Agriculture reveal that 94 percent of Americans aren't getting an adequate daily dose of dietary fiber.[10]

Plant-based diets have also been shown to reduce the risk of developing two of the world's deadliest diseases:[11] type 2 diabetes[12] and cancer.[13]

Environmental Impact

There are many environmental benefits to eating mostly plants, including significantly reducing[14] your carbon footprint to combat planetary climate chaos,[15] saving groundwater (especially in places where millions-year-old aquifers are on the verge of depletion[16]), and preserving oceans that can support marine life.[17] Globally, the production of meat and dairy products uses 83 percent of the world's agricultural land to produce just 18 percent of the world's calories. When you eat lower on the food chain, you help save soil, land, water, and ecosystems.[18] Plant-based diets allow for far more efficient land use, which can combat world hunger and promote economic justice for the most vulnerable humans.[19] Shifting from an omnivore to a plant-based diet could also significantly curb greenhouse gas emissions.

Quite simply, adopting a plant-based diet could be the most potent single step any of us can take to contribute to a more sustainable human presence on Earth, and to leave a better legacy for future generations.

Ethical Considerations

The vast majority of animals killed to feed humans are raised in factory farms that deny these creatures their freedom, physical and emotional health, and full life span. Many never see the sun or a blade of grass in their entire lives. You don't have to be a vegetarian, or an "animal rights person," to be appalled by the conditions in modern factory farms—and to choose not to support them with your dollars. While there is controversy about exactly how much better "cage-free," "free-range," and "grass-fed" really are, there's no doubt that a plant-based diet can lead to far less animal cruelty. Many people feel good about themselves when they make this choice.[20]

Will This Really Work for *You*?

If you're plant-based, or you're thinking about moving in that direction, you might worry about whether you need meat to get enough protein, dairy to get enough calcium, or fish to get enough omega-3 fatty acids. You might have heard the research telling us that micronutrients like zinc and iodine, and some vitamins like A and B_{12}, are easier to source from animal-derived foods.

I wrote this book to make healthy eating simple. Not as simple as "just eat lots of plants and you'll be fine" or "take these twelve expensive daily supplements and you can eat anything you want." In this book we're going to step away from all the hype, marketing, and dogma. Instead, we'll dig into the helpful truths that can help you optimize your diet in your real-world, everyday life. We'll discover that you can thrive without animal-derived food and you don't necessarily need lots of supplements to get the nutrients you need.

Healthy eating can be simple when you understand which key nutrients are often lacking in modern diets (I call them "notable nutrients") and how to get them in sufficient quantities from easy-to-find sources.

What Are the "Notable Nutrients"?

The big nutritional debates of our time (or at least the ones that are most often shouted about on social media) focus on what are called macronutrients: protein, fat, and carbohydrates. These are the nutrients in food that provide the energy we need to stay alive.

But it's the essential micronutrients (vitamins and minerals) that many people end up deficient in, as well as dietary fiber. When going plant-based, it's also important to be aware of omega-3 fatty acid food sources. And while most people eating a modern industrial diet get plenty of protein, we sometimes see folks getting insufficient protein when they shift to a plant-based diet—not because plants don't provide enough protein, but because people are oftentimes unsure how to replace the meat, eggs, and dairy on their plate.

These are the building blocks of our cells; the components of the chemicals that transmit messages between our cells, tissues, and organs; and the catalysts for critical biological processes. They allow our bodies to maintain health in an ever-changing environment. Getting enough of these essential nutrients is crucial for growth, maintenance, and repair. If you don't have enough of one or more of them, the quality of your health (and your life) can be diminished. At worst, deficiencies can even be life-threatening. That's why these are the "notable nutrients."

What about Supplements?

If these notable nutrients are so important, shouldn't we just take supplements to make sure we get enough of all of them? Many people take this approach, and in some cases it isn't without merit. But it brings a few problems. For one thing, the supplement market isn't well regulated, and it's quite possible that the dosage on the packaging is far lower or higher than what is in the actual product.

In fact, there are countless cases of independent labs finding that a particular product doesn't contain *any* of its supposed active ingredients.[21] Even worse, some supplements have been found to be contaminated with lead, cadmium, aluminum, and other harmful substances. Even if you find a supplement that's rigorously and regularly tested by an external lab, and you feel confident it contains exactly what's on the label and nothing more, that still doesn't mean it is the way to go. That's because nutrients in supplement form rarely work the same way they do when we get them from whole foods.

For example, scientists can synthesize or extract lycopene (the key antioxidant responsible for many of the health benefits of a tomato) and put it into a pill, but the lycopene found in the actual tomato works together with thousands of other compounds, creating a whole that is much greater, more complex, and ultimately more beneficial than the sum of its parts.

This has real implications for health. There have been several famous instances where nutrients that are known to be beneficial when we consume them from food actually harmed people who took them in supplemental form. One example is vitamin E, a poster child for supplementation gone wrong. A study published in 1993 in the *New England Journal of Medicine* found a significant relationship between vitamin E intake from food and lower risk of cardiovascular disease in women.[22] As a result, supplement makers immediately started marketing vitamin E capsules and processed food

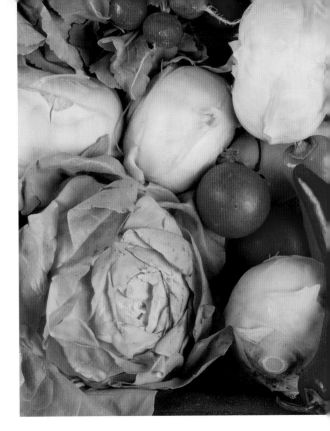

manufacturers began fortifying their products with vitamin E.

When researchers looked for benefits from this supplementation, they came up empty. Vitamin E in supplemental form didn't show evidence of lowered risk for any of the conditions it could prevent when consumed from food: cardiovascular diseases, cancer, diabetes, cataracts, and chronic obstructive lung disease.[23] Not only that, but the people who took vitamin E supplements were actually more likely to die (researchers like to call it "all cause mortality") than those taking a placebo.[24]

The same thing happened when researchers put beta-carotene supplements to the test.[25] One study of almost 30,000 Finnish smokers showed that beta-carotene supplements, which were supposed to help prevent cancer,

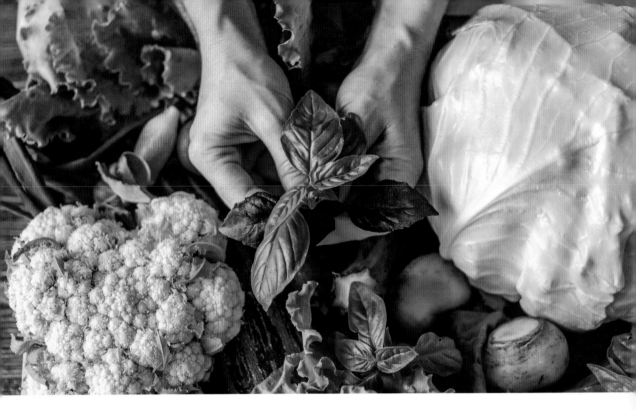

increased cancer risk by 8 percent in the group taking it.[26]

This isn't true of all nutrients, however. Not all supplementation is bad. There are some instances where certain people will derive benefits from supplemental beta-carotene, vitamin E, and other nutrients. Even so, the takeaway from these examples is that the best way to get nutrients is usually not from pills but from food.

What about Depleted Soil?

Many people believe that modern industrialized agriculture is producing crops that are so nutrient-deficient that we can no longer rely on food to meet our nutritional needs. I'll be the first to agree that modern industrialized agriculture has some huge problems: The overuse of synthetic fertilizers and toxic pesticides is harmful to farmworkers and to our soil, air, and water. And there is reliable data[27] showing that today's fruits and vegetables may be less nutrient-dense than those eaten by previous generations.

But here's the thing: current research still shows awesome health benefits from eating lots of plant foods. Even though plants may not be as loaded with nutrients as they once were, they're still the best option we have for getting the nutrients our bodies need. In fact, I'd go so far as to argue that soil depletion is a reason to eat an even more plant-forward diet. A generation ago, folks who got 50 percent of their calories from processed foods could likely get away with it because the plants they did eat provided the recommended amounts of key nutrients. But with the less nutritious crops of today, we can't afford to dilute our diets with poor-quality fare. Now more than ever, it makes sense to go for the healthiest foods we can access.

Can You Really Get the Nutrients You Need on a Plant-Based Diet?

It's true that some nutrients are more easily sourced from animals than plants. For some people, that's proof that plant-based diets are inferior, or even unnatural. It's also true that you could construct a vegan diet that is nutritionally inadequate, particularly if you're eating lots of vegan processed foods (I'm looking at you, French fries and donuts!). With the newfound popularity of plant-based meat and cheese alternatives, it's easier than ever to be vegan and never touch an actual vegetable— and be nutrient-poor.

Of course, that's also true of omnivorous diets that include animal products.

If, however, your plant-based diet mainly consists of whole foods—that is, as close to their natural state as possible—with lots of vegetables in the mix, you can get the vast majority of your nutrients from food with no need for animal products or supplements.

The first half of this book will introduce you to the notable nutrients that can determine your health status. There are, of course, many nutrients that are essential to your well-being, but the ones we are going to cover are most relevant to those eating a largely or wholly plant-based diet. These nutrients are of concern to omnivores as well—especially people who aren't eating a lot of fruits, vegetables, whole grains, beans, nuts, and seeds.

In the first nine chapters, you'll discover which plant-based foods are the best sources of these nutrients. We'll include taking a hard, science-based look at some nutrients that even the healthiest diets might be lacking and offer suggestions for both food and supplemental forms of these nutrients.

The second half of this book contains recipes to help you put your knowledge into action where it counts: in your kitchen. You'll find dozens of easy and delicious recipes that include the foods and ingredients richest in notable nutrients. You won't find these anywhere else—they're all originals cooked up (pun totally intended) by Food Revolution Network's Lead Dietitian Nutritionist and recipe developer extraordinaire, Nichole Dandrea-Russert, RDN.

Each of these recipes is designed to make you fall in love with delicious foods that actually love you back. (Requited dietary love is a beautiful thing!) And in today's busy world, even the most delicious dishes aren't going to get made if they take too long. That's why we have prioritized making them fast and easy. Most of the recipes in this book can be prepared in 30 minutes or less!

So whether you're a seasoned, card-carrying vegan (actually, I don't think there is a card), want to become more plant-based, or just love taking care of your health, this book will guide you to get the nutrients your body needs from foods your mouth will adore.

Ready to jump in? Let's do this.

PART I

NOTABLE NUTRIENTS

CHAPTER 1

PROTEIN

About 25 years ago, I started working out with my dad. He'd been working out for a few years already, so he was stronger than I was. I thought to myself, *Well, I'll catch him soon, because Father Time has a way with everyone. Everyone's muscles deteriorate with age.*

Now, I'm the age he was when we started—and he still lifts more weight than I do on every single piece of gym equipment. He's actually getting stronger, setting personal records at age 76. My new goal is to surpass him in strength before he hits 100, and I'm not entirely confident about achieving it.

So what's going on? Is he some kind of genetic freak? (If so, then presumably so am I.) Is he just lucky? Or is his remarkable strength at the age when many people become increasingly feeble the result of his dietary and lifestyle choices?

It's easy to rule out genetics; his own father—my grandpa, Irv Robbins—was diagnosed with type 2 diabetes and headed toward early death when his cardiologist recommended a book about the link between lifestyle and disease called *Diet for a New America* (which, in one of life's great ironies, was authored by his son—my dad—John Robbins). And luck? Well, I wouldn't call it lucky that my father contracted polio as a child, spent time in a wheelchair, and struggled with serious disabilities for much of his early years—and in fact seriously struggles with post-polio syndrome, or PPS, today.

So that leaves diet and lifestyle, which is what I'm betting on. We know that muscles are built in the gym, not the kitchen, so obviously my dad's commitment to lifting weights was key to his strength and physique. (And in

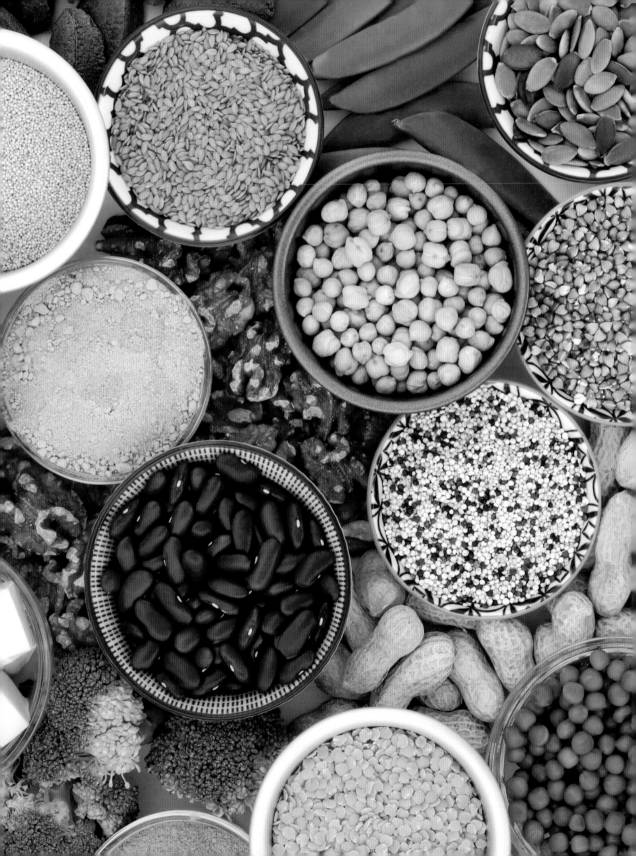

all candor, he does spend considerably more time in the gym than I do, although in my defense, I spend a good deal more time typing on the computer, and that really should count for something.) But in terms of the longevity of his strength into an age when most people are rapidly losing muscle mass, the workouts don't explain everything. Researchers at Baylor University found that the average life span of a professional male bodybuilder is just 47 years[1]—at that age, my dad had barely even started pumping iron.

So what about diet? What role did it play, not just in his getting strong in his 50s but getting stronger well into his 70s?

The conventional wisdom among people who care about big, strong muscles is that it's really important to consume lots of protein. And this makes sense: protein is an essential nutrient for the building, maintenance, and repair of almost all the tissues in your body, including your bones, blood, hair, nails, organs, and muscles. In our modern world, protein is often considered the most important nutrient. This may have started with the macronutrient's naming by a Dutch chemist, Gerhard Johannes Mulder, who discovered it in 1839.[2] Mulder was so taken by the role of protein in sustaining life that he dubbed it *protéine* in French, from the Greek *prōteios*, meaning "of prime importance."

These days, the word *protein* has become more or less synonymous with animal protein, or meat. That's why everyone who has ever gone vegetarian or vegan has to deal with *The Question* over and over again: "Where do you get your protein?"

Taken together, these two beliefs—that protein is the most important nutrient for health and that you get it from animal products—mean that many people who eat plant-forward diets worry about being protein-deficient. In response to that worry, two plant-based camps have emerged: the "supplement vigorously" crowd and the "don't worry about it" faction.

Those who advocate gulping protein supplements by the smoothie-load express concern that plants are low in protein compared to rich sources like beef, chicken, and fish. Even if you can technically meet your RDA (recommended dietary allowance) with plant-based proteins, they aren't as readily absorbed as proteins from meat. And while the notion of "complete protein" is a bunch of hogwash (every single one of the amino acids that make up protein is found in every whole plant food), it is possible to be deficient in specific amino acids if your total protein consumption is close to the line.

People who dismiss protein-deficiency concerns in plant-based eaters argue that plants have plenty of protein—after all, that's where the strongest and largest land animals, like gorillas and elephants, get all their protein. Many plants are richer in protein (as a percentage of calories) than animal products, and most of the building blocks of proteins in our body are recycled with an efficiency that would make Henry Ford jealous.

So what's the truth? Can people get the protein they need entirely from plant-based sources without needing to supplement? Is more protein always better, and does the source of the protein matter?

In this chapter we'll look closely at protein: what it is, what it's made of, what our bodies do with it, and where it comes from. We'll investigate the latest science—rigorous studies using precise measurements—to inform our protein intake requirements.

After all, getting this right is of "prime importance" if I want to live long enough and get strong enough to bench press more than my dad.

What Is Protein?

Your body needs protein to build, maintain, and repair just about all its tissues—but there's much more to it than that. Protein can also provide energy to your body. Consuming it helps reduce hunger and cravings, and boosts your metabolism.

Symptoms of protein deficiency include the following:[3]

- Weakness and fatigue
- Slow healing of wounds
- Frequent infections
- Thinning hair or hair loss
- Brittle nails
- Dry skin
- Swelling of the hands, feet, and legs (edema)
- Increased susceptibility to bone fractures
- Poor concentration
- Muscle wasting and loss of muscle mass
- Mood swings, depression, and anxiety

- Stunted growth in children
- Hunger and cravings for protein-rich foods

In terms of structure, protein is made up of building blocks called amino acids. Your body requires 20 different amino acids to function optimally, but since it can synthesize 11 of them on its own, there are 9 so-called "essential" amino acids that you can get only from food or supplements. (For children, there's technically a tenth essential amino acid, since young mammals can't make arginine themselves and must get it from their diets.)[4]

If you're seeking to remember the nine essential amino acids, you might find the acronym PVT TIM HALL (or "Private Tim Hall") helpful. It's a mnemonic medical students use to recall phenylalanine, valine, threonine, tryptophan, isoleucine, methionine, histidine, arginine, leucine, and lysine when cramming for their Biochemistry 101 exams.

How Much Protein Do You Need?

This is best explained by two different but related questions. The first is about your total protein requirements, and the second is about getting enough of each of the PVT TIM HALL amino acids. Let's tackle the first question first.

Total Protein Requirements

The official daily RDA of protein is 56 grams for adult men and 46 grams for adult women. These calculations are based on the Food and

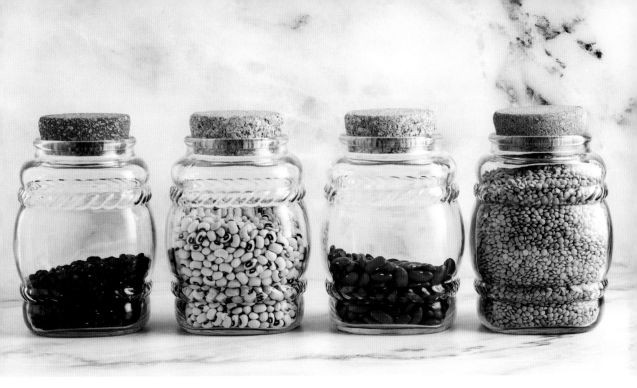

Nutrition Board of the National Academy of Sciences target recommendation of 0.36 grams of protein for every pound of body weight.[5] (Leave it to Americans to use the metric system for weighing nutrients and the imperial system for weighing ourselves.) For example, a 150-pound man aiming for 0.36 grams of protein for each pound of his body weight would need almost 56 grams of protein per day. A 120-pound woman would require closer to 43 grams per day.

A few words about these numbers. First, the RDA represents a level that should deliver enough protein for around 98 percent of the population,[6] meaning that for most people, it may be enough. Second, your protein needs may vary based on a variety of factors unique to you, including your weight, your level of physical activity, the amount of physical or emotional stress you're experiencing, whether you're pregnant or lactating, and your age. Let's look more closely at these factors below.

Weight

Bigger bodies need more protein for several reasons. Since protein is vital for the maintenance, repair, and growth of tissues, heavier individuals have more tissue and require more protein for their body's upkeep. Larger individuals often have a higher metabolic rate, meaning they burn more calories, even at rest. Protein can help meet their increased energy needs. Protein can also promote satiety, helping with weight management.

Physical Activity

The more wear and tear your body experiences, the greater the turnover of amino acids and the higher the intake needed to replace them. And

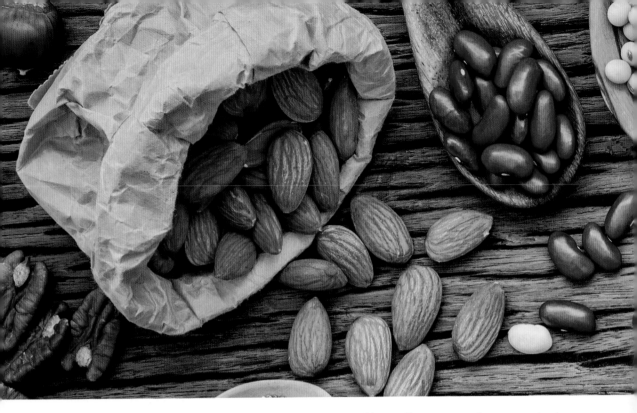

if you're an athlete trying to build muscle, you need extra protein to form those larger traps, quads, pecs, and buns of steel.

Stress

During periods of stress, the body's metabolic rate increases. This leads to a more rapid turnover of proteins in the body, increasing the need for dietary protein to replace what's been used. Stress, especially physical stress from an injury or illness, can lead to tissue damage. Proteins are essential for tissue repair and regeneration; hence, the body's requirement for protein increases when it's stressed.

Stress can also lead to hormonal changes, especially an increase in cortisol, a hormone that can lead to muscle breakdown. To counteract this, the body needs more protein to help preserve muscle mass.

Additionally, proteins play a crucial role in the immune system. During periods of stress, the immune system works harder, which can increase the body's demand for protein.

Pregnancy and Lactation

Pregnant and lactating women require more protein to keep themselves and their children healthy. During pregnancy the fetus grows and develops using nutrients sourced from the mother's body. Protein is a crucial building block for this development, especially for the baby's brain and other organs.

During pregnancy and breastfeeding, a woman's body undergoes considerable changes and growth. Additional protein is required to support physical changes like the enlargement of the uterus and the development of the placenta. Proteins are essential components of red blood cells, and more protein is needed to allow for a pregnant woman's blood plasma to increase by up to 50 percent. Lactating women need additional protein to produce breast milk, which in turn provides the baby with nutrients essential for growth and development.

And since protein plays a vital role in the immune function, higher protein intake can help a pregnant or breastfeeding woman maintain a strong immune system to keep herself and her baby healthy.

Age

There are a few reasons why older adults may require more protein. Muscle mass tends to decrease with age in a process known as *sarcopenia* (a word whose Greek origin means, vividly, "impoverished flesh"), and protein helps maintain and rebuild muscle. Also, extra protein can help slow the rate of bone loss and decrease the risk of fractures.

As people age, their immune function naturally declines, and a higher protein intake can help support immune health. Protein is also critical for wound healing and recovery from illness. Since older adults might experience longer recovery times, greater protein intake can support this process.

Older adults tend not to absorb protein as efficiently due to changes in metabolism or to digestive issues. Research suggests that protein requirements may be higher in older adults, and some experts recommend .5 to .6 grams of protein per pound of body weight.[7] Seniors may also eat less than when they were younger and so need more protein to compensate for their decreased consumption.

How Much Protein Is Enough for Folks Who Need More?

The Mayo Clinic recommends that folks under great stress and pregnant and lactating women consume 0.45 grams of protein per pound of body weight per day. That's 113 grams for someone weighing 250 pounds and 70 grams for a 155-pound non-senior adult experiencing a lot of stress or hitting the gym hard (or both). If a 120-pound woman is pregnant, her requirement jumps from 43 to 54 daily grams of protein. And they suggest anyone over the age of 65 should get between 0.5 and 0.6 grams of daily protein per pound of body weight.[8] That comes out to roughly 75 to 93 grams for a 155-pound senior citizen.

DAILY PROTEIN REQUIREMENTS

Athletes	1.4 to 2.0 grams per kilogram per day
Pregnant and Lactating (all ages)	71 grams per day
People over 65	.5 to .6 grams per pound per day

As we'll see below, plant-based eaters may want to increase these targets by about 10 percent.

Essential Amino Acid Requirements

Total protein deficiency is extremely rare in people who are consuming enough calories to avoid starvation mode. Medical professionals in the industrialized world read about symptoms of protein deficiency in textbooks and case studies, but they almost never see them in their practices. One reason is that, as I mentioned earlier, your body is really good at recycling amino acids from proteins that your digestive system has already broken down.

That said, if you don't get enough total protein, the deficiency of certain specific amino acids will likely impact you before total protein deficiency does. There are a few essential amino acids that tend to be harder to get from a plant-based diet—most notably lysine, methionine, and tryptophan. If you get enough total protein in your diet and it comes from a variety of sources, you should be fine. But that's another reason for plant-based eaters to aim for over the minimum intake to be safe. The alternative—tracking your consumption of individual amino acids—isn't my idea of a fun way to spend the day.

For example, while lysine concentrations are lower in plants than in animals, there are a number of plant foods that are particularly rich sources, such as pumpkin seeds, tofu, lentils, almonds, navy beans, quinoa, and cauliflower.[10]

Is Animal Protein Superior to Plant Protein?

Even if you can hit your recommended protein intake numbers (for both total protein and for each of the essential amino acids) from only plants, there's a misconception out there that you still must carefully combine plant-based protein sources to get the right combination of amino acids at every meal. This idea originated in research from the early 1900s showing that baby rats grew better on a meat diet than on one composed of plants.[11] The myth that foods of animal origin are "complete" proteins, while plant proteins are "incomplete" was popularized with the publication of *Diet for a Small Planet* in 1971. This myth has been thoroughly debunked. Every plant food contains all nine essential amino acids, so no combining is needed. If you're eating plenty of protein overall from a variety of whole plant foods, none of these specific amino acids is likely to be a problem.

Even in a domain where meat is still widely considered superior to plants—the weightlifting gym—there's plenty of evidence that plant protein is just as good at supporting muscle growth as beef and chicken. A 2023 study[12] compared the strength-training adaptations between lacto-ovo-vegetarians (who consume some eggs and dairy but avoid meat and fish) and meat eaters who both supplemented their diets with extra protein. After 12 weeks of strength training, both groups showed similar increases in muscle thickness, strength, lean body mass, and body composition, even though the vegetarians consumed significantly less overall protein.

For folks consuming a plant-based diet with few or no products of animal origin, it is prudent to get a little more protein than what's recommended for the general public. This is not because plant protein is deficient or inferior but because the extra fiber in a plant-based diet can actually block some protein absorption.[13] But that doesn't mean you should cut down on fiber—it's one of the most important nutrients, and most modern people don't get nearly enough. Instead, if you eat a largely or wholly plant-based diet, simply increase your protein RDA by 10 percent.

However, a small 2023 study suggested that vegans may need even more. Researchers carefully measured protein intake and outflow (through a process called "nitrogen balance") in 18 minimally active vegan men over the course of five days.[14] The researchers found that some of them were losing protein even while consuming the RDA. They recommended that vegans aim for a 25% increase, to 0.45 grams of protein per pound of body weight rather than the typical 0.36. That puts them in roughly the same category as athletes, elders, those under great stress, and pregnant and lactating women. And if a vegan is also an athlete, elder, under stress, or nourishing a baby directly, then it stands to reason that their protein RDA should rise yet again.

Where Can You Get Your Protein as a Plant-Based Eater?

Just about every plant food contains protein, but some are richer sources than others. Here are 10 high-protein plant foods that can make it easy to meet your daily requirement:

- Tempeh: 16 g per ½ cup
- Lentils: 9 g per cooked ½ cup
- Edamame: 9 g per ½ cup
- Chickpeas: 7 g per cooked ½ cup
- Black beans: 7 g per cooked ½ cup
- Hemp seeds: 10 g per 3 tablespoons
- Quinoa: 4 g per cooked ½ cup
- Tofu: 9 g per 3 ounces
- Peanut butter: 8 g per 2 tablespoons
- Almonds: 6 g per ounce
- Soy milk (unsweetened): up to 12 g per cup
- Sunflower seeds: 5 g per ounce

How Much Protein Is Too Much?

Protein is different from other macronutrients (like carbohydrates and fat) in that your body can't store extra for later use. Your liver hangs on to carbohydrates in the form of glycogen so it can release it when you need energy to power your muscles. Your fat cells collect fat for longer-term storage. But protein is either used, excreted, converted into energy, or turned into fat in a complicated process that can strain your kidneys and liver.

Research suggests that high-protein diets (specifically those including large amounts of animal protein) may be as bad for your health as smoking. In a 2018 study[15] published in the *International Journal of Epidemiology*, researchers followed 81,337 participants for 6 to 12 years. The researchers looked at the

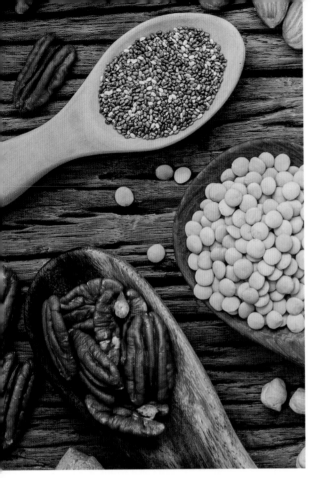

if your body makes too much of it, increase the risk of cancer, heart disease, and many age-related diseases.

That might begin to explain why my dad keeps getting stronger as he ages. Not only is he stressing his muscles through exercise so they keep growing and adapting but he's also avoiding foods (like ultraprocessed foods, added sugars, and animal products) that can rob us of health and vitality as we age. In other words, he's getting all the benefits of protein without the costs.

What about Protein Powders?

As long as you're consuming a variety of foods (especially good sources of protein like legumes, nuts, seeds, and whole grains) so that you're meeting your individual needs, you very likely don't need to worry about protein.

But if you're in one or more of the groups that might need more—maybe you're large, highly stressed, an athlete, elderly, pregnant and/or nursing a baby—should you supplement with more-refined protein supplements to add protein to your diet? Well, maybe. But there are some reasons to be concerned. Many protein powders on the market contain added artificial sweeteners, flavorings, fillers, preservatives, and gums, some of which could be associated with a range of health problems. For example, not only do some artificial sweeteners train the brain to crave more sweetness but some studies also show that they may contribute to obesity and cardiometabolic disease.[16] Gums are added to manufactured foods to help emulsify the ingredients, and while most

percentage of protein that came from animal and plant sources for these participants. What they found was that the risk of cardiovascular death steadily climbed with higher consumption of meat protein—but fell steadily with increased consumption of protein from nuts and seeds.

Overconsumption of protein, especially from animal sources, is associated with higher rates of cancer, renal disease, liver function disorders, and coronary artery disease. But the effect has been found only when the protein comes from animal sources. One theory is that animal protein in particular causes higher levels of insulin-like growth factor 1 (IGF-1), a hormone that affects tissue growth, and may, gums are generally regarded as safe (GRAS) by the FDA, some people experience gastrointestinal discomfort when ingesting gums. Fillers, preservatives, and flavorings can be chemically derived (anything but whole food!) and probably not what you intend to pay for when purchasing protein powder. Conventional protein supplements are also often made with whey, a dairy protein, rather than a plant-based source.

Even if you can find a "clean" protein powder, you still may be consuming harmful substances that aren't listed on its label. In 2018 the Clean Label Project tested 134 of the most popular protein powders on the market. They found that virtually all these products contained detectable levels of at least one heavy metal, and more than half tested positive for the harmful endocrine disrupter chemical BPA.[17] Furthermore, some of the worst offenders were the plant-based and organic protein powders.

So if you're going to use a protein powder, you might want to opt for a simple one that doesn't have additives or flavorings, and seek out a manufacturer that's third-party tested for heavy metals or that's California Proposition 65 compliant (since the state of California has especially rigorous heavy metal testing requirements).

And probably better yet, you could add hemp seeds, flaxseed meal, peanut butter, unsweetened soymilk, or chia meal to your diet and get not only an abundance of protein but also extra fiber, and potentially omega-3 fatty acids and several other essential nutrients that you'll read about in the coming chapters.

Conclusion

Protein is critical for maintaining optimal health and supporting physical strength and longevity. It's important to get enough protein for your weight, physical activity level, and stage of life. And while protein has long been associated with meat, there's no evidence that animal protein is superior to plant protein. In fact, there's a lot of evidence that the opposite is true: plant protein builds muscle and enables bodily repair without the harmful effects of large quantities of animal protein.

Because a whole-food, plant-based diet is rich in fiber, protein requirements on this diet are a bit higher than those on a standard omnivorous diet high in animal products and processed foods. Fortunately, it's not difficult to meet your protein requirements with plants. You don't need to keep a Google spreadsheet in your kitchen or stress about combining complementary proteins—and you probably don't need to supplement with protein powder either. There are many natural, whole, plant-based foods high in protein that can not only meet your overall protein needs but those for each of the essential amino acids as well.

CHAPTER 2

FIBER

Fiber is the ultimate underestimated nutrient. It's long been thought of as nothing more than "roughage" that cleans your digestive tract, about as wonderful and glamorous as the broom wedged against the wall of your utility closet. While many vitamins come with exciting origin stories (who can forget the swashbuckling tales of Vitamin C and the Mystery of Scurvy or Vitamin B$_3$ and the Case of the Disappearing Pellagra?), and phytonutrients fuel the quest to double the human life span, fiber has always just been there, overlooked as researchers dig deeper into the biochemistry of health and wellness.

Part of fiber's problem is a matter of marketing. It's just too widely available to be bottled and sold for large profits. With nobody to profit from selling it, who's going to pay for advertisements?

Yet fiber is more closely associated with a long life span than just about any other nutrient. Studies show that for every 10 grams of fiber you consume per day, you cut your risk of dying by a whopping 10 percent[1]—that's how powerful a disease fighter it is. (Statisticians assure me that this does *not* mean that 100 grams of daily fiber guarantees eternal life—but rather that it can contribute to a longer and healthier one.)

Fiber benefits us comprehensively, far beyond providing the roughage needed to keep things moving through our digestive tracts.

Before we get to the other benefits, I do want to pause to just appreciate how great it is to poop regularly and magnificently. A story comes to mind: In 2013 my dad and I led a white-water rafting trip on the Klamath River. It was one of those "leave no trace" trips,

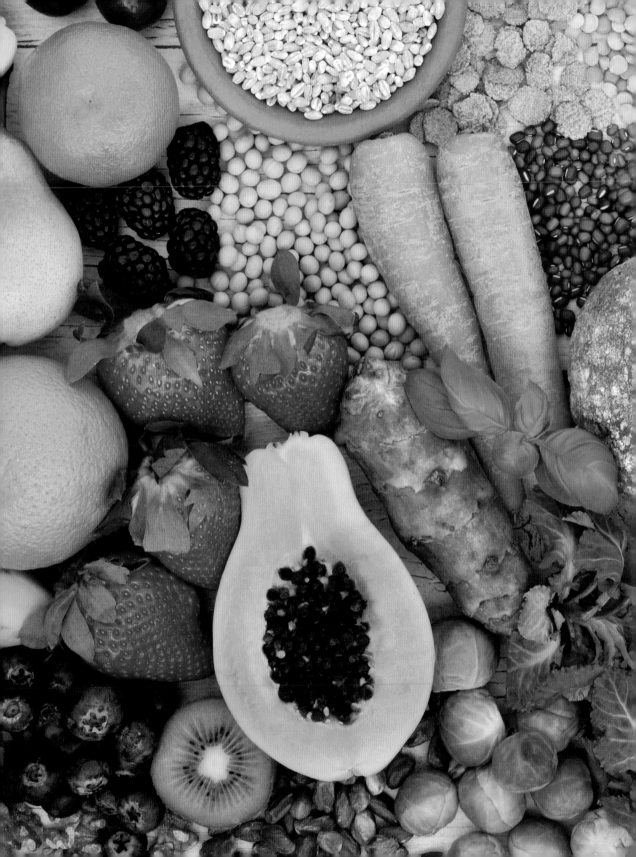

which meant pooping in five-gallon buckets (with very tight-fitting lids) and hauling those buckets with us as we paddled down the river.

The rafting company we hired to coordinate the trip had been leading these tours for almost 20 years. They had everything down to a science—the right amount of food, the time it would take to navigate from campground to campground, the number of canisters of cooking gas, that sort of thing. As well as the number of porta potty buckets required to handle the fecal material of a given number of participants.

As it turned out, our group of plant-based eaters blew their toilet-bucket projections out of the water (so to speak). After the first night, our guides informed us that we had filled roughly twice as many buckets as any prior group, and it became apparent that the 10 buckets they had brought were not going to do the job. And that's why one of the guides found himself on an emergency mission to town, to purchase 10 additional buckets to accommodate this oddly "productive" group.

For my money, that's enough of a reason to make sure you get plenty of fiber. Constipation is no fun! And regular and healthy bowel movements can absolutely contribute to a healthy life.[2] But that's just the tip of the iceberg, to abruptly shift visual imagery.

What Are the Health Benefits of Fiber?

Most famously, of course, fiber helps you poop.[3] Regular bowel movements are really important; constipation is not only uncomfortable but may increase your risk for chronic diseases like cancer, hormonal imbalances,[4] and cardiovascular disease. But there's so much more. For one, fiber helps your digestive system remove toxins from your body. It can also speed potential carcinogens through your digestive tract more quickly, reducing the exposure time and preventing damage that could lead to full-blown cancer. And fiber can help you eliminate spent hormones that might otherwise hang around and cause harmful imbalances that can lead to osteoporosis, mood disturbances, erectile dysfunction, unwanted hair growth or loss, and a myriad of other symptoms.[5]

Getting enough fiber also has a significant impact on the composition of your microbiome. As researchers continue cracking the secrets of the gut microbiome, they've come to appreciate that certain types of fiber—indigestible by humans—are actually the main food source for the beneficial bacteria that live in your large intestines.[6] A diverse microbiome composed of multiple strains of beneficial bacteria can keep harmful bacteria populations in check. (More on those good gut critters and the good things they do for you later in this chapter.)

Fiber can also help regulate your blood sugar, which is why many dietitians and other lifestyle medicine practitioners recommend that people with type 2 diabetes consume fiber-rich beans and other legumes.[7] These high-fiber powerhouses help slow the absorption of glucose while also regulating blood sugar and preventing sugar spikes over time.

Eating lots of fiber can help you feel full, which can discourage overeating that can cause weight problems.[8] Dietary fiber may also

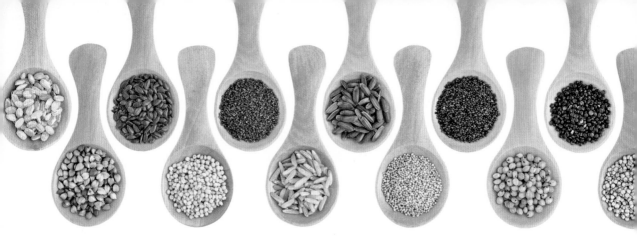

help reduce systemic inflammation associated with cardiovascular disease. Soluble fiber can lower your cholesterol levels and has been shown to reduce your risk of cardiovascular and coronary artery disease.[9]

How Much Fiber Do You Need?

The World Health Organization recommends a minimum of 25 grams of fiber per day for adults,[10] while the Institute of Medicine suggests 14 grams of fiber per every 1,000 calories consumed[11]—which comes out to as much as 51 grams per day if you eat as much as the average American does (and more like 32 grams per day if you have a caloric intake that's aligned with common nutritional recommendations).

Even though they're eating more total calories than ever, members of industrialized societies, on average, don't even come close to meeting this requirement.[12] There is no fiber in meat, dairy, or eggs. You won't find fiber in sugar or oil. There's hardly any fiber in processed white flour. If you base your diet around processed foods and animal products, it's easy to wind up deficient. How easy? Only 6 percent of Americans get their recommended amount of fiber.[13] And fewer than 1 out of 10 adults in the U.K. achieves the minimum suggested fiber intake.[14]

There's evidence that even the recommended amounts may be suboptimal, and that higher fiber consumption can equate to better health. The Physicians Committee for Responsible Medicine recommends aiming for at least 40 grams of fiber per day.[15] That number may seem daunting, but there are many groups around the world that surpass it with ease. One example is the hunting and gathering Hadza people of Tanzania, who average about 150 grams of fiber a day, the majority of which come from tubers and baobab fruit. Scientists attribute their incredibly diverse gut microbiome to their fiber-rich diet.[16]

You don't have to give up your day job and spend your time foraging for roots and fruits to get lots of fiber. All it takes is eating a variety of whole or minimally processed plant-based foods on a regular basis.

Fiber is found in the cell walls of plants, where it provides structure, functioning a lot like a plant skeleton. Biochemical researchers have historically ignored and/or underestimated the nutritional power of fiber: humans can't actually digest it because we lack the enzymes for the job. All that roughage passes through our digestive system unabsorbed, seemingly just the packaging for the "real" nutrients contained in plant foods. We can't even convert fiber into calories for energy. But science has discovered in the 21st century that much of this "indigestible" fiber does get digested inside our bodies, just not by "us" as we commonly think of the term. The beneficial bacteria in our gut love the stuff and digest it gleefully (at least I like to think they're smiling broadly and rubbing their little tummies when we eat plants).

Types of Fiber

There are two main categories of fiber—soluble and insoluble—and they perform different jobs in your body.

Soluble fiber dissolves into a gel with the addition of water in your digestive tract. This gel slows down digestion,[17] which helps balance blood sugar and cholesterol and aids in the absorption of nutrients. Soluble fiber is found in abundance in foods like whole grains, beans, and nuts and seeds, as well as fruits like figs and apples, and vegetables like carrots, sweet potatoes, and broccoli.

Insoluble fiber adds bulk to your stools and works to clean out your digestive tract. It promotes healthy bowel movements and helps with insulin sensitivity. You can find insoluble fiber in whole grains, vegetables such as potatoes and kale, and wheat bran.

You may have heard health and wellness advocates praising the use of prebiotics and probiotics—from both foods and supplements. Prebiotics fall under the soluble fiber umbrella and also act as food for your gut's natural bacteria. While probiotic-rich foods and supplements have received a lot of attention, there's a problem with eating them on top of a fiber-poor diet: they can't survive without their own food. You can consume 60 billion beneficial probiotic bacteria from a capsule, but if you neglect to feed them, you'll just eliminate 60 billion dead bacteria in your next stool.

Prebiotic-rich foods include things like legumes (beans, peas, and so on), leafy greens,

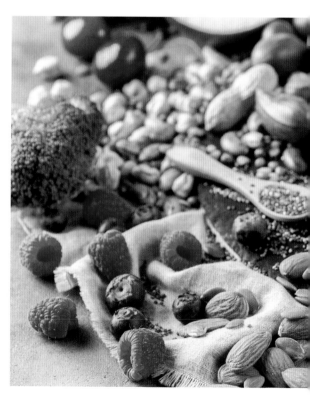

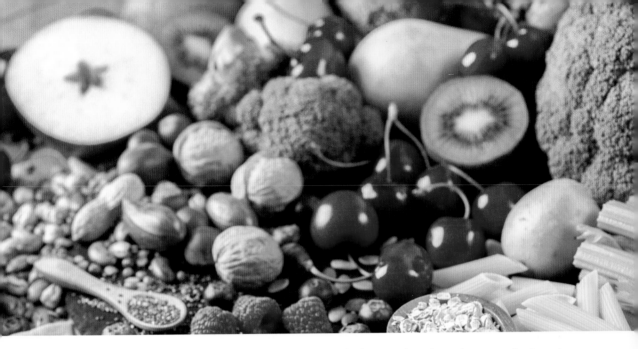

members of the allium family (onions and garlic), and jicama, a juicy root vegetable that looks like the love child of a potato and a water chestnut.

Resistant starch is a type of fermentable carbohydrate that is also a prebiotic. Since it's not digestible, it belongs in the fiber family. Whole grains, potatoes, and green bananas are all good sources of resistant starch. Like other types of prebiotic fiber, this type of starch improves insulin sensitivity and produces short-chain fatty acids in the gut that keep your immune system healthy. These fatty

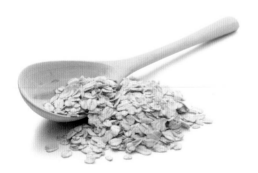

acids also circulate throughout your body and can minimize inflammation (a major contributor to just about every chronic disease) and help your cells and tissues communicate with each other.

How to Get Enough Fiber

We've just talked about soluble fiber, insoluble fiber, and resistant starch. But the reality is, there are other subcategories of fiber too—including glucomannan, beta-glucans, pectin, inulin, and many others. And when it comes to nourishing a healthy gut microbiome, they're all pretty awesome. In short, the best way to get enough fiber is to eat a wide variety of minimally processed plant foods so you'll get all the types.

The American Gut Project is the largest human microbiome study ever undertaken, involving more than 10,000 people from 45 different countries. In this study, the people who ate more than 30 different types of plants per week had gut microbiomes that were far healthier than those who ate 10 or fewer types of plants per week.[18] It's clear that the diversity and number of plants you eat will determine the diversity and number of bacteria that grow in your gut.

Here are 10 high-fiber plant foods to include in your diet on a regular basis that makes hitting your fiber target easy and delicious:

- Oats: 2.5 g per cooked ½ cup
- Split peas: 8 g per cooked ½ cup
- Lentils: 9 g per cooked ½ cup
- Black beans: 7.5 g per cooked ½ cup
- Lima beans: 4.5 g per cooked ½ cup
- Chickpeas: 6.5 g per cooked ½ cup
- Almonds: 3.5 g per ounce
- Chia seeds: 10 g per ounce
- Raspberries: 8 g per cup
- Avocado: 9 g per fruit

Conclusion

Fiber is a vital nutrient that doesn't receive the attention it deserves, despite that fact that it offers a multitude of health benefits. It promotes regular bowel movements, regulates blood sugar levels, and even reduces the risk of chronic illnesses such as cardiovascular disease. And it doesn't just feed you; it's also a favorite food of the beneficial bacteria in your gut that can have a huge impact on your health and your mood.

The evidence is clear that incorporating a wide variety of fiber-rich foods into your daily diet, such as beans, legumes, whole grains, vegetables, and fruits, can significantly contribute to your overall health and well-being.

And with recipes like the ones you'll find in this book, doing so can be easy and delicious.

CHAPTER 3

OMEGA-3 FATTY ACIDS

Our next nutrient of concern, omega-3 fatty acids, should be on everyone's radar. They're associated with seafood, so you might think that people who eat a lot of fish have nothing to worry about here. But it's a bit more complicated than that, as we'll soon see. For now, let's find out why these omega-3s are so important.

To begin with, omega-3s are part of the "essential fatty acid" family, meaning that your body can't make them—so you've got to source them from your diet. They appear in the forms ALA, EPA, and DHA. The following are just a few of their benefits.[1]

Omega-3s protect against heart disease by lowering LDL cholesterol, triglycerides, and blood pressure. People with coronary artery disease who consume enough omega-3s have a lower risk of death than those who do not. And these fatty acids are particularly important in preventing sudden death caused by cardiac arrhythmias.[2] They can also raise HDL ("good") cholesterol, reduce inflammation, and prevent coronary artery blockages by inhibiting the formation of blood platelets.[3]

Omega-3s are also critical for early brain development[4] and lifelong cognitive health.[5] Getting enough omega-3s is

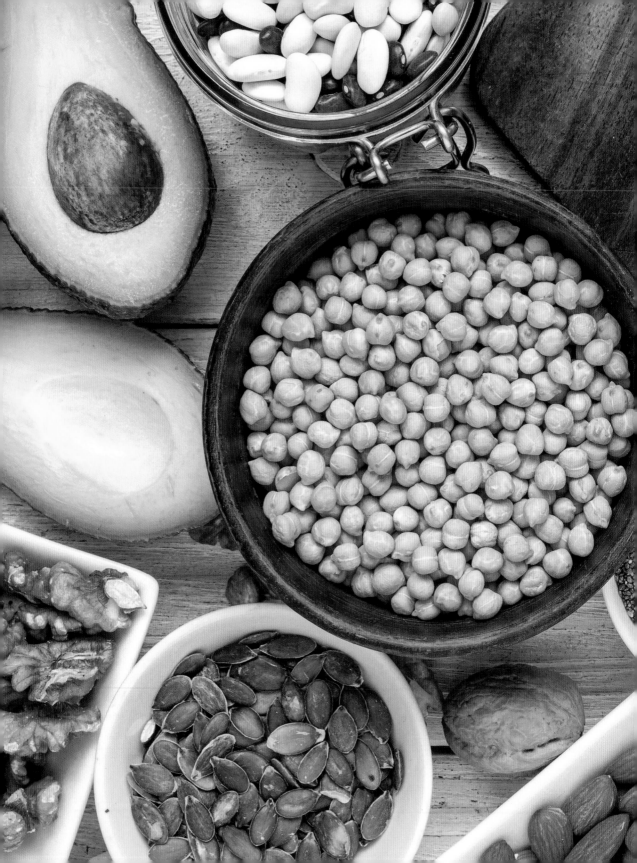

particularly essential early in life, as the brain grows and develops. Thanks to their potent anti-inflammatory and antioxidant effects in the brain, they may also benefit people with mild cognitive impairment by slowing the rate of cognitive decline and reducing the risk of major depression. One form of omega-3, EPA, appears to reduce depressive symptoms, while another, DHA, may reduce suicidal thoughts and lower the risk of suicide.

Omega-3s are highly anti-inflammatory not just in the brain but throughout the body. In addition to combating dementia,[6] they can help suppress inflammation that could contribute to cardiovascular disease, autoimmune diseases like rheumatoid arthritis, and other serious conditions.[7]

At the same time, your body needs omega-3 fats to keep your immune system firing on all cylinders. (That's a metaphor; science has not discovered any actual cylinders in the human body.) They're considered immunonutrients,[8] meaning they play an essential role in the cellular structure and signaling of the immune system. DHA is anti-inflammatory, which means it can bring down chronic inflammation in the body so the body can "rev up" in response to dangers without being in constant overdrive (who knew we could have so much fun with automobile metaphors!)—but it actually appears to boost the actions of the beta immune cells, leading to healthier and more calibrated immune responses.[9]

Omega-3 fatty acids also support eye health. Having enough omega-3s circulating in your body may help prevent age-related macular degeneration (AMD), a common eye condition that can result in vision loss.[10]

What Are Omega-3s?

Omega-3s are a type of polyunsaturated fatty acid (known by the acronym PUFA, which sounds like a Teletubby or an extremely comfortable chair). If you have an interest in chemistry, you may already know that "omega-3" signifies that the double bond in its carbon chain is located at the third carbon from the end of the carbon chain. (I like to imagine the double bond asking directions and being told, "If you reach the end of the chain, you've gone too far.")

As we've seen, there are three types of omega-3s: ALA, EPA, and DHA. Let's demystify that chemical alphabet soup.

ALA (alpha-linolenic acid) fats are needed for energy and are mostly metabolized in your intestines and liver. Your body can also convert ALA into the other two long-chain omega-3s, EPA and DHA.[11]

EPA (eicosapentaenoic acid) and DHA (docosahexaenoic acid) are long-chain omega-3 fatty acids. In addition to getting EPA and DHA from the conversion of ALA, you can also get them directly from food and supplements.

You might think that since our bodies can convert ALA into EPA and DHA, we can keep it simple and just focus on getting enough ALA. Unfortunately, for most people, it isn't that simple at all.

Harvard Health puts it this way: "The main problem with ALA is that to have the good effects attributed to omega-3s, it must be converted by a limited supply of enzymes into EPA and DHA. As a result, only a small fraction of it has omega-3's effects—10%–15%, maybe less. The remaining 85%–90% gets burned up as energy or metabolized in other ways. So in terms of omega-3 'power,' a tablespoon of flaxseed oil (with 7,000 mg of ALA) is worth about 700 milligrams (mg) of EPA and DHA."[12]

Also, the conversion rate can vary significantly between people, depending on factors like genetics, age, and overall health status. Studies suggest that women may be better at this conversion than men, thanks to higher estrogen levels.[13]

The good news is: Your body can likely convert EPA to DHA and DHA to EPA with pretty high efficiency. Also, many people can get enough ALA from that single tablespoon of flaxseed oil to end up with sufficient EPA and DHA, even with that inefficient conversion percentage.

However, there's another factor that can affect your body's ability to synthesize EPA and DHA: your consumption of a different group of PUFAs called omega-6 fatty acids. Researchers surmise that some omega-6s compete for the same enzymes that turn ALA into the other omega-3s.[14] Omega-6s can promote inflammation, countering many of the positive effects of omega-3s in the body. That's not to say that omega-6s are bad and omega-3s are good; both types are essential for your health. The issue is getting them in the right proportions.[15] And the modern industrialized diet, high in processed vegetable oils, isn't your friend here.

While you can find omega-6s in most vegetable oils, sunflower, corn, soybean, safflower, and cottonseed oils are particularly

rich sources. The optimal ratio of omega-6 to omega-3 is somewhere between 4:1 and 1:1. In Western diets, it's estimated to be as high as 16:1.[16] So getting enough of the right mix of omega-3s likely means reducing omega-6s as well.

How Much Omega-3 Do You Need?

The National Institutes of Health recommends that adult females consume 1.1 grams of ALA per day, and that males consume 1.6 grams.[17] Since our bodies can convert ALA into EPA and DHA, only ALA is technically essential. But since the conversion rates are low and can be compromised in several ways, this is a rare nutritional instance where consuming more than the recommended daily amount is probably better.

That said, it may also be beneficial to consume EPA and DHA directly and not have to rely on your body to synthesize them from ALA. Research suggests that your combined EPA and DHA intake should be at least 250 to 500 milligrams per day, depending on how much ALA you're taking in and how efficiently your body converts it. And as we've seen, lowering your omega-6 intake by limiting your consumption of most vegetable oils is also a key part of the strategy to get enough EPA and DHA.

What about Fish?

For many nutrition and health influencers, omega-3s are synonymous with fish or fish oil

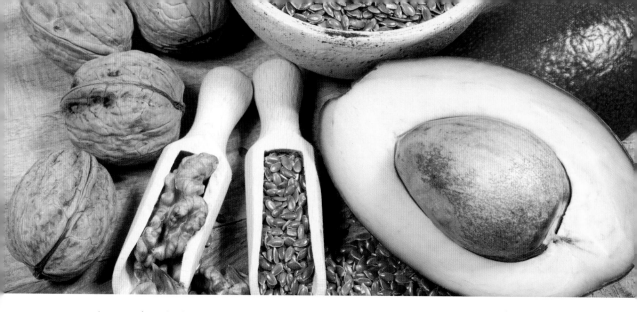

supplements (partly due to effective marketing by the fish oil industry, which earned almost $13 billion worldwide in 2022).[18] Certain kinds of fish, including sardines, anchovies, herring, and salmon, are especially high in DHA and EPA. And indeed, a large body of research has linked consumption of fish with improved health incomes, at least compared to other foods in the modern industrialized diet. For instance, the ongoing Adventist Health Study has so far found that vegetarians outlive omnivores, vegans outlive vegetarians, and pescatarians—people who avoid all animal products except for fish—appear to have the longest life expectancy of all.[19]

But there are some significant problems with using fish as your main source of omega-3s too. For one thing, modern research is quite clear that fish feel pain. For those who prioritize animal welfare in their food choices, eating (and killing) fish could be a nonstarter. Additionally, the rampant overfishing and destructive techniques employed by the fishing industry are depleting fish stocks and disrupting marine ecosystems. Commercial fishing industries are harvesting over 160 billion pounds of sea life out of the ocean every year—that's nearly half a billion pounds every single day. And if fishing rates continue at this pace, nearly all of the world's fisheries will collapse in the next 30 years.[20]

On the other hand, fish farming, or aquaculture, presents its own set of problems. Despite being touted as a solution to declining wild fish populations, aquaculture often relies in part on wild fish harvested from the ocean, and it contributes to pollution, disease, and the use of harmful chemicals. The conditions in which farm-raised fish are kept often necessitate the use of antibiotics and pesticides, raising public health concerns about antibiotic resistance and the consumption of contaminated fish.[21]

And all ethical and environmental concerns aside, there are health concerns with eating fish too. Most fish are at the top of long food chains, and they tend to bioaccumulate not just omega-3 fatty acids but also mercury, PCBs, and other toxins. And a study published in 2022 found that eating fish regularly could

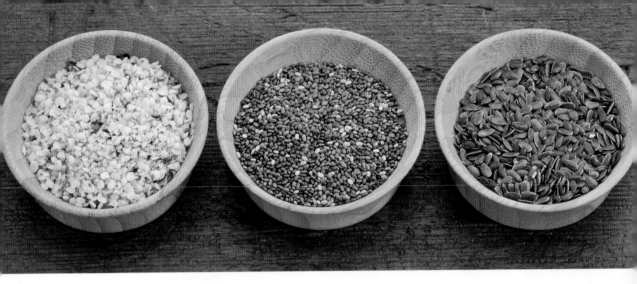

increase your risk of developing melanoma by 22 percent.[22]

Plant-Based Sources of Omega-3s

If you want plenty of omega-3 fatty acids and you don't want to eat fish, I've got good news. While fish are a rich source of omega-3s, they are not the only source. As the saying goes, you are what you eat. For fish to contain omega-3s, they must themselves consume omega-3s—in their case from the nutrient-rich aquatic plants they eat.

There are many plant-based sources of omega-3s. Some of my favorite sources are flaxseeds (containing 6,000 milligrams of omega-3 per ounce of seeds), chia seeds (5,000 milligrams per ounce), and hemp seeds (2,600). These are easy to add to your diet. Hemp seeds are ready to go right out of the bag, while with flaxseed or chia seeds it's best to buy them whole and then grind some up in a coffee grinder and refrigerate the ground meal. You can sprinkle your omega-3 rich seeds on just about anything—smoothies, salads, stir-fries, pizza, or soup, to name a few.

Hemp seeds have a special bonus feature. They're high in a form of ALA, stearidonic acid,[23] which your body converts to EPA and DHA more efficiently than other forms of ALA.[24] As an added bonus, hemp seeds are also high in protein.

Some nuts are also a good source of ALA. Walnuts in particular are rich in the nutrient, delivering 2,500 milligrams per ounce. And flaxseed oil, while not a whole food, is a very rich source of ALA that your body can convert to DHA and EPA. (Note that flaxseed oil must be consumed raw. It goes rancid quickly, so keep it refrigerated and buy only what you'll use within a month or two.)

While the only form of omega-3s in most plant foods is ALA, there are a few that provide EPA and DHA directly. Sea vegetables and seaweed both contain varying amounts of DHA and EPA—up to 130 milligrams per ounce.[25] There are lots of ways to enjoy sea vegetables. You can make sushi rolls using sheets of dried nori; add dulse or wakame flakes to salads and main dishes for a unique flavor and texture; or enjoy leafy sea vegetables in miso soup.

And, while not huge sources of DHA and EPA, spirulina and chlorella powders deserve an honorable mention as they contain some too.

When You Might Want to Supplement

Especially if you don't consume any fatty fish or large amounts of flax, chia, and hemp seeds, you may want to consider an omega-3 supplement. Pregnant women and people over the age of 65, who are at greatest risk of deficiency, should especially consider taking a supplement just to be on the safe side. A simple blood test can give you a baseline to see if your EPA and DHA levels are adequate.

Fish oil supplements are made from real fish and come with all the health and environmental drawbacks we've already looked at. Fortunately, you can find vegan omega-3 supplements that are made from algal oil. Studies tell us that they are at least as efficiently absorbed as fish oil–based supplements but without the toxins found higher on the aquatic food chain or the environmental harms.

A word of warning about EPA and DHA supplements, however: In 2023, researchers at George Washington University published a study in the *Journal of Dietary Supplements*. The researchers analyzed 72 omega-3 supplements and found that 32 percent of the flavored supplements and 13 percent of the unflavored ones were in fact rancid. The rates were probably higher with the flavored ones because flavoring can mask the rancidity.[26] Now, this is a problem because rancid omega-3s can actually be worse than useless, causing a host of new health problems.

So if you are going to take DHA or EPA supplements, and there's good reason to do so, it's best to aim for unflavored forms and to be on the lookout for an "off" taste, which could be an indication of rancidity. Also, keep them in the fridge, and don't stock up on large quantities. You might want to aim to get them on a subscription, auto-shipped to your door, or from a store that keeps them refrigerated.

Conclusion

It can be challenging to get enough omega-3 fatty acids in a modern diet. Fish are the most common food source, but they come with significant ethical and environmental concerns—as well as a sizable dose of heavy metals and increased risk of melanoma. If you don't eat fish, look for ways to add nuts and seeds—especially flax, chia, and hemp—to your diet on a daily basis. Consider adding sea vegetables, and cut back on or eliminate high omega-6 vegetable oils. You can get your blood levels for EPA and DHA checked, and you might well want to take a fresh and unflavored omega-3 supplement, especially if you are pregnant or over 65. Vegan supplement options appear to be just as effective as fish oil–based supplements.

However you do it, make sure your diet includes omega-3s for a healthy heart, a well-functioning brain, and limber, pain-free joints.

CHAPTER 4

SELENIUM

Selenium is what's known as a trace mineral. Your body needs it only in very small amounts.

If you're an etymology fan, you might recognize the root word *selene* in the nutrient—it means "moon" in Greek. In early 19th-century Sweden, industrial chemists in a sulfuric acid factory originally mistook it for another recently discovered element, tellurium, which means "earth element." When it turned out that selenium wasn't the same as tellurium—the similarity was limited, apparently, to the fact that both smelled strongly of horseradish when burned!—the chemists simply named it after the next nearest heavenly body, the moon.[1]

What Does Selenium Do in the Body?

Your body needs selenium to convert two common amino acids, cysteine and methionine, into two uncommon ones, selenocysteine and selenomethionine, respectively. These unusual amino acids are called "noncanonical" because they aren't among the 20 standard amino acids that are commonly found in proteins.[2]

Selenium creates molecules called selenoproteins when it replaces your body's natural sulfur in those proteins. Selenoproteins perform important functions in your body, like protecting against heart disease and cancer, supporting the immune system, and helping with

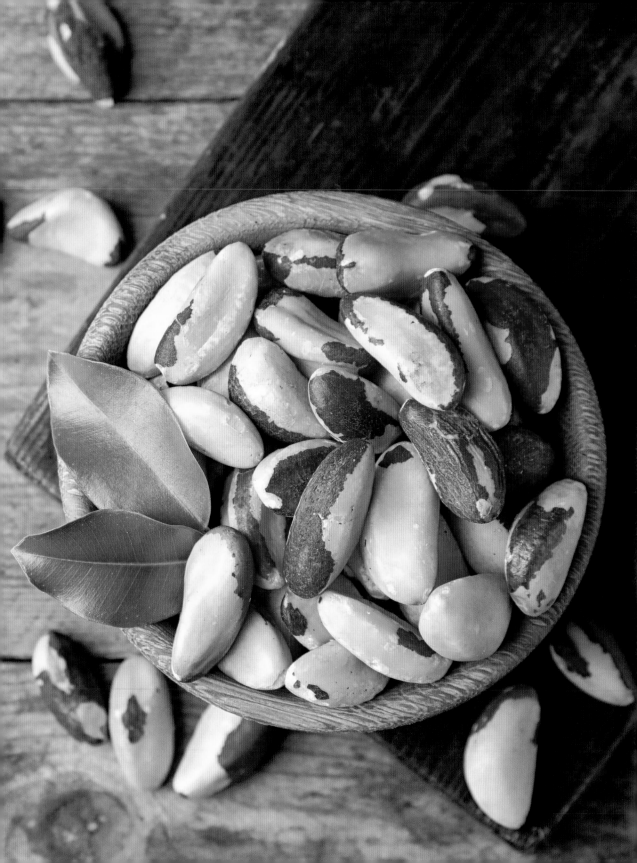

development and growth.[3] Pregnant women in particular need to meet their selenium needs, as a deficiency can lead to their child developing cretinism,[4] a condition that can include stunted growth, intellectual disabilities, and developmental delays.

Your thyroid gland requires selenium to properly metabolize iodine (see Chapter 9), which is in turn needed to create the hormones that regulate your metabolism and support other important bodily functions. Symptoms of what appears to be iodine deficiency can actually be caused by a lack of dietary selenium.[5]

Selenium gets incorporated into proteins that primarily function as antioxidants. They help prevent and repair injuries to your DNA caused by free radicals and keep other cells throughout your body healthy and free from damage. In this way, selenium can be helpful in stopping the progression of cancer. You also need selenium to fight off infections (including viral ones), reduce excess or chronic inflammation, and support proper immune function.

We're still learning about how selenium works to keep us healthy, but we do know that there are lots of other functions that selenium is involved in, including male fertility, cognition, and a happy and healthy microbiome.[6] It's important to get enough of this vital nutrient.

How Much Selenium Do You Need and Where Can You Get It?

As I mentioned, selenium is a trace element, so you only need, well, a trace of it. The recommended amount for adults is 55 micrograms (mcg) of selenium per day, unless you're pregnant (in which case it rises to 60 mcg) or lactating (where it goes up to 70 mcg).[7]

How much is that? Well, a microgram is one-millionth of a gram, and a gram is about the weight of a paperclip. So imagine a paperclip cut into a million pieces—one of those pieces is as much selenium as you require daily.

You wouldn't think that anyone would have trouble achieving that daily intake, but the problem is that plants get selenium from the soil they grow in, and selenium is not distributed evenly in the earth's soil.[8] Unfortunately, it's not as simple as looking up a food—a banana, say, or a cup of cooked lentils—and assuming that the selenium content measured in some lab will apply to the banana or lentils sitting in front of you.

That said, here's the average selenium content of some foods grown in North American (Canadian) soil[9] that are high in the mineral:

- Firm tofu: 17.4 mcg per 3.5 ounces
- Mushrooms: 18.5 mcg per cooked ½ cup
- Couscous: 21.5 mcg per cooked ½ cup[10]
- Long-grain brown rice: 7.5 mcg per cooked ½ cup
- Baked beans: 7 mcg per cooked ½ cup
- Cooked oatmeal: 6.5 mcg per cooked ½ cup
- Sunflower seed kernels: 22.5 mcg per ounce
- Lentils: 3 mcg per cooked ½ cup
- Frozen spinach, boiled: 6 mcg per ½ cup
- Dry roasted cashews: 3 mcg per ounce

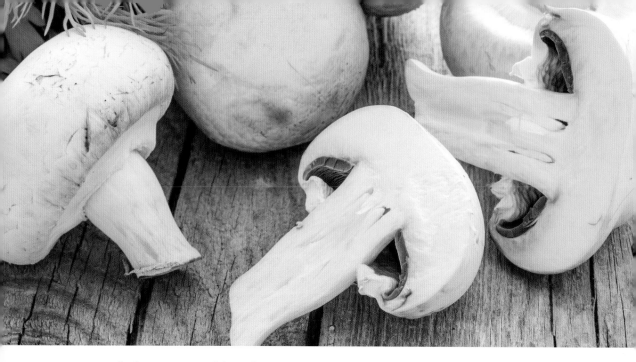

With the exception of the tofu, none of these are going to get you most of the way to 55 mcg, let alone 60 or 70. So if these foods aren't showing up regularly in your diet, and if you don't eat fish, ham, pork, beef, turkey or chicken (all of which contain sizable amounts of it), there's a chance that your selenium levels may not be optimal. But don't worry about having to adopt the "baked bean and sunflower seed" diet, or starting your day with a cup and a half of couscous in order to ensure sufficient quantities of this seemingly elusive nutrient. For dramatic effect, I omitted one food from the above list that blows all the others out of the water when it comes to selenium.

- Brazil nut: 67–91 mcg per nut

That's right: a single Brazil nut grown in Bolivia, the world's leading exporter, contains around 70 to 90 mcg of selenium, enough to meet (and likely exceed) your needs. So here's the punch line of this entire chapter: if you eat a single Brazil nut every day, you will most likely never have to worry about selenium again.

Can You Get Too Much Selenium?

Having too much selenium in your body, a condition known as selenosis, can cause a host of health problems. The first sign is often metallic, garlicky breath, followed by hair and nail loss or brittleness. Continued excess can bring about gastrointestinal issues, skin rashes, fatigue, and nervous system abnormalities. In severe cases, it can lead to acute respiratory distress syndrome, kidney failure, cardiac failure, and even death.

Tolerable Upper Intake Level (UL) for selenium varies by age and gender. In general, adults should keep their intake below 400 mcg per day.

Unless you regularly enter couscous-eating contests, if you're a plant-based eater, the only way to approach this limit with food is to eat too many Brazil nuts—say, more than 4 or 5 per day (less than an ounce). It's easy to over-consume them if you think of them as food because they're delicious (at least I think so) and very "snackable." For that reason, I recommend putting Brazil nuts in the mental category of "super healthy real food supplement" rather than a staple food.

Should You Take a Selenium Supplement?

Because it's so easy to get enough but not too much selenium from a single Brazil nut a day, most people won't need to take a supplement. If you have a condition that impairs your absorption of some nutrients (like gastrointestinal or malabsorption syndromes) talk with your health care professional about whether you would benefit from a nonfood source of selenium.

Conclusion

Selenium is a crucial trace mineral that your body needs to survive and maintain health. While concentrations in food can vary greatly depending on the soil in which the plants were grown, you can probably source it from a variety of everyday plant-based foods, including tofu, mushrooms, baked beans, and brown rice. And for an insurance policy, a single Brazil nut every day will almost certainly more than meet your selenium needs.

But too much selenium can be as dangerous as not enough, so unless you can't source your requirement from a daily Brazil nut, supplementation probably isn't necessary and generally isn't recommended. If you do take a supplement, it's probably best to make sure it's just a small amount.

CHAPTER 5

ZINC

Like selenium, zinc is also a trace mineral that your body needs to stay well. After iron, zinc is the next most abundant micronutrient in your body.[1] It is stored mostly in your bones and skeletal muscles.

Zinc has a similar chemical structure to a couple of other essential minerals, like calcium and magnesium, that allows it to bind easily with lots of the proteins in your body. Researchers estimate that some 2,800 human proteins[2] require zinc to function properly and support important processes like facilitating chemical reactions, building tissues, and maintaining homeostasis (a stable internal balance in the face of a constantly changing external environment).

You also need zinc for a variety of crucial bodily functions, including fighting off bacteria and viruses, growing new cells,[3] healing wounds, and synthesizing and repairing your DNA. It's crucial for fertility, metabolism, and protecting the brain and nervous system from harm. Zinc also helps prevent processes that can harm the cardiovascular system, such as inflammation and atherosclerosis (blockages of the arteries).[4]

It also appears to play a role (one not yet fully understood by researchers) in your sense of smell and taste—a connection that scientists discovered as they searched for treatments for COVID-19.[5] It also works alongside vitamin A and other antioxidants to support eye health and normal vision.[6]

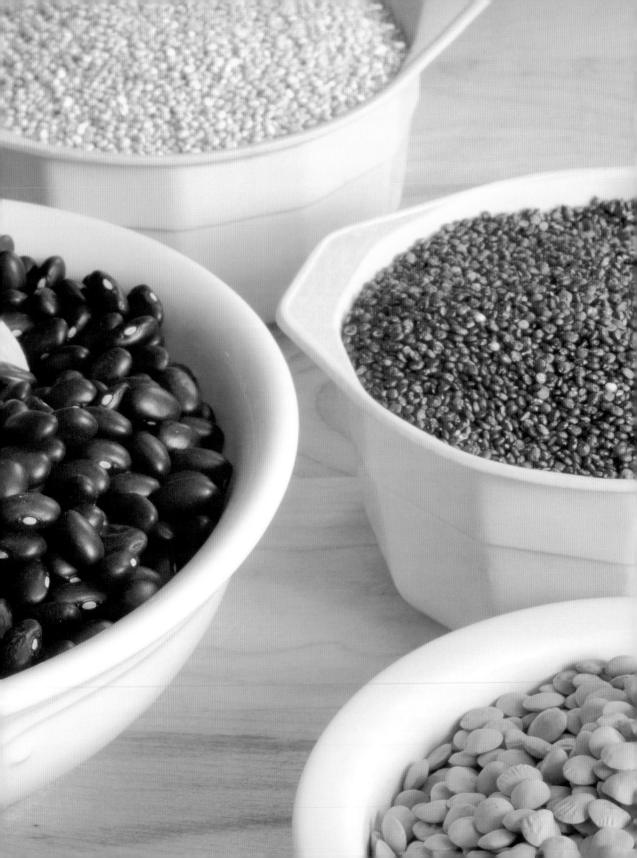

How Much Zinc Do You Need?

The U.S. Recommended Daily Allowance (RDA) of zinc is 8 to 13 milligrams per day, which is less than the weight of an eyelash or a single grain of sand. Women generally need a little less than men, except when pregnant or lactating, when they require a bit more.

Below are the RDAs for zinc based on age group:

- 0–6 months: 2 mg
- 7–12 months: 3 mg
- 1–3 years: 3 mg
- 4–8 years: 5 mg
- 9–13 years: 8 mg
- 14–18 years: 9 mg (girls), 11 mg (boys)
- 18+ years: 8 mg (women), 11 mg (men)
- Pregnancy: 11–12 mg
- Breastfeeding: 12–13 mg

As you can see, that's not a lot of zinc, so it should be pretty easy to meet your daily requirements, right?

Actually, that depends on the content of your diet. Animal-derived foods tend to be higher in zinc than plant-based ones, with oysters packing the biggest punch with about 25 mg of zinc per ounce. If you don't eat animal foods, you may have to put a bit of effort into including zinc-rich foods in your diet.

Plants get zinc from the soil and tend to store it in their reproductive organs: seeds, nuts, and grains. Consuming whole foods in those three categories is a good strategy for ensuring enough zinc.

Here are some other plant foods that are good sources of zinc:

- Tofu: 1.7 mg per 3 ounces
- Lentils: 1.2 mg per cooked ½ cup
- Hemp seeds: 3 mg per 3 tablespoons
- Wild rice: 1 mg per cooked ½ cup
- Oatmeal: 0.65 mg per cooked ½ cup
- Pumpkin seeds: 2 mg per ounce
- Quinoa: 1 mg per cooked ½ cup
- Black beans: 1 mg per cooked ½ cup
- Peas: 0.5 mg per cooked ½ cup
- Shiitake mushrooms: 1 mg per cooked ½ cup

There's a bit of a catch, though: the zinc in plant-based foods is not as bioavailable as the zinc found in some animal products. This is probably because many zinc-rich foods, like beans and whole grains, are also high in compounds called phytates. Phytates are sometimes known as "antinutrients" because they can inhibit the absorption of certain nutrients, including zinc. Even so, I don't recommend avoiding phytate-containing foods, since research overwhelmingly shows that the benefits of these foods far outweigh any potential downsides. Instead, here are some strategies that allow you to have both phytates and zinc.

How to Get Enough Zinc from Food

First, consume enough zinc. Some nutritionists recommend that vegetarians and vegans double the RDA when calculating their daily intake.[7] If you avoid animal products and find that you're constantly catching colds, suffering from frequent diarrhea, have brittle hair or hair loss, and have cracking skin around the corners of your mouth, you may be able to resolve all of these issues by increasing your consumption of the zinc-rich foods listed above.

You can also reduce the phytate content of grains and legumes by soaking, sprouting, fermenting, or simply cooking them before eating. (I hope you're already cooking your beans and grains prior to consumption; if not, I don't want to see your dental bills.)

Finally, consider adding other foods that can boost your zinc absorption. Research shows that consuming zinc along with protein increases the usable amount absorbed by your body. (An exception is casein, the main protein found in milk, which inhibits zinc absorption.[8]) Citrate, a compound found in vitamin C–containing foods like citrus fruits, may also help enhance zinc absorption.[9] So having some orange slices for dessert or squeezing lemon juice on your pilaf, rice, and beans can help you get the zinc you need.

Who Might Need to Supplement?

People with digestive disorders (such as ulcerative colitis or Crohn's disease) may not be able to absorb sufficient amounts of zinc from their diets alone. Pregnant and breastfeeding women may want to consume a little extra from a supplement to ensure enough zinc for their growing baby.

Most people get plenty of zinc, and some get too much. Plant-based eaters may occasionally benefit from a zinc supplement, particularly if they find themselves getting sick often or if they experience any of the other symptoms of mild deficiency I mentioned

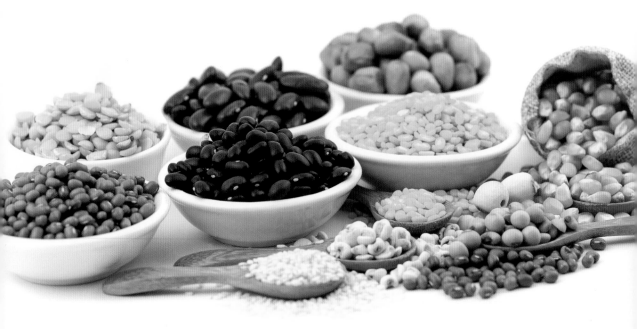

earlier. Also, some plant-based eaters over the age of 65 may find it worthwhile to consider supplementing prophylactically.

The Dangers of Too Much Supplemental Zinc

It's possible to overdo zinc; even with all its uses and benefits, too much is just as bad as not enough. Scientists discovered this after a tragic case study where a man with schizophrenia ingested 461 pennies and died of zinc toxicity. It turned out that so-called "copper" pennies minted after 1981 are actually 97.5 percent zinc. The mineral slowly interacted with the man's stomach acids and caused multisystem organ failure.[10] So just in case you were considering going on the penny diet (which I hear is pretty affordable, as diets go) . . . don't do it.

While it's practically impossible to experience zinc toxicity from food alone (unless you're committed to an all-oyster diet), you can experience zinc toxicity if you take overly high doses of zinc supplements.[11]

Signs that you're getting too much zinc may include nausea, vomiting, loss of appetite, diarrhea, stomach cramps, and headaches. If you ingest too much zinc over a long period of time, you can experience additional problems like decreased copper levels, reduced immunity (for instance, getting sick more often), and sometimes reduced levels of HDL ("good") cholesterol.

How much is too much? At 100 mg of zinc per day, you're no longer doing yourself any favors. And you'd likely start noticing serious symptoms at 1 to 2 grams per day, which is roughly 100 to 200 times the recommended dose.[12]

Also, keep in mind that supplemental zinc can interact with certain drugs and medications. For example, some antibiotics, penicillamine (a drug for the management of rheumatoid arthritis), diuretics, and even other mineral supplements can interact with zinc or cause absorption issues. It's probably wise to speak with your health care provider before taking a zinc supplement, especially if you're taking other medications or mineral supplements.[13]

Conclusion

Zinc is a vital trace mineral that your body needs to function properly. This mineral plays several crucial roles in keeping you healthy, including facilitating chemical reactions, building tissues, and maintaining internal balance. It also helps fight off bacteria and viruses, supports cell growth and wound healing, and is involved in DNA synthesis and repair. Zinc protects the brain, nervous system, and cardiovascular system. Additionally, zinc works together with vitamin A and other antioxidants to promote eye health and normal vision.

While the richest sources of zinc are foods of animal origin, it's not difficult to get more than enough zinc from plants, especially if you prioritize eating nuts, seeds, legumes, and grains. Consume them regularly, or take a small amount in supplemental form, to make sure you're getting enough of this essential nutrient.

CHAPTER 6

IRON

"Pumping iron" is a great way to build muscle and stay in shape. Ironing is an effective way to eliminate wrinkles from your clothes. And irony can be a humorous way to get people to consider new ideas. But what about the kind of iron inside your body?

Iron is not only useful but essential for life—and getting the right amount of iron from your diet is extremely important. But it's a "Goldilocks" nutrient: Not enough or too much can both be harmful. You've got to get it just right.

In this chapter we'll explore how much iron you need and the best places to get it. We'll cover the two different forms of iron you can get from food and how they differ. We'll see why iron— in the preferred form—is crucial for health, and why too much of the other, not preferred, form can lead to all sorts of problems.

Why You Need Iron for Health

We call someone "red-blooded" when they're healthy, vigorous, and maybe even a bit lusty. It's a good thing, right? Blood itself looks red because of the iron that sits in the middle of each hemoglobin molecule it contains. Hemoglobin is the body's transport mechanism for getting the oxygen you breathe into your organs, muscles, and other tissues—actually, into every single one of your body's roughly 40 trillion cells.[1] Iron is crucial for DNA metabolism, a necessary process that replicates cells, repairs damaged DNA, and transcribes DNA into the RNA that codes the synthesis

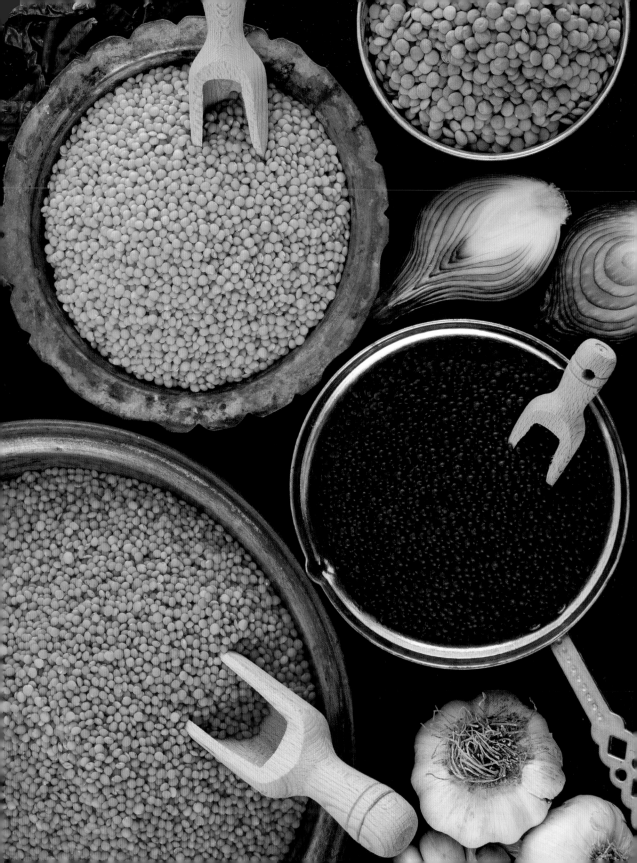

of the proteins you need to stay healthy.[2] Iron is also necessary for the proper functioning of your mitochondria, the "powerhouses" that generate the chemical energy for every cell in your body.

The Two Kinds of Iron

In foods, iron occurs in two forms: heme and nonheme.

Heme iron is found only in animal-derived foods, while nonheme iron comes from plants. Technically, meat contains some nonheme iron, but not a lot.[3]

If "heme" reminds you of hemoglobin (found in animal blood), that's a good way to remember which is which. You, as an animal, are full of heme iron, so named because it's found in the hemoglobin protein that carries oxygen to red blood cells.

Nonheme iron is found mostly in plants. Meat may contain small, negligible amounts of nonheme iron if the animal it is sourced from recently ingested some from plants. Since plants don't have blood, there's no heme or hemoglobin, and there are no red puddles on your cutting board when you chop broccoli or zucchini. (An exception would be bioengineered plant-based foods like Impossible Burger, which contains heme iron made from soybean DNA and inserted into yeast cells for mass production.[4])

The big difference between heme and nonheme iron, functionally speaking, is that heme iron is easier for our bodies to absorb. You might reasonably assume that's a good thing, and for someone with severe iron deficiency anemia, it might be. The problem is

that sources of heme iron are also associated with cardiovascular disease, type 2 diabetes, and some cancers. To reduce your risk of these outcomes, limit your consumption of heme iron and focus on ingesting significant plant-based sources of iron.

Heme iron doesn't take "no" for an answer, even if your body already has enough iron. Because of its chemical structure, it can "force" itself in, whether it's needed or not.[5] Nonheme iron, by contrast, makes it much easier for your body to decide how much it needs to absorb. And since it's critical that your iron stores are in the "just-right" range—not too low and not too high—consuming heme iron can mean risking dangerously high concentrations of iron in your tissues.

Why Too Much Iron Is a Problem

If you've ever owned a cast-iron skillet or worked with iron nails, you're familiar with this big problem: rust. Exposure to oxygen and water can weaken and corrode the metal over time, leading to structural damage. The same thing can happen inside your body in a process called oxidation that negatively impacts your health.

While antioxidants like vitamin C and polyphenols from plants can protect your body, prooxidants, including iron, can speed up oxidation. Oxidation, or oxidative stress, is implicated in many chronic diseases and is thought to be one of the main drivers of the aging process.[6] So while getting enough iron is crucial to your health, it's just as important to keep iron levels in the low-normal range to decrease cellular damage and defer aging.

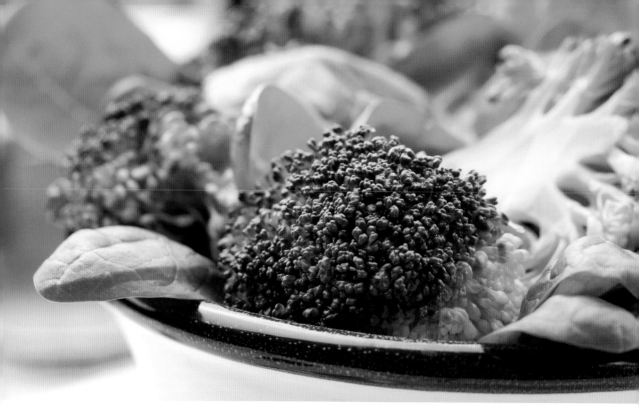

In industrialized populations, more people may be suffering (and even dying) from problems caused by too much iron than from too little. Heme iron in particular appears to be problematic. Higher iron stores from the overconsumption of animal-derived foods may translate into greater risk of heart disease, worse insulin sensitivity, progression of certain cancers, and acceleration of neurodegenerative diseases like Alzheimer's and Parkinson's.[7]

Studies show that heme iron increases the risk of developing plaque buildup in your arteries.[8] One Swedish study from 2013 found that the more heme iron consumed by men with no history of cardiovascular disease, the higher their risk of having a stroke.[9] A 2014 meta-analysis of six studies (that included over 130,000 participants) found that a person's risk of developing coronary heart disease increased by 27 percent for every 1 milligram of heme iron consumed per day.[10]

High consumption of heme iron from animal products appears to increase the risk for type 2 diabetes as well. Interestingly, non-heme iron and even supplemental iron had no such harmful effect.[11]

Heme iron consumption also appears to contribute to your risk of developing colon and rectal cancers, which, when combined into a single category, represent the third most common cancer worldwide.[12]

Studies show that while most vegans and vegetarians consume the same amount of iron as their omnivore counterparts,[13] they typically have lower iron stores (in the form of ferritin, a protein that stores iron and releases it as needed) in their body than meat eaters.[14] In general, that might not be a bad thing.

How Much Iron Do You Need?

The daily RDAs for adults who include meat in their diets are as follows:[15]

- Men: 8 mg
- Menstruating women (ages 19–50): 18 mg
- Non-menstruating women: 8 mg
- Pregnant women: 27 mg
- Lactating women: 9 mg

If you're a vegetarian or vegan, the recommendation is to multiply those numbers by 1.8 to get your RDA (since nonheme iron tends to be less readily absorbed). That comes out to:

- Men: 14.4 mg
- Menstruating women (ages 19–50): 32.4 mg
- Non-menstruating women: 14.4 mg
- Pregnant women: 48.6 mg
- Lactating women: 16.2 mg

Because iron is such an important nutrient, and because it can cause severe problems both in excess and with insufficiency, you may want to request a blood test as part of your annual health care checkup. If the test reveals a problem with your iron stores, your health care provider can offer guidance and may suggest more frequent testing.

How to Get Enough Iron

The condition of not having enough iron—technically, being short on healthy red blood cells and hemoglobin—is called anemia. Symptoms include fatigue, weakness, shortness of breath, dizziness, irregular heartbeat, and cold extremities.[16] If you are predisposed to anemia (based on age, gender, overall health, and in some cases, genetics), you'll need to pay attention to the amount of iron you're getting from your diet.

One reason nonheme iron from plants tends to be absorbed less fully by the body is because of the presence of so-called "antinutrients" (like phytates and oxalates) that may inhibit the uptake of iron.[17] If your iron levels tend to be too low, you can prepare foods containing these antinutrients in ways that lower their concentrations. Examples include soaking beans, grains, nuts, and seeds prior to cooking or eating, and cooking dark leafy greens to reduce their oxalate levels.

Calcium can interfere with iron absorption, a phenomenon mostly seen with calcium from supplements and dairy products. If you take supplemental calcium or consume dairy and you want to increase your iron intake, avoid those calcium sources while eating iron-rich foods or taking iron supplements.

Tannins, caffeine, and polyphenols (a trio of compounds found in coffee, tea, and cacao) can also interfere with iron absorption.[18] If you're looking to increase your iron levels, avoid consuming them from one hour before until two hours after an iron-rich meal.

There are more strategies to increase your absorption of iron. If you have 25 to 100 mg of vitamin C along with iron-rich foods, you can increase absorption by up to 400 percent. Some of the foods highest in vitamin C include bell peppers, citrus, kiwi fruit, and broccoli. Combining vitamin A–rich foods (red and orange fruits and vegetables and leafy greens such as kale and spinach[19]) with grain-based meals likewise increases the amount of iron that will make it into your cells.

You can also get your dietary iron from a surprising source: cast-iron cookware. Encouraging people to heat their food in cast-iron pots and pans is one of the strategies promoted by public health officials for reducing anemia in developing countries.[20]

Finally, you can get more iron from foods rich in the mineral when you consume them along with vegetables from the allium family: onions, garlic, leeks, scallions, and so on.[21]

Getting enough iron is not hard to do on a varied plant-based diet. Here are some good plant-based sources:

- Lentils: 3.5 mg per cooked ½ cup
- Tofu: 4 mg per 3.5 ounces
- Chickpeas: 2.4 mg per cooked ½ cup
- Pumpkin seeds: 2.3 mg per ounce
- Tempeh: 2.2 mg per ½ cup
- Edamame: 1.8 mg per ½ cup
- Cashews: 1.9 mg per ounce
- Leafy greens: 1–4 mg per cup
- Dried apricots: 0.8 mg per ¼ cup

How to Avoid Too Much Iron

Hemochromatosis is a genetic disorder characterized by the excessive absorption and accumulation of iron in the body. It is a condition that can take decades to diagnose due to the slow buildup of the mineral. This iron overload is extremely dangerous, causing damage to organs such as the liver, heart, and pancreas.[22] Roughly one out of every 300 to 500 white, non-Hispanic people have this hereditary disorder, with lower rates among other ethnic groups. If you have this condition, in addition to regular blood removal (either by donating or as a medical treatment) and medical monitoring, you can also limit the iron you ingest by reversing the strategies from the previous section.

In this case, you may want to drink coffee or tea alongside any iron-containing meals. Avoid citrus fruits and their juice while eating iron-rich foods. Don't cook out of cast iron (especially acidic foods such as tomatoes and tomato sauce). And take advantage of the plant "antinutrients" and other compounds that inhibit iron absorption by getting most or all of your dietary iron in nonheme form, from plants.

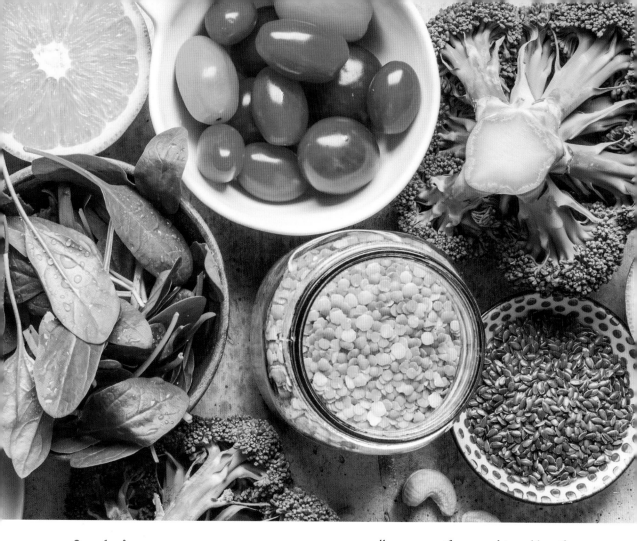

Conclusion

Iron is another one of those nutrients that you need enough of, but not too much. For most people, the best way to ensure healthy but not excessive levels is to get it from plants in its nonheme form. This enables your body to naturally get more if you need it and less if you already have plenty. If you have trouble absorbing iron, there are many ways to increase the amount you get from food—most notably by incorporating some vitamin C–rich foods. If excess iron builds up in your body, you can reverse those tactics to reduce your intake.

CHAPTER 7

MAGNESIUM

In the same way plants often struggle to get enough nitrogen despite its abundance in the atmosphere, we humans often don't get enough magnesium—even though it is the seventh most common element on our planet. Magnesium is absolutely essential for good health, and many people aren't consuming an adequate amount.

To add to the irony (or "magnesium-y"), your body doesn't even need that much. If you could weigh every atom of magnesium in your body, it would come to somewhere around 25 grams, or about the weight of a double-A battery. A little more than half resides in your bones, with the rest doing its thing in your soft tissues.[1]

Unfortunately, many people aren't ingesting enough magnesium to maintain even this relatively modest requirement.

Researchers estimate that somewhere between 10 and 30 percent of people around the world suffer from magnesium deficiency.[2] And it's even more dire in the U.S., where a majority of residents don't get enough.[3]

While the problem is serious, magnesium deficiency doesn't show up with obvious warning signs, unlike some other nutrient deficiencies. Instead, subclinical deficiency (revealed only by biochemical changes evident in lab tests rather than physical symptoms) may be a silent contributor—and a big one—to the epidemic of cardiovascular disease in the industrialized world.[4]

When I first learned about this, my initial questions were "What foods are rich in magnesium?" and "Am I eating enough of these magnesium-rich foods?" If you're wondering the same thing, here's the spoiler

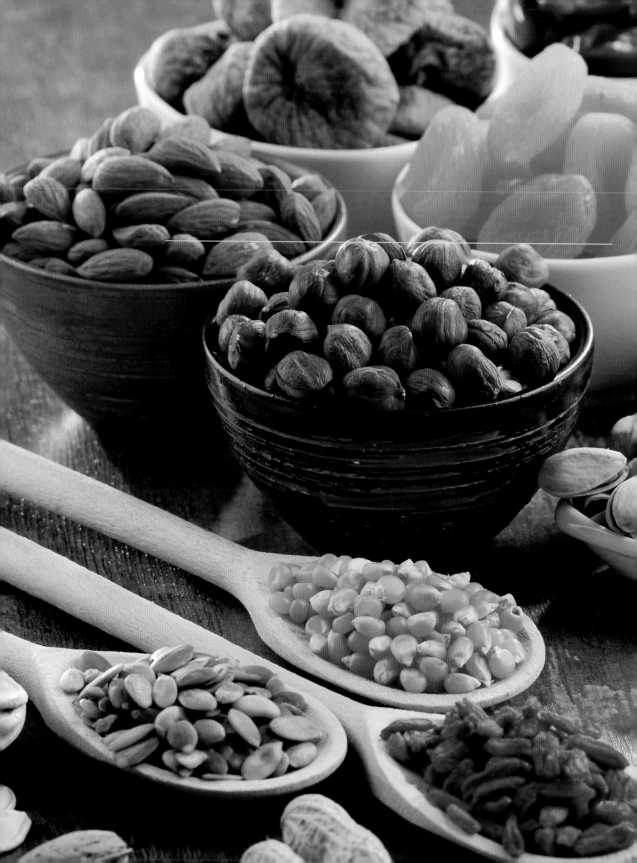

for this chapter: You can get magnesium only from plants; it's virtually nonexistent in animal-derived foods. So the U.S.'s poor showing in the Are You Getting Enough Magnesium? game can be pinned directly on the standard American diet, which is high in processed and artificial foods and animal-derived products like meat, dairy, eggs, and fish, and low in whole plant foods.

By the end of this chapter, you'll understand how magnesium functions in your body, why it's important for many aspects of your health, and what happens when you don't get enough. We'll identify magnesium-rich foods and look at strategies to maximize absorption. We'll also consider who may want to take a magnesium supplement as an insurance policy against deficiency.

What Is Magnesium?

Magnesium is a mineral needed to support a number of critical functions in your body. It helps maintain normal blood pressure, keeps your bones strong through the metabolism of calcium and potassium, and helps keep your heartbeat steady. It's also a cofactor involved in over 300 enzyme systems that regulate biochemical reactions.[5] These include important tasks such as DNA and RNA synthesis, muscle contraction and relaxation, and the firing of nerve cells.

As if that weren't enough, your body also needs magnesium in order to turn food into energy.[6] One of its cofactor roles plays a part in the breakdown of carbohydrates, proteins, and fats, along with your body's enzymes.

Magnesium is involved in the synthesis and storage of ATP (adenosine triphosphate), the primary molecule used for energy transfer in cells, and it's required for the structural integrity and proper functioning of your mitochondria, the microscopic power stations operating inside all your cells.

Magnesium is also an electrolyte, which means it carries an electric charge when dissolved in bodily fluids, like blood. When your blood levels of the mineral are low, the concentrations of other crucial electrolytes such as potassium and calcium can also take a hit.[7] Since less than 1 percent of your body's magnesium is in your bloodstream, those stores must be carefully controlled within that tight margin for error. Your kidneys are the main organs in charge of this task, deciding on a moment-by-moment basis how much magnesium to either excrete from the body in urine or to send back into the bloodstream for further use.

What Are the Symptoms of Magnesium Deficiency?

Symptoms of early magnesium deficiency can include constipation, fatigue, loss of appetite, and weakness, all of which can eventually lead to more severe complications. Muscle contractions, seizures, low blood levels of calcium and potassium, abnormal heart rhythm, personality changes, and numbness in the limbs can develop. Long-term, untreated magnesium deficiency can result in high blood pressure, type 2 diabetes, osteoporosis, and heart disease.

What Are the Health Benefits of Magnesium?

Instead of focusing only on the health consequences of magnesium deficiency, let's look at just a few of the wonderful, positive things that can happen when you have enough. (Since magnesium is required by so many bodily systems, a comprehensive list would literally fill an entire book—if not multiple volumes.)

Healthy blood magnesium levels support your cardiovascular health, significantly lowering your risk of developing high blood pressure and heart disease.[8] Supplemental magnesium can even increase survival and recovery prospects for people about to undergo heart surgery. Giving intravenous magnesium or injecting it directly into muscles helps reduce the incidence of postoperative atrial fibrillation. This in turn can lower the risk of blood clots, stroke, heart failure, and other complications from surgery.[9]

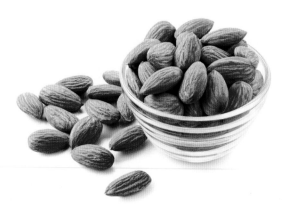

Getting enough magnesium can also reduce your chances of developing type 2 diabetes. A 2016 review of clinical trials including over half a million people found that for every 100 milligrams of magnesium consumed daily, the risk of type 2 diabetes dropped by about 10 percent.[10]

Magnesium and calcium work together to keep your bones strong and healthy, so it makes sense that getting enough of these minerals can help slow or prevent the skeletal weakening that often accompanies aging. Getting enough magnesium in the diet can also help maintain musculoskeletal health as you age and prevent osteoporosis and bone fractures.[11]

Magnesium is known to have a calming effect for many people, which may help improve sleep. Given that roughly half of all older adults suffer from some degree of insomnia, up-leveling their magnesium intake could make a big difference to their health and mood (and the moods of people who spend time with them!). In addition to aiding relaxation, magnesium can also reduce symptoms of restless leg syndrome, a condition whose treatment is also crucial for improving sleep duration and quality.[12]

This one will be of particular interest to migraine sufferers: having enough magnesium can help prevent these debilitating headaches.[13] Magnesium deficiency can contribute to something called cortical spreading depression, which is basically a sudden increase in brain cell activity followed by a period of decreased activity—picture a tsunami wave rather than a gently rolling surf. It's thought that this phenomenon is partly responsible for migraine pain, as well as the visual disturbances so familiar to those prone to migraines. Not having enough magnesium also changes how your brain and nervous system perceive and interpret pain—which can make migraines incredibly painful. And low magnesium stores can also constrict blood flow to the brain via a nasty process known as platelet hyperaggregation.

Some migraine sufferers find that taking large doses of magnesium at the first onset of symptoms can avert the worst of their symptoms.[14] Others, however, experience abdominal pain and diarrhea from these large doses and prefer to focus on prevention by consuming moderate amounts of magnesium on a regular basis.

Finally (for the purposes of this chapter, anyway), getting enough magnesium may help uplift your spirits and combat depression. A 2017 study found that six weeks of daily supplementation significantly lowered depression scores in outpatients with reported mild-to-moderate depression. Half of the participants said they experienced enough benefit to their mood to continue taking magnesium supplements after the study ended.[15]

How Much Magnesium Do You Need?

Most people eating a modern, industrialized diet don't get enough magnesium. But that doesn't mean it's hard to meet your daily requirement through food. So how much magnesium should you be aiming for? The Recommended Dietary Allowances (RDA) for magnesium are as follows:[16]

- Men 19+ years: 400–420 mg
- Women 19+ years: 310–320 mg
- Pregnant women: 350–360 mg

There isn't any known danger from eating too much magnesium from food. The more relevant concern is not getting enough, since only about 30 to 40 percent of the magnesium you get from your diet ends up getting absorbed by your body. As we've already seen with iron and zinc (and as we'll soon encounter with calcium), there are often nutrients and compounds in plants that can interfere with magnesium absorption—the so-called *antinutrients*. So let's look at how you keep your magnesium absorption rate as high as possible.

One of the antinutrient compounds that makes it harder for your body to absorb magnesium is phytic acid—found naturally in many plant foods like nuts, seeds, legumes, and grains. Sprouting, soaking, and fermenting the grains helps lower their phytic acid content. You can also mitigate the effects of phytic acid on magnesium absorption by eating foods rich in vitamin C (like, as we've discussed, citrus, red bell peppers, and broccoli). It turns out that vitamin C—even in the relatively modest quantities found in half a cup of strawberries or broccoli, or a third of a bell pepper—essentially neutralizes phytic acid.[17] (Maybe vitamin C, also known as ascorbic acid, should be renamed "absorbic acid"! Okay, maybe not.)

If you use calcium supplements (which we'll look at in the next chapter), don't take them within two hours before or after eating. Avoid high-dose zinc supplements (refer

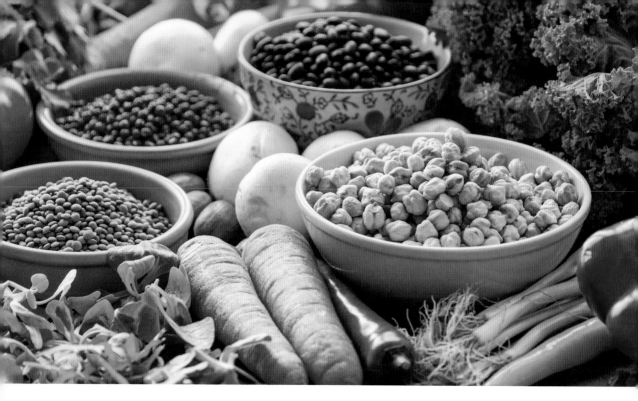

to Chapter 5), and make sure you get enough vitamin D (see Chapter 9).

What Foods Are Good Sources of Magnesium?

In general, the best way to get magnesium in the right amount, and in a form your body can recognize and absorb efficiently, is through your diet.

Some of the best sources include nuts and seeds, especially almonds, cashews, and peanuts (technically a legume, but a very nutty one), as well as nut butters and nut milks. Whole grains are excellent sources, especially quinoa and whole wheat flour.[18]

Beans and legumes pack a magnesium punch, as do lightly processed soy products such as tofu and tempeh. Boiled dark leafy greens, including kale, spinach, collard greens, turnip greens, and mustard greens, are magnesium powerhouses,[19] as are cauliflower, potatoes, and avocados. And bananas, despite being more famous for their potassium content, are also good sources of magnesium. And if you're into chocolate, you can bolster your magnesium stores if you choose dark chocolate that contains a high cacao or cocoa content.

To give you a sense of how you can achieve your 300 to 400 milligrams per day, here are some foods and their magnesium content:

- Pumpkin seeds: 156 mg per ounce
- Chia seeds: 111 mg per ounce
- Almonds: 80 mg per ounce
- Spinach: 79 mg per boiled ½ cup
- Cashews: 83 mg per ounce
- Peanuts: 52 mg per ounce

- Soymilk: 51 mg per cup
- Black beans: 46 mg per cooked ½ cup
- Potatoes: 43 mg per 3.5-ounce potato
- Brown rice: 38 mg per cooked ½ cup
- Dark chocolate, 70-85 percent: 65 mg per ounce

What about Magnesium Supplements?

Because magnesium deficiency is so rampant, supplements can be helpful for those who find it difficult to achieve their RDA through food alone.

There are several health conditions that can contribute to magnesium loss, including digestive disorders such as celiac disease and chronic diarrhea. Taking medications like diuretics or proton pump inhibitors can also lead to deficiency. And just plain old getting older can take a toll, as your body's ability to absorb magnesium wanes with age.[20]

If any of those descriptors fit you, you may want to consider taking a magnesium supplement. The recommended upper intake from supplements is 350 milligrams per day.

Conclusion

There's a good chance you're not getting enough magnesium if you aren't consuming a diet rich in whole plant foods. This deficiency, although often lacking obvious warning signs, can cause lots of health problems indirectly, including increasing your risk of cardiovascular disease, type 2 diabetes, and osteoporosis. The good news is that most people can meet their magnesium needs through a varied and healthy plant-based diet. If you still have reason to worry about deficiency, you can focus on the highest-magnesium foods, optimize absorption by combining them with vitamin C–rich foods, and take steps to minimize phytates in your diet. In more rare cases, it may be helpful to consider a supplement to ensure an adequate supply of this vital nutrient.

CHAPTER 8

CALCIUM

If you're of a certain age, you may remember using classroom chalk. Before dry-erase boards and smelly markers, teachers used chalk to write homework assignments on a slate chalkboard, and troublesome kids would be forced to write, "I will not talk in class" (or, if they're Bart Simpson, "I will not waste chalk") 100 times as punishment.

Chalk is a form of calcium-rich limestone, and the name calcium comes from the Latin *calx*, meaning "lime" (the inorganic material used for making plaster and mortar, and for raising the pH of agricultural soil). In 1808, when British chemist Sir Humphry Davy ran an electric current through some metal oxides to isolate the mineral, he named it calcium.[1] (Davy, quite the busy chap, also managed to isolate magnesium, which we just discussed in the previous chapter, using that technique in the very same year.)

While calcium-rich chalk and plaster can break and flake easily, calcium inside your body is associated with considerably more robust objects: bones and teeth. The dairy industry spends tens of millions of dollars[2] every year to remind us that we need calcium for strong bones, which is true. (They also tell us that we need milk to get that calcium, which, as we'll see, is not necessarily true.)

There's more calcium in your body than any other mineral. In addition to its role in keeping bones strong (and also supple), calcium enables your nerves to carry messages between your brain and the rest of your body.

Your blood vessels need calcium for structural integrity and flexibility; insufficient

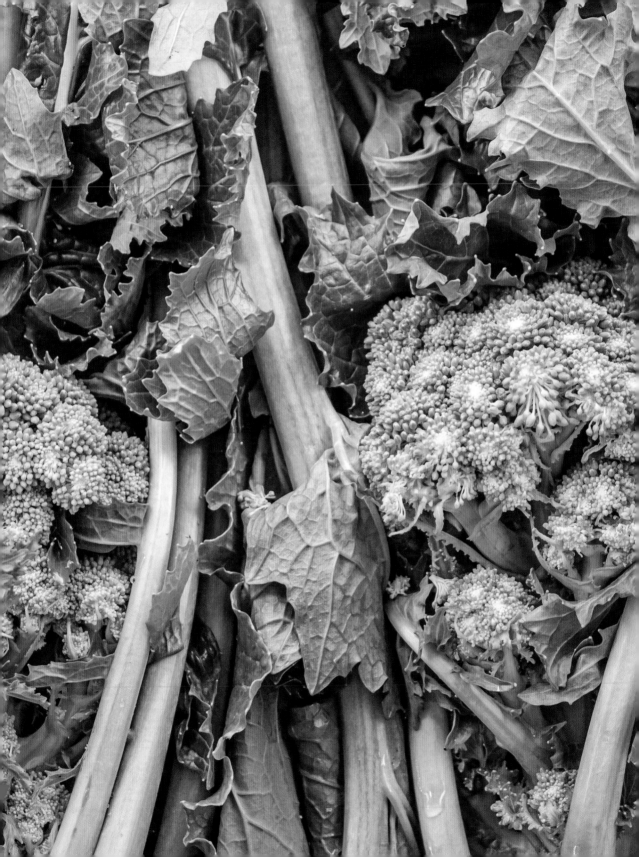

calcium can lead to unhealthy blood pressure levels. Calcium is required to transport various enzymes and hormones through your blood to where they're needed.[3]

Your muscles need calcium to contract and relax, meaning that without calcium, you could not move. And since your heart is a muscle, it needs calcium for every beat.[4]

How Much Calcium Do You Need?

The Recommended Dietary Allowance for adults 18 years and older is 1,000 to 1,200 mg of calcium per day.[5] That increases to 1,300 mg per day during teenage years, pregnancy, and lactation—all periods of extra bone growth. The Food and Nutrition Board also recommends that postmenopausal women increase their calcium intake to combat bone loss and reduce the risk of fractures.[6]

That may not be the final word on the subject, however. The National Health Service of Britain recommends considerably less calcium per day—only 700 mg.[7] And the World Health Organization goes even lower, setting the bar at 500 mg. So what accounts for the differences?

It's probably not that Americans say "tomāto" while Brits say "tomäto," or that the rest of the world calls it "football" instead of soccer. Rather, I suspect that the powerful influence of dairy industry lobbyists[8] and political campaign financial contributions,[9] which are much more prevalent in the U.S. than in other countries, may account for the gap. It is also worth noting that U.S.-recommended levels are based on short-term studies that have since been contradicted by more rigorous research.[10]

Do You Need Dairy to Get Enough Calcium?

Dairy *is* high in calcium, but studies haven't always found a correlation between high dairy consumption and healthy bones.[11] In fact, the countries with the highest rates of osteoporosis (that is, weak and brittle bones) are the same ones where people consume the most dairy: the U.S., Finland, Sweden, and the United Kingdom.[12] And in dairy-avoidant countries, such as those in sub-Saharan Africa, bone fractures are relatively rare.[13]

Of course, there are other factors, besides calcium consumption, that also influence bone health. Perhaps the most prominent one is exercise. Physical activity plays a crucial role in developing robust bones during youth and is vital for preserving bone density in older age. Since bones are living tissues, they evolve based on the physical demands exerted on them. Engaging in consistent exercise prompts your bones to increase in mass and become more dense.

So when it comes to strong bones, dairy isn't the whole story—and we aren't even absolutely sure if it's helpful. And there are other problems with high dairy consumption, including increased risk of several cancers, such as prostate,[14] breast, lung, and ovarian.[15] This may be due to high concentrations of sex hormones like estrogen and other growth factors that are naturally present in milk.[16]

Dairy also contains lactose, a form of sugar that about two-thirds of people worldwide lose the ability to digest after weaning. In fact, the ability to consume the milk of a different species into adulthood appears to have developed as an evolutionary adaptation in people of European descent relatively recently in human history.[17]

Additionally, factory-farmed dairy could be less healthy than the milk and cheese people were consuming even just a hundred years ago. Modern dairy products can often deliver worrying concentrations of contaminants and antibiotics.[18]

Plant-Based Sources of Calcium

Fortunately, you do not need to drink milk or eat cheese to get enough calcium. There are plenty of plant-based sources that provide sufficient amounts of the nutrient. Here are a few examples, with their calcium content per serving size:

- Broccoli rabe: 516 mg (1 bunch, cooked)
- Sesame seeds: 280 mg per ounce
- Chia seeds: 179 mg per ounce
- Black beans: 23 mg per cooked ½ cup
- Lentils: 19 mg per cooked ½ cup
- Almonds: 76 mg per ounce
- Collard greens: 162 mg per cooked ½ cup
- Kale: 128 mg per ½ cup (frozen, cooked)
- Tofu: 128 mg per 3 ounces

- Orange: 75 mg (1 large orange)
- Fortified plant-based milk: 300 mg per 8 ounces

If you struggle with maintaining adequate calcium levels, the problem may not stem only from the amount consumed in your diet; you may not be absorbing it well. There are several factors that can interfere with your calcium absorption. Eating too much salt can increase calcium loss, especially on a high-calcium diet.[19] And smoking and other forms of tobacco intake can contribute to calcium loss, reduce bone density, and increase the risk of fractures.[20]

And while we're on the topic, getting your calcium from dairy appears to reduce absorption as well, compared to plant-based sources. For example, one study found that calcium in Brussels sprouts was absorbed at 64 percent, cauliflower at 69 percent, and kale at 50 percent,[21] while calcium in cow's milk reached only 32 percent.[22]

Calcium is a team player in your body, not a solo superstar. For your body to absorb and use calcium properly, you need other nutrients like vitamins D, C, K, and E, as well as magnesium and boron.[23] You can also increase your absorption by incorporating regular, moderate exercise into your routine.[24]

Finally, keep in mind that some leafy greens that are technically rich in calcium provide less than you might think. That's because they contain a class of compounds called oxalates, which can inhibit calcium absorption. Examples of oxalate-rich foods include spinach, rhubarb, beet greens, and Swiss chard. These can't be relied upon for their calcium content (though they do contain many other healthy nutrients!). Be sure to eat other calcium-rich foods, like the ones listed above, to ensure you get what you need.[25]

Should You Take a Calcium Supplement?

For many people, calcium supplements seem to do more harm than good. For one thing, they can increase your risk of kidney stones[26] (which are a lot less entertaining than The Rolling Stones). Calcium supplements may also increase blood calcium, which can cause stiff arteries and increase blood pressure. In one study, postmenopausal women were randomized to receive either a calcium supplement (1,000 mg) or a placebo over five years. Those who took calcium supplements experienced more heart attacks, strokes, and other unwelcome cardiac events.[27]

Calcium supplements can also prevent certain medications from working. Specifically, they can reduce the absorption of certain antibiotics, anticonvulsants, and—ironically enough—medications used to treat osteoporosis.[28]

Many plant-based milks are fortified with calcium, sometimes containing at least as much of the nutrient as (or even more than) cow's milk. If you consume plant milk, check the label, as the calcium content can vary between varieties and brands. It can be a way to boost calcium intake in addition to getting plenty of calcium from whole plant-based foods.

Conclusion

Calcium plays a crucial role in maintaining strong bones and teeth, and it enables your nerves, blood vessels, and muscles to function properly. It also aids in the important transport of enzymes and hormones within your body.

To ensure you're getting enough calcium, it's essential to include calcium-rich foods in your diet. While the U.S. dairy industry promotes milk as the primary source of calcium, there are plenty of other options available. Foods like leafy green vegetables, tofu, nuts, and legumes can provide sufficient calcium if you include them in your diet on a regular basis. And remember, maintaining adequate calcium levels is not just about consuming enough of it but also ensuring proper absorption. Factors like vitamin D intake (more on that in the next chapter), physical activity, and overall diet quality can influence calcium absorption.

I make no bones about it: prioritizing your calcium intake from whole plant foods can serve your skeleton, your muscles, and your overall well-being.

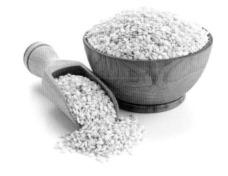

CHAPTER 9

SUPPLEMENTS AND OTHER KEY NUTRIENTS

In addition to the notable nutrients we've already explored, there are a few other key nutrients that may require special attention, especially if you follow a plant-based lifestyle. In this chapter, we'll look at four vital nutrients that may be challenging to obtain in sufficient quantities for everyone, and perhaps especially for exclusively plant-based eaters: iodine and vitamins K, B_{12}, and D. We'll explore why they're essential for overall health and well-being, describe the roles they play in your body, and discuss if and when supplementation might be appropriate.

Iodine

In the first decades of the 19th century, France was engaged in a series of bloody wars against many neighboring countries. One of the most in-demand substances was saltpeter, an essential ingredient in gunpowder. Saltpeter manufacture required sodium carbonate, which at the time was sourced from seaweed beds on the coasts of Normandy and Brittany.[1] After extracting the sodium carbonate, workers would get rid of the giant piles of waste by pouring sulfuric acid on them, a process that generated violet vapors that crystallized into violet solids.

A French chemist, Bernard Courtois, whose father was a saltpeter manufacturer, was the first to suspect that this violet stuff was a yet-to-be-discovered chemical element. When he confirmed the discovery of this new element, it was named iodine, after the Greek word for violet: *ioeidēs*.

What Are the Health Benefits of Iodine?

Iodine is a pretty rare element on Earth, where the greatest concentrations are found in oceans. It's crucial for the health of all vertebrates because it supports the thyroid gland—a small, butterfly-shaped organ located in the front of the neck. The thyroid gland needs iodine to produce the hormones thyroxine (T4) and triiodothyronine (T3), which play several critical roles in your body. T4 and T3 are important for metabolism, the body's process for turning food into energy. They help maintain the body's temperature, heart rate, and energy levels. They're also needed for proper bone and brain development during pregnancy and infancy.

Iodine can be the limiting factor in the thyroid's hormone factory. When you don't get enough iodine, your thyroid can become underactive, a condition known as hypothyroidism.[2] This can lead to symptoms like fatigue, weight gain, and depression.

Insufficient iodine can also lead to goiter, or enlargement of the thyroid.[3] When your pituitary gland notices a shortage of thyroid hormones, it sends a message to the thyroid to increase production. The thyroid gland tries to compensate by increasing its activity. In the absence of sufficient iodine, however, this increased activity cannot bring the hormones to their proper levels and causes a visible swelling in the neck that can make it difficult to swallow and breathe.

On the other hand, too much iodine can cause the thyroid gland to go into overdrive, a condition called hyperthyroidism.[4] Symptoms of this condition include weight loss, increased heart rate, and anxiety.

(If you find yourself getting confused about hypo- and hyperthyroidism, here's a quick Greek lesson. *Hypo* means "too little." For example, hypothermia means "too little heat." *Hyper*, on the other hand, means "too much." For instance, hyperactivity describes overly active behavior.)

How Much Iodine Do You Need?

Fortunately, you need only trace amounts of iodine to provide all that your thyroid gland requires. Here are the recommended daily amounts for adults:[5]

- Adults: 150 mcg
- Pregnant women: 220 mcg
- Breastfeeding women: 290 mcg

The main sources of iodine in the modern diet include fish and other seafood, dairy products, and eggs.[6] And perhaps most significantly, since the 1920s, many brands of table salt have been "iodized" (that is, fortified with iodine) in order to combat iodine deficiency on a population level.[7]

If you eat an exclusively plant-based diet and you cook and season your food with iodized salt, you probably don't have to worry about your iodine levels. If you avoid salt

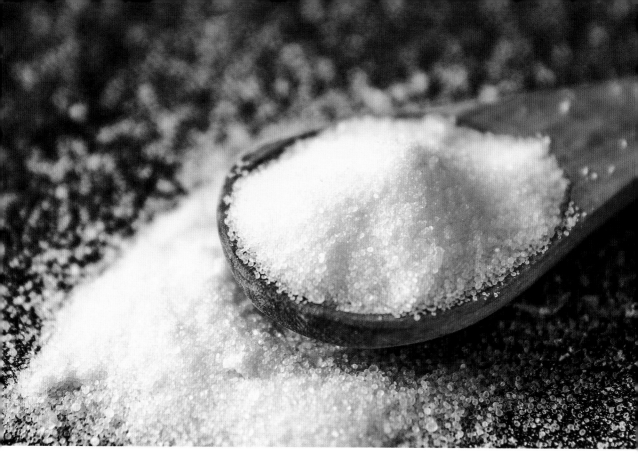

completely as part of an "SOS-free" diet (one that excludes salt, oil, and sugar and is sometimes recommended for people with heart disease) or use only "high-quality" non-iodized salt like Himalayan or Celtic sea salt, you may be at risk of deficiency.

Luckily, there's a plant-based source of iodine that can give you all you need: sea vegetables (also known as edible seaweed).[8] Abundant sources include wakame, nori, dulse, and arame. You can think of these as plant-based iodine supplements.

Some forms of sea vegetables are so rich in iodine that you should be careful not to overconsume them and risk hyperthyroidism. In fact, some species of kelp (such as kombu)

are generally not recommended because their iodine content is so high. Most people should stay below an average of 300 mcg/day on a regular basis, and definitely below 1,100 mcg/day, which is the daily tolerable upper limit for people without thyroid disease. Since a single tablespoon of dried kelp may contain up to 2,000 mcg of iodine, even modest amounts of this sea vegetable on a regular basis could cause problems.

On the bright side (if you're trying to make sure you don't get too much iodine), cooking significantly reduces the amount of iodine you get from sea vegetables. For example, boiling kombu for 15 minutes can make it lose up to 99 percent of its iodine content.[9]

Much of that iodine may be released into the water, however. If you're cooking sea vegetables and then drinking the broth, you are likely still getting a hefty dose of iodine.

One class of plant compounds called goitrogens can inhibit your uptake of iodine. These so-called antinutrients are found in cruciferous vegetables (such as cauliflower, cabbage, kale), as well as other healthy plant-based foods such as millet, soybeans, flaxseeds, and sweet potatoes. If you're getting and absorbing enough iodine, goitrogens don't appear to be a problem. But if you are already low on iodine or suffering from hypothyroidism, you may want to consider cutting back on consumption of these foods. (Since these foods are generally super healthy, getting the support of a qualified health care professional could be important if you have hypothyroidism. Hopefully, if you do find it necessary to eliminate goitrogen-rich foods, you can do so temporarily, as you don't want to solve one problem but create a bunch of new ones.)

What about Iodine Supplements?

Iodine supplements on the market usually come in the form of potassium iodide or sodium iodide. Many multivitamin-mineral supplements also contain iodine. For most people, small amounts of sea vegetables can provide the same benefits without having to take a pill.

Vitamin K

Vitamin K is primarily involved in blood clotting, bone metabolism, and building proteins.[10] It does its work in your liver and other tissues—including your brain, pancreas, heart, and skeletal system. The Danish researcher who discovered this nutrient in 1929 named it in honor of its main function in blood clotting. He called it the "koagulation" vitamin (using the German spelling), or vitamin K.[11]

Vitamin K is a fat-soluble vitamin, which means your body can retain it for long-term use. Whatever you don't use right away gets stored in your liver and fatty tissues. Vitamin K and other fat-soluble vitamins are best absorbed when consumed along with some dietary fat.

There are actually two types of vitamin K: K_1 and K_2.

Vitamin K_1, or phylloquinone, is primarily found in cauliflower and leafy green veggies like spinach, kale, and cabbage. If you're a fan of the cruciferous family, you'll likely find it easy to get enough K_1.

Things aren't so straightforward when it comes to K_2. Also known as menaquinone, it's made predominantly by bacteria found in the intestines of humans and animals. You can also find moderate amounts in certain fermented foods. If you don't consume animal-derived foods (the richest animal-based sources of K_2 include egg yolks, organ meats, and high-fat dairy), you may either need to make friends with fermented plant-based foods or consider a supplement. Some of these fermented plant-based dishes include sauerkraut and kimchi, lacto-fermented pickles (not the supermarket dill or sweet kind), as well as tempeh. The most K_2-rich food of all is a fermented soybean paste called natto.

What Are the Health Benefits of Vitamin K?

Both K vitamins are critical for blood clotting, which is nature's way of keeping you from bleeding to death from a small cut or internal injury. Many of the proteins responsible for triggering coagulation in the presence of an open wound are dependent on vitamin K for their formation and function.[12]

Vitamins K_1 and K_2 may also help with regulating calcium balance, which maintains skeletal strength. Clinical trials have shown that vitamin K_2 supplementation can reduce the risk of spinal and hip fractures in postmenopausal women.[13] High doses of vitamin K_2 have also been used to prevent further bone mineral loss and to reduce the risk of fractures in patients with osteoporosis.[14]

K_2, specifically, may also help keep your heart healthy. Studies have found that it may keep your arteries free of the calcium buildup associated with atherosclerosis, a risk factor for heart disease.[15]

K_2 is involved in processes that help protect your brain as you age. It plays a role in the production of compounds called sphingolipids, which are responsible for much of the cell signaling that goes on in the brain (and sound like a lot of fun!). Changes in sphingolipid metabolism have been linked to neurodegenerative diseases like Alzheimer's.[16] Vitamin K_2 can also protect against oxidative stress and inflammation and may influence psychomotor behavior and brain function.[17]

K_2 also has potential anticancer benefits. Men with higher levels of the vitamin had a significantly reduced risk of advanced prostate cancer. In a randomized clinical trial, men with liver cancer who received 45 milligrams of a supplemental form of K_2 called menatetrenone had much higher survival rates than those who didn't. Three years after the surgical removal of their livers, all the non-menatetrenone patients had died, while almost 60 percent of those who got the supplemental K_2 were still alive.[18]

How Much Vitamin K Do You Need?

Vitamin K is obviously doing some important work in your body, so how much should you be getting? Currently, most health authorities focus on K_1 specifically, which is a shame because it seems that K_2 is also super important for long-term health.[19] For most people, getting enough vitamin K_1 is not a problem.[20] If you eat enough total calories, you're very likely getting more than the recommended amount.

Here are the recommended daily requirements for vitamin K_1 from food, according to the National Academy of Medicine:[21]

- Women: 90 mcg
- Men: 120 mcg

In my opinion, K_2 deserves more attention. Very few health authorities have created a separate recommendation for it, but studies suggest that its health benefits are best seen with a daily intake of between 10 and 45 mcg.[22]

One reason researchers have prioritized K_1 intake is because your body has the natural ability to convert K_1 into K_2. This conversion happens mainly in the intestines. So if you get enough K_1, which as we've seen is found abundantly in veggies, you may be set.

But if K_1 and K_2 were to share their relationship status on social media, they would definitely describe it as "complicated." Researchers don't yet know how efficient the conversion process is and what factors affect it. There's no consensus on whether other tissues in the body, in addition to intestinal gut bacteria, participate in the process. And it's still unclear if the conversion is one way or if the body can turn K_2 back into K_1 if needed. If things weren't confusing enough, there's no blood test available to accurately assess your K_2 status.

One of the countries where plant-based eaters don't seem to be at any risk of K_2 deficiency is Japan. This is likely due to the popularity of natto, a fermented porridge-like dish that provides 50 mcg of K_2 in a single teaspoon.[23]

What about Vitamin K Supplements?

If you aren't a fan of organ meats, egg yolks, full-fat dairy, or natto (which, to be fair, many people find to be an acquired taste), you might consider adding a K_2 supplement to your daily regimen. The most effective way to take it is in combination with vitamin D; some formulations contain both for convenience. Or you can simply eat a half teaspoon per day of natto—which could be a taste worth acquiring.

Vitamin B_{12}

Of all the known vitamins, vitamin B_{12} has the largest and most complex structure. (Think of it as the vitamin equivalent of Ken Follett's historical fiction.) Like all other B vitamins, B_{12} is water-soluble. This means your body uses what it needs and excretes the rest through your urine. Vitamin B_{12} can be stored in the liver for a long time (up to four years), but it's important to get a regular supply in order to prevent deficiency.

Vitamin B_{12} contains the metallic chemical element cobalt, which is why B_{12} compounds are also known as cobalamins. Your body requires B_{12} to form red blood cells, keep your brain functioning properly, and synthesize DNA. B_{12} also plays an essential role in folate (vitamin B_9) metabolism, which is a critical nutrient for reproduction. In other words: no B_{12}, no life.

What Are the Health Benefits of Vitamin B_{12}?

B_{12} supports brain health and a positive mood. Vitamin B_{12} deficiency appears to be a hidden factor in as many as one in three cases of clinical depression.[24]

Vitamin B_{12} can help protect against heart disease by reducing levels of homocysteine, a by-product of protein metabolism.[25] High levels of homocysteine have been linked to a higher risk of heart disease, stroke, and dementia.[26] This ability to bring down homocysteine levels benefits not only your cardiovascular system and your brain but your eyes as well. Elevated homocysteine levels can increase the risk of a number of eye-related diseases, including macular degeneration, cataracts, and some forms of glaucoma.[27]

Adequate levels of B_{12} in pregnant women can also protect against certain serious birth defects. While we most often hear about the importance of folate for preventing neural tube defects in developing children, vitamin B_{12} also plays a crucial role. Fetuses of mothers with low levels of vitamin B_{12} are at a higher risk for birth defects like spina bifida and anencephaly.[28]

Vitamin B_{12} also helps make sure you have enough red blood cells in circulation. This is a good thing, since that's how oxygen gets transported from your lungs to every cell in your body. In fact, having enough B_{12} in the blood may be a performance-enhancing secret weapon for athletes. A 2020 study looked at the relationship between athletic success and blood levels of B_{12} in over 200 track-and-field athletes over six years—concluding that winning performance was associated with a B_{12} concentration of 400 to 700 picograms per milliliter.[29]

Vitamin B_{12} has antioxidant properties that enable it to protect your cells from damage caused by free radicals and reduce your cancer risk. If Jeff Goldblum had gotten more B_{12}, *The Fly* might have been a very different (and much less scary) movie.

How Much B_{12} Do You Need?

Here are the daily intake recommendations for vitamin B_{12}:

- Adults (14+ years): 2.4 mcg
- Pregnant women: 2.6 mcg
- Lactating women: 2.8 mcg

B_{12} is made only by certain bacteria and single-celled organisms. Before modern agriculture, these critters were all over the place, including in the soil (and on foods grown in soil), and could readily be obtained from most produce. In our current industrialized food system, which relies on synthetic chemicals instead of decaying organic matter for fertility, the bacteria that make B_{12} often can't survive.

Before the advent of modern sterilization practices, you might have also gotten B_{12} by drinking well or river water. These days, many of us drink chlorinated tap water, which kills nasty pathogens that can cause cholera, typhoid, and dysentery but also destroys good B_{12}-producing bacteria. Over time, modern society has developed a collective fear of dirt and germs. While there are undeniable public health benefits to our antimicrobial efforts (see mention of cholera, typhoid, and dysentery), there are serious negative side effects as well, including a lack of bioavailable B_{12} in our environment.

For most people, the main dietary source of B_{12} is meat and other animal products.

So if you don't eat meat, dairy, or eggs, you might have a harder time getting sufficient quantities in your diet. Some advocates of meat-eating point to this fact to argue that plant-based diets are unnatural. But it turns out that many omnivores are also deficient in B_{12},[30] suggesting that the problem originates in soil that no longer supports a healthy bacterial population, and not in individual dietary choices. Also, animals raised as livestock are routinely given B_{12} supplementation,[31] so even people eating a meat-only "carnivore diet" are likely getting the majority of their B_{12} from this supplemental form (albeit with a middle-man, or "middle cow," as the case may be).

That said, there are a few plant-based sources of B_{12}. Dried shiitake mushrooms (these are technically fungi, but let's think of them as plants for our purposes) may contain almost 6 mcg per 100 grams.[32] Some sea vegetables are decent sources; green laver, also known as nori (the sheets that are used for sushi) can contain up to 64 mcg of B_{12} per 100 grams (though 100 grams would be 40 sheets of nori, so that's an awful lot of sushi!). B_{12} levels in tempeh, a fermented product made from soybeans, vary widely—and some may contain up to 8 mcg per 100 grams.[33] You can also get some from B_{12}-fortified foods such as plant milks and nutritional yeast.

Some root vegetables, such as carrots, potatoes, and turnips, might have once been decent sources of the nutrient, thanks to their excellent ability to extract it from the surrounding soil. But because the nutrient and microbial content of so much agricultural soil

has degraded over time, today these foods are not reliable sources of B_{12}.

There's one other potential source of vitamin B_{12} that's very close at hand—or should I say, close at belly. That is, it's actually possible that some of your very own gut bacteria are taking care of your needs completely.[34] Many people have natural B_{12}-producing bacteria in their gut's microbiome. Others who may have gastrointestinal disorders, however, may not, and when combined with any natural difficulty absorbing the vitamin, this can put them at risk of a B_{12} deficiency.[35]

What about B_{12} Supplements?

Given the importance of adequate levels of B_{12}, relying on plant foods and your gut microbiome is a bit risky, and this nutrient is too important to leave to chance. And considering that even omnivores could be at risk of deficiency, this is a case where supplementation is a good thing to consider for just about everybody. If you follow a plant-based diet, you may want to get your levels checked on a regular basis. (A vitamin B_{12} test can be done at the same time as other general labs at a wellness checkup. But because it's not a standard test, you will likely have to request it. Also of note, a different test, called methylmalonic acid (MMA for short), seems to be a better indicator of B_{12} status than serum B_{12}.)[36]

Supplemental vitamin B_{12} comes in two main forms: cyanocobalamin and methylcobalamin. Cyanocobalamin, the synthetic formulation, is the more common of the two, mainly because it's cheaper and more stable to manufacture. It also may be more easily absorbed by your body. However, methylcobalamin, the natural form (that is, the kind found in food sources), may be retained better than cyanocobalamin.[37]

Overall, available research around vitamin B_{12} suggests that the differences in bioavailability between these two forms may not be enough to suggest one over the other for most people. Instead, factors that affect the absorption of vitamin B_{12}, like age and genetics, may be more influential than the form of the supplement itself.

B_{12} deficiency is probably the most common serious nutrient deficiency that vegans run into. Don't mess around with this one. If you aren't getting your blood levels checked regularly, and you're a plant-based eater, I urge you to take some form of B_{12} supplement at least every other day.

Vitamin D

Your skin's ability to convert UV rays from the sun into a hormone essential for health is one of the coolest tricks your body can pull off. The hormone created during this process, calcitriol, is also known as vitamin D. (Vitamin D is not technically a vitamin because your body can still synthesize it without needing an external source, but let's just stick with the

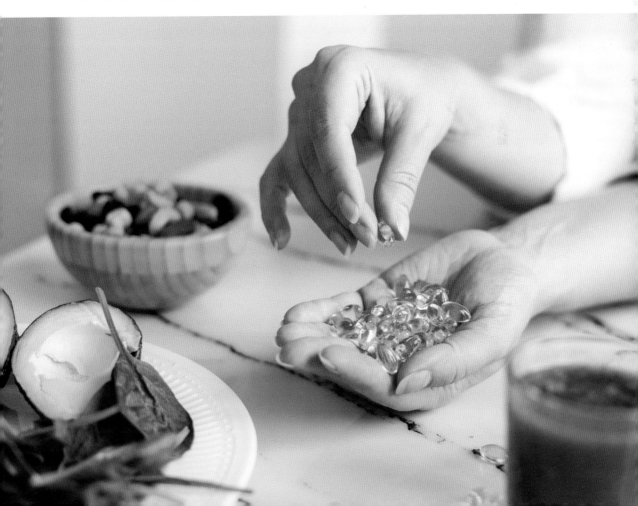

common lingo.) The active form of calcitriol is D_3, or cholecalciferol. This more scientific name indicates that it is calciferous (carries calcium around) and a sterol (a type of steroid hormone).[38]

In addition to direct sun exposure, you can also get vitamin D from a few foods or from dietary supplements. It's a fat-soluble compound, so your body can store unused vitamin D in fatty tissues throughout your body and save it for a rainy day (literally). That also means that if you take it orally, you'll need to consume it with at least some fat for the best absorption.[39]

Vitamin D helps your gut absorb calcium from food and helps you maintain healthy serum calcium (the level of calcium present in your blood) and phosphate concentrations. Vitamin D also works with vitamin K to regulate calcium metabolism, which is essential for heart health. It plays a key role in skeletal health and bone strength. Also, it reduces inflammation and regulates processes like cell growth, neuromuscular and immune function, and glucose metabolism.

What Are the Health Benefits of Vitamin D?

Vitamin D is good for your bones and muscles. You need vitamin D in order to absorb calcium, which is necessary to grow and maintain strong bones. People who are vitamin D–deficient may have compromised skeletal integrity.[40] In addition to bone health, vitamin D is also needed for the normal development and growth of muscle fibers— the thousands of muscle cells that are tightly wrapped together to form your muscles. Not having enough vitamin D can lead to muscle weakness and pain.[41]

Having higher serum levels of vitamin D may reduce your risk of developing cancer. A meta-analysis of 16 studies involving over 100,000 participants found that for every 20 nmol/L (that's nanomoles per liter, in case this gets turned into an audiobook) increase in serum vitamin D levels, the chances of developing cancer dropped by 7 percent.[42] Other studies have linked adequate vitamin D to lower incidence of colorectal and ovarian cancers.[43] In addition to guarding against cancer, vitamin D can also protect the health of your heart. Studies show that people with higher serum vitamin D levels experience fewer heart attacks and strokes.[44]

Not having enough vitamin D is a risk factor for multiple sclerosis, a progressive autoimmune disease in which the insulating covers of nerve cells in the brain and spinal cord are damaged.[45] Researchers are continuing to discover links between vitamin D deficiency and other autoimmune diseases as well.[46]

For people with type 2 diabetes, getting enough vitamin D can be helpful in managing the disease. Giving diabetics supplemental vitamin D has been shown to lower their insulin resistance, the hallmark symptom of type 2 diabetes.[47] Also, low vitamin D levels are associated with an increased risk of hyperglycemia, or uncontrolled high blood sugar, regardless of whether a person is diabetic.[48]

Recently we've come to appreciate how vitamin D contributes to the strength of the immune system, especially when it comes to fighting off viral infections. In 2020 researchers compared the average vitamin D levels among populations from 20 European countries to their rates of COVID-19 infection and mortality. The lower the vitamin D levels, the more people became ill and the more people died of the virus.[49] Vitamin D supplementation has also proven effective in reducing the severity of COVID-19 once contracted. Data shows that patients in a Spanish hospital who were treated for COVID-19 with supplemental vitamin D, an immunosuppressant, and an antibiotic were admitted to the ICU in smaller numbers and had a higher survival rate.[50] The immune benefits of vitamin D also extend to other viral illnesses, like seasonal influenza.[51]

Finally, low vitamin D levels have been linked to depression and other mood disorders. This is likely due to the fact that many parts of the brain, including those that regulate our mood, contain crucial vitamin D receptors in their neurons and glial cells.[52] Women with depression and anxiety who were given high doses of vitamin D each week reported mood improvement after six months of treatment.[53]

How Much Vitamin D Do You Need?

The most common way to get "the sunshine vitamin" is, unsurprisingly, from sunlight. The sun's ultraviolet B (UVB) rays interact with a protein called 7-DHC in your skin, resulting in vitamin D_3 production. But how much sunlight do you need to get optimal levels of vitamin D?

There are several factors that impact the amount of sunlight you need, but a big one is your skin tone. While official recommendations range from 7 to 30 minutes per day over a large portion of your body, people with darker skin pigmentation may need up to six times more sun exposure than lighter-skinned people. For most of human history, getting enough sunlight was not a problem. Today, because so many of us spend most of our time indoors and/or with our skin covered in clothing, typical sunlight exposure may be insufficient to meet our vitamin D needs. And that's especially true the farther you get from the equator and during the fall and winter months, when sunlight hours are limited.

One way to determine if you're getting enough vitamin D from the sun is to get a blood test. Recommended blood levels of D_3 are generally in the 30 to 60 ng/mL range (that's "nanograms per milliliter" for the audiobook narrator).[54]

Other than a supplement, sunlight is probably your best bet, since there are very few foods that naturally contain vitamin D; the ones that do are fatty fish and dairy products (though dairy products don't contain much of it naturally—it's usually added to them through fortification). If you don't include these in your diet, you can ingest some vitamin D from fortified foods and beverages (it's added to most plant milks) or by eating mushrooms that were exposed to UV light while growing.[55]

What about Vitamin D Supplements?

Many people around the world (including omnivores) are deficient in vitamin D, or at least are working with suboptimal levels that keep them from feeling and functioning at their best.[56] The most reliable way to raise low vitamin D levels is to take a supplement. There are two main supplement forms, D_3 and D_2. Of these, D_3 is the more effective.

Most D_3 supplements come from animal products such as lanolin, which is a greasy substance found in sheep's wool. Still, vegan vitamin D_3 supplements are becoming more widespread. These are made from lichen, an organism that arises from algae or cyanobacteria.

While many vitamin D supplements come in gel, oil, or capsule form, there are also liquid dropper options called micellized vitamin D_3. Micellization of vitamin D_3 appears to improve its solubility, absorption, and bioavailability. This explains why that form of vitamin D_3 is shown to be more effective in raising serum vitamin D levels than a fat-soluble version. (I'd love to explain to you what micellization is, but when the first definition I found online stated, "Micellization is a dynamic phenomenon in which n monomeric surfactant molecules S associate to form a micelle Sn,"[57] I decided that I didn't need to know that badly, and you probably don't either.)

You may want to pair a vitamin D_3 supplement with a vitamin K_2 supplement. Here's why: Because it's a fat-soluble compound, D_3 can accumulate in your body. And too much vitamin D can lead to excessive calcium in your blood, which contributes to calcification of blood vessels. Vitamin K_2 helps make sure that the calcium in your body is used to fortify your bones and teeth instead of ending up in your arteries where it doesn't belong and where it can do serious damage.[58] Bottom line: You don't want to be deficient in vitamin K_2 if you're taking vitamin D—and especially if you're also taking calcium. For this reason, it may be advisable to take vitamins D and K_2 together.

For adults up to age 70, a reasonable daily dose of supplemental vitamin D is 15 mcg, or 600 IU (which stands for International Units, the metric you'll find on most supplement labels). After age 70, the recommended daily amount rises to 20 mcg, or 800 IU.

Studies have shown that, on average, each additional 100 IU of vitamin D_3 you consume per day will raise your blood vitamin D levels by 2.5 nmol.[59] Many people find they get best results with 2,000 IU per day, and depending on their needs, some go as high as 10,000 IU per day. But you can get too much, so getting a blood test periodically and working with your doctor to determine the best dose for you is a great idea if you plan to supplement.

Speaking personally for a moment, I started taking a 5,000 IU vitamin D_3 supplement daily about 10 years ago. I've found that this seems to be the perfect amount to get my blood levels where I want them. Before I started taking vitamin D_3, I got colds about two to three times per year (like most people do). Since I started taking it, I've averaged a cold every two to three years, if that. And most of the colds I've gotten have occurred at times when I had, for one reason or another, slacked on my D_3 supplementation. Personally, I'm convinced that it's been great for my immune health.

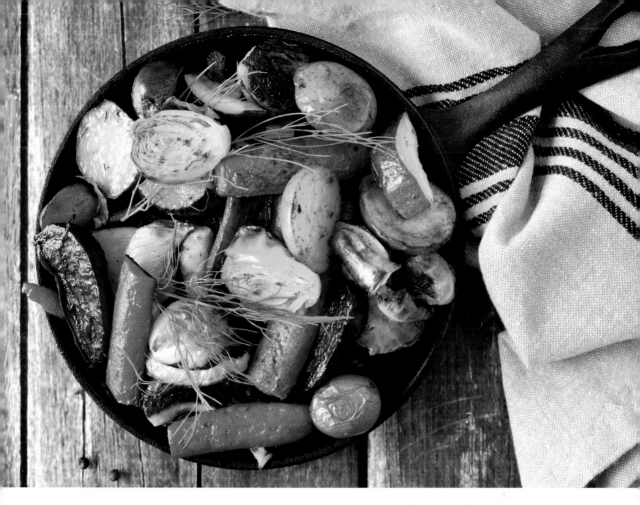

Conclusion

There are certain individual factors that can increase your risk of vitamin D deficiency.[60] The most obvious one is not getting enough outdoor sun exposure directly on your skin. And yes, it has to be outdoors; studies have shown that you don't get enough UVB rays through a window. As we saw, having high melanin levels in your skin, which generally accompanies dark skin pigmentation, can reduce the amount of vitamin D you can synthesize from sunlight. Being of advanced age is also a risk factor for deficiency, as is obesity. Certain medical conditions that limit fat absorption can also lower your vitamin D levels.

If you have any of these risk factors, checking your vitamin D levels is especially important. Fortunately, this is a fairly simple test compared to many other lab tests. The vitamin D assay can be accomplished with a pinprick at a doctor's office, a testing lab, or even at home. And if your blood levels are less than optimal, this could be a great place for an appropriate form of D_3 supplementation.

PART II

RECIPES

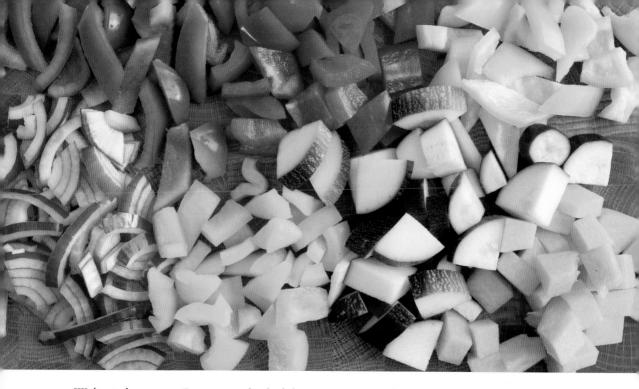

We live in busy times. Between work schedules, kids' schedules, exercise schedules, and caring for our pets, many of us barely have time to watch a half hour of Netflix (important stuff), let alone prepare *and* cook a meal. Our fast-paced world has resulted in an interesting wave of consumer demands that include quick, convenient foods that promise more energy, less stress, and better health—all for low prices, while delivering great taste. While the ease of readily available processed foods can be tempting, the best approach to nutrition is getting nutrients, as much as possible, from whole foods.

The first part of this book armed you with the information you need to eat a healthy and varied plant-based diet. And now comes the fun part. It's time to put what we've been learning into delicious and nutritious action. These quick and effective recipes (most of which can be completed in 30 minutes or less) are here to guide you.

Each of the 65 recipes in this section lists the notable nutrients included per serving, options for ingredient substitution, food storage tips, and more. Before you get cooking, here are some tips to cut down on cooking time, boost the nutritional content of the recipes, and maximize your enjoyment of these delicious plant-powered meals!

Time-Saving Tips

Precut, Canned, and Frozen Fruits and Veggies

Most of the time, plant-based foods require some sort of manipulation to get them from their whole-food form to edible bite-size forms (unless gnawing on crunchy kale leaves plus the fibrous stems is your jam). In each of the recipes, you'll see the whole-food ingredient and how it should be cut. For example, you may see chopped onions, diced tomatoes, or minced garlic—I promise not to ask you to make pretty flowers out of cucumbers. Oftentimes you can prepare these while other ingredients like grains or legumes are cooking on the stovetop to save time. But if that is still too time-consuming or if you just don't want to chop your vegetables, purchasing precut, canned, or frozen produce is certainly an option. This can also save time because they're typically prewashed. If you're purchasing canned goods, look for a BPA-free can to avoid harmful chemicals leaching into your food. Frozen food deserves a special, approving nod because it's often frozen immediately after harvesting, making it an even more nutritious option than the fresh version of that same food. Plus it will last a long time in the freezer, making it less likely to go "bad" than food that's stored in the back of the refrigerator.

I like to keep canned beans on hand for times when I forget to soak dry beans overnight and need something quick. While canned beans and legumes work well in a pinch, the dried versions have their own benefits. Simply put, you have more control over the beans when you cook them from scratch. Soaking and cooking dried beans softens their texture while reducing the compounds that create gas, easing any digestive discomfort. You can also add other ingredients to the cooking liquid, like onions, garlic, and spices, to create delicious flavors that will knock the socks off canned options. Preparing dried beans is doable when you plan ahead for soaking time.

Lentils and split peas deserve some recognition for their quick cooking time (about 20 minutes) without needing to be soaked.

You can cook lentils and quinoa together for a nourishing grain bowl mix that's ready to go! They both cook in about 20 minutes and require a 3:1 ratio of liquid to legume or grain Add veggies and a plant-based sauce for a yummy, nutritious meal.

Precooked Grains

Some grains come precooked in vacuum packaging (or precooked and then dried) so they take considerably less time to make. Also, there are raw grains that require very little time to prepare, like fonio (less than 5 minutes), bulgur (15 minutes), quinoa (20 minutes), and buckwheat (cooking is optional. You can soak it overnight, drain it, and toast it over the stovetop for a few minutes before adding it to salads or using it in grain bowls). Other grains, like farro, einkorn, and sorghum, require soaking and 45 to 60 minutes to cook.

Tofu and Tempeh

Tofu and tempeh can add texture and protein to recipes, creating super satisfying plant-based meals. I like to press tofu to remove excess moisture and to achieve a firm texture, but this step is optional if you're short on time. Firm or extra-firm tofu is your best bet if you plan to skip the pressing step. Note that without pressing, the result will be a less firm (but softer and more silky) texture in your dish.

Unlike tofu, which can be added into dishes raw (silken tofu can be blended into soups and dressings right out of the package to give them a thick and creamy consistency), tempeh should generally be cooked before it's consumed. Straight out of the package, it can have a slightly bitter taste. To remove its bitter-tasting compounds, steam or boil the tempeh for 10 to 15 minutes before proceeding with the recipe.

Prep Your Kitchen and Ingredients Ahead of Time

While some culinary advice entails chopping, slicing, dicing, or otherwise preparing each ingredient in a recipe before moving on to the directions, this book is a little different. Instead of suggesting you precut everything, I will have you cooking grains on the stovetop or baking tofu in the oven first and then preparing your ingredients while these first items cook. This can save a lot of time, but it works only when you have all your ingredients on hand before getting started.

One time-saving tip is to wash and then dry your produce before storing it in your fridge. Placing a paper towel beneath washed foods catches any excess water and preserves their shelf life. Be sure to store them in the proper refrigerator bins or drawers to further manage moisture—a key component to keeping produce fresh.

Another tip is to batch-cook your ingredients. Having cooked grains and beans ready to go for the week is a game changer when it comes to preparing food quickly. Once you have a grain and legume base ready to go, it's easy to add prepared veggies to a plant-based sauce (that you've hopefully made ahead of time and stored), creating a nourishing meal in minutes. If you have a little extra space in your refrigerator, you can also portion out your batch cooking into individual containers (this is often referred to as meal prepping) so all you need to do is heat and serve!

One-Pot, One-Pan, and No-Cook Meals

One-pot meals place all the ingredients into (you guessed it) one pot, and everything cooks together at the same time. Quick and easy! One-pan meals place everything on a single baking sheet to bake or roast.

Also consider the time-saving advantage of no-cook meals, like the Morning Zen Buckwheat Muesli (page 102) or Lettuce Go to the Farmers Market Salad (page 118) in this book. You need no heating elements and very few cooking utensils.

Time-Saving Kitchen Equipment

Let's start with the basics: a good ole (sharp!) chef's knife and wooden cutting board are key before you start any plant-based culinary journey. It may sound counterintuitive for a knife to be sharp and safe; however, keeping your knife sharp prevents it from slipping and makes chopping, dicing, slicing, or any other cuts you're making go smoothly and quickly. One good chef's knife is really all you need to get started. Rather than purchasing one online, visit a store in person to feel it in your hand and try cutting with it (a rib of celery is often the victim here). You'll want to enjoy using it because you'll be using it often! Wooden cutting boards are preferred over plastic or glass since wooden boards are nontoxic and won't slip.

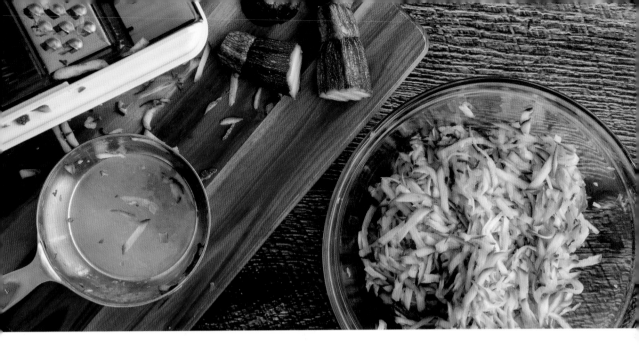

Next in line is a kitchen tool that has saved me countless tears and many minutes of time—a mandoline. Probably one of the most dreaded veggies to cut of all time is the onion, through no fault of its own. In fact, we should thank the onion for its ability to make us cry because the compounds that create those intense fumes are part of what gives onions their claim to health fame. A mandoline can slice an onion in record time and keep your crying at bay. Finally, you can return to fully appreciating the onion and all it has to offer! Look for a mandoline set that allows you to slice and shred.

I could stop there, but there are so many more pieces of equipment that can save you time if you have the space and the financial means to purchase them.

Next up in importance, right beside the mandoline, is a high-speed blender. Plant-based creations often require lots of blending for making plant cheese, sauces, dips, and more. A high-speed blender, like a Vitamix or Blendtec, will make blending a cinch by cutting blend time down significantly and resulting in the creamiest textures.

A food processor is great for blending things that don't need liquid, like hummus or nut or seed butters. They come in a variety of sizes. If you plan to make things in bulk and store them away for later, the 12-cup size might serve you best. If you prefer individual portions, opt for the 4- or 8-cup size food processor. If you skip the mandoline purchase but still want something to do the chopping for you, consider a food processor with a chopping blade option.

I mentioned slow cookers' role in one-pot meals; the pressure cooker also has this capability. Electric multifunction cookers, designed around pressure cooking, are all the rage right now and include multiple other functions, like slow cooking, sautéing, yogurt making, and more. If you plan to be in the kitchen lots and enjoy experimenting with all the ways to cook, it may be worth purchasing a multifunction unit. Pressure cookers can also save you lots of time! For example, cook chickpeas in 25 minutes instead of an hour on the stovetop, or make a stew in 30 minutes instead of 60. The time to cook varies depending on the food and other ingredients, so it's best to check manuals and specific recipes for the type of pressure and time to cook.

Air fryers are another hot kitchen item (pun not intended at first, but I'm taking credit anyway) at the time of writing. People love the crispy textures and intense flavors you can get from cooking food in an air fryer, and I appreciate that I can get those textures and flavors without any added oil.

Silicone spatulas, both big and small, will come in handy when stir-frying or making soups (big spatulas) or scraping every last bit of plant-based sauce or smoothie from your blender (small spatulas). Silicone and stainless steel are generally preferred materials since they're nontoxic.

Speaking of nontoxic, investing in a set of glass or stainless steel storage containers is key, especially if you plan to batch-cook (in fact, better make it two sets of storage containers!) or have leftovers. The material matters as chemicals from plastic containers can leach from the plastic into your food.

Keep an eye out for the "Time-Saving Tips" in the Chef's Notes section of the following recipes. They will offer advice for preparing ingredients or components for the specific recipe ahead of time.

Money-Saving Tips

Healthy eating often gets a bad reputation for being expensive. Sure, if your shopping cart is filled with brands that make plant-based cheese and meat alternatives, you may gasp at the size of the bill. But if you stick to whole plant-based foods, you'll most likely notice a reduction in your grocery costs. As of this writing, in the U.S. a pound of ground beef will cost you $5.23. But a pound of dried beans will cost you about $1.50 (and make six cups of cooked beans).

Then there's the recurring question: Is organic food worth the extra cost? Supporting organic farming practices means supporting practices that protect farmers' health, consumers' health, and the health of the planet. Organic farming also uses fewer toxic pesticides. Unfortunately, organic produce can be more expensive than conventional produce; therefore, eating it is not always financially possible. Or perhaps your local grocery store doesn't carry many organic offerings. If organic produce is out of your price range, it's still better to eat more conventional veggies and fruits than none at all. If purchasing conventional produce is what works best for you and your family, simply wash it well before consuming. (One trick for removing most pesticide residues is to use a mixture of 1 ounce of baking soda with 100 ounces of water (about 12 cups) and soak the produce for 12 to 15 minutes.)

You could also inform your organic produce purchasing based on the Environmental Working Group's Dirty Dozen list, which identifies the 12 produce items found to contain the highest amounts of synthetic pesticides. They publish the list annually, along with their Clean Fifteen list, which includes conventional produce that contains the lowest concentrations of synthetic pesticides (at least from those that they tested).

You can save money by cutting out waste (the average American family wastes more than $2,000 per year on food that goes "bad" before it gets eaten), buying in bulk, making your own foods more often (with recipes like you'll find in this book!), minimizing prepared "convenience" and restaurant meals, and eating more plant-based foods.

One final cost-saving tip that also helps the planet is to purchase foods in bulk, using your own packaging. Be sure that you store excess foods appropriately to prevent spoilage, which would defeat the purpose of saving your hard-earned money.

Global Recommendations

You may notice similar ingredients in recipes, such as tofu and cashews: two staples in a plant-based diet. There are some general guidelines to follow with some of these similar ingredients to help ensure your dish turns out with the right consistency and flavors. There are also tricks you can use in the kitchen to expedite the preparation or cooking times of recipes. Below are some of our top recommendations to make your plant-based recipe creations successful and efficient.

Air frying: If you own an air fryer, you can use a general rule of thumb for recipes that call for baking, which is to decrease the temperature by 25° and reduce the cooking time by 20 percent when using an air fryer.

Chia and flax eggs: Both chia seeds and flaxseed meal turn into binding agents or "eggs" when mixed with water. Whole chia seeds get very gelatinous in water, while flaxseeds are typically ground before adding water. To replace one egg in a recipe, combine one tablespoon of chia seeds or flaxseed meal with three tablespoons of water. Either flax or chia eggs are good not just for binding but also for adding moisture to baked goods.

Chopping fruits and vegetables: To expedite the preparation time of chopping fruits and veggies, you can chop veggies in a food processor with a chopping blade, purchase pre-chopped fruits or veggies, or chop them ahead of time and store them in the refrigerator for up to two days.

Dressings and sauces: To save time, most dressings and sauces can be made ahead of time and stored in an airtight container in the refrigerator for five to seven days.

Kala namak: We occasionally recommend the sulfurous salt kala namak when trying to achieve an egg-like flavor in recipes. This salt originates from India and Pakistan. Also known as Himalayan black salt, it is a kiln-fired rock salt with a sulfurous, pungent smell that gives vegan dishes traditionally made with eggs an eggy aroma and flavor. You should be able to find it in specialty food markets, Indian food markets, or online.

Lemon and lime juice: We use them both a lot as they can really brighten up a dish! We always recommend freshly squeezed instead of store-bought bottled lemon or lime juice.

Maple syrup and date paste: We typically use maple syrup and date paste to sweeten dishes that need a little sweetener. Whenever we mention maple syrup, we mean pure maple syrup. The only ingredient on the food label should be maple syrup, with no other added sugars or additives. Date paste can be made by soaking pitted dates in hot water (enough to cover them) for at least 30 minutes. Then drain them and blend them in a food processor into a paste. If the mixture is dry, add 1 tablespoon of water at a time until you reach a paste-like consistency.

Nut-free: For recipes that call for nuts in their whole form, consider using sunflower seeds, pumpkin seeds, hemp seeds, or chia seeds in their place. For recipes that call for blended cashews to make a creamy sauce, cheese, or dressing, consider using raw sunflower seeds or silken tofu instead. Where nut butters are used, try tahini instead.

Oil-free sautéing: Fats are important from a culinary perspective because they help to carry other flavors to the palate, balance flavors, and add smoothness and richness to dishes. So, why oil-free? The main goals of oil-free sautéing are maximizing the nutritional value of meals and minimizing lifestyle-related health risks. Using whole-food forms of fat whenever possible will give you much more nutrition. For example, you can make

salad dressings creamy by blending a whole avocado with vinegar or lemon juice and any other ingredients, rather than using just the avocado oil. Or you can create creamy sauces by blending whole cashews into a creamy base instead of using oil or plant-based milk. There are three essential practices when it comes to successful oil-free sautéing:

- Make sure the pan is nice and hot.
- Stir constantly to prevent sticking.
- Keep a bit of water or vegetable broth by the stovetop for deglazing, if needed.

Organic reduced-sodium tamari or coconut aminos: Both of these condiments are wonderful for adding umami flavor to dishes, and you'll see them used often throughout this book. We suggest using organic tamari since it's made from soy, and we recommend choosing organic soy whenever possible. We also suggest using reduced-sodium tamari because regular tamari is high in sodium, though reduced-sodium tamari is still high (about 470 mg sodium per tablespoon). Coconut aminos is an alternative that has slightly less sodium (about 270 mg per tablespoon), which is why you'll see it used in the pages that follow.

Reducing gassiness from beans: First, if beans are new to you, go slow. Enjoy them in small doses and maybe try one variety a week before moving on to the next bean. Second, there are ways to reduce those gas-causing compounds in beans. If you're using canned beans, rinse them well before adding them to a recipe. If you're cooking beans from scratch, make sure to soak them in water overnight or for up to 24 hours, changing the soaking water after 12 hours. Use fresh water to cook them. You can also add fennel seeds, cumin seeds, or a piece of kombu seaweed to the cooking water to help reduce the gas-forming compounds. Also remember to drink plenty of water when consuming beans and any fiber-rich food (plants!) as water helps move the fiber through the gastrointestinal tract.

Salt: You'll notice that salt is always an optional ingredient. Just a touch of salt can be a game changer from a culinary standpoint as it can help balance flavors like sweetness and minimize overly bitter flavors. It can also enhance the flavors of spices in a dish. Therefore, we do recommend adding the recommended amount of salt (we don't use much!). However, if you are on a sodium-restricted diet, feel free to omit it altogether.

Pressing tofu: In recipes that use tofu in its whole form (rather than blended), where it's typically baked, grilled, or stir-fried, you may see a suggestion to drain and press it. Pressing the water out of tofu before you cook it creates a firm and crispy texture. To do this, wrap the tofu in paper towels or a clean tea towel, and set something heavy on it, like a cast iron pan or a few heavy books. Let it press for 20 to 60 minutes, if possible. Pressing is optional if you're short on time. Selecting firm or extra-firm tofu is your best bet if you skip the pressing step. If you happen to find super-firm tofu, you don't need to press it as this type of tofu already has much of the water content removed.

Soaking cashews: If you're low on time, skip soaking altogether; however, the end consistency may not be as smooth.

Soaking grains: Soaking whole grains helps increase the bioavailability of minerals like iron, zinc, and calcium and also helps decrease the cooking time. Soak grains by covering them with a generous amount of water for 6 hours or overnight and then draining and rinsing them before using them in a recipe. If you don't have time to soak grains, you can simply rinse and cook them. They may take from 5 to 30 minutes longer to cook. Cook to your desired level of tenderness, adding liquid if needed. More detailed information about soaking times can be found in Food Revolution Network's handy Whole Grains Cooking Guide on page 241.

Whole-food sweetener: If you prefer to use a whole-food sweetener in place of maple syrup, you can use date paste. However, you may need to increase the amount of date paste by one-third to reach your desired consistency and sweetness.

Whole grains: Whole grains are very versatile and can easily substitute for each other in recipes. That said, their cooking times and the grain-to-liquid ratio can vary quite a bit. Before substituting grains, consider the amount of liquid to add and their cooking time. Check Food Revolution Network's helpful Whole Grains Cooking Guide on page 241 for more specific guidance on various whole grains' cooking times and liquid amounts.

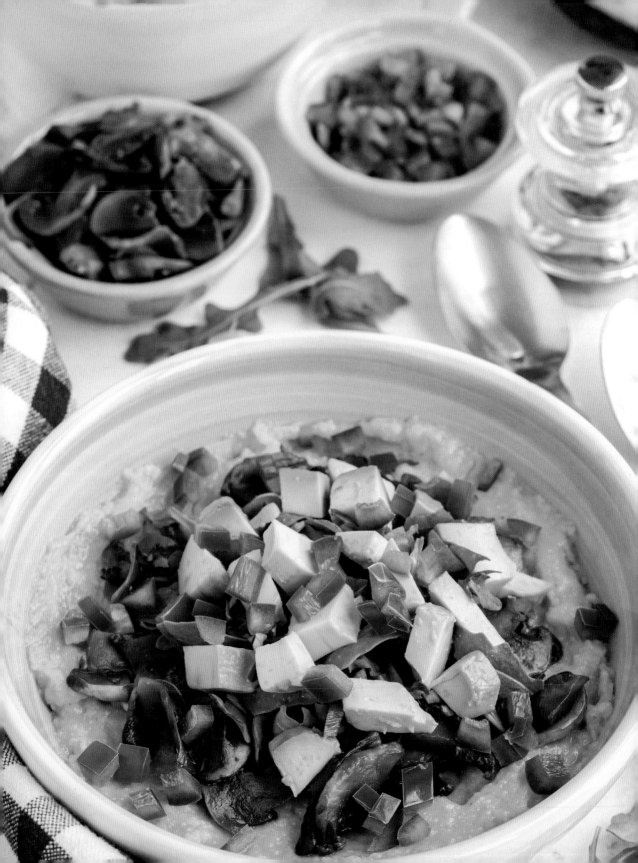

BREAKFASTS

THREE-GRAIN PEACHES AND CREAM BREAKFAST BOWL

Just about all the notable nutrients we've discussed are present and accounted for in this hearty breakfast bowl. An ideal blend of satisfying plant protein, filling fiber, and healthy fats in the form of omega-3s, this dish is the true breakfast of champions. The optional addition of plant-based yogurt does double duty to provide a creamy texture and a dose of gut-nourishing probiotics.

Serves: 2 **Prep time:** 10 minutes **Cooking time:** 15 minutes

¼ cup dry quinoa, rinsed

¼ cup dry millet, rinsed, soaked, and drained (see page 242)

¼ cup dry buckwheat, rinsed, soaked, and drained (see page 241)

1 pinch salt, optional

1 cup plain, unsweetened plant-based yogurt

Sweet and Savory Pecan Topping

3 tablespoons maple syrup

1 teaspoon vanilla extract

1 teaspoon ground cinnamon

1 pinch ground nutmeg

¼ teaspoon salt, optional

2 cups halved raw pecans

Peach Topping

1 cup frozen and thawed or fresh peaches, cubed

2 tablespoons maple syrup

1 teaspoon ground cinnamon

1. Preheat the oven to 350°F. Line a baking sheet with parchment.

2. In a medium saucepan over medium-high heat, bring 1½ cups of water, all the grains, and the pinch of salt to a boil.

3. Reduce the heat to low, cover, and simmer for 15 minutes or until the grains are tender. Remove from the heat but leave the lid in place for 10 minutes.

4. While the grains are cooking, make the Sweet and Savory Pecan Topping: In a medium bowl, combine the maple syrup, vanilla, cinnamon, nutmeg, and salt. Add the pecans and mix until well coated.

5. On the baking sheet, spread out the pecans evenly and bake for 15 minutes, tossing and turning them halfway through to ensure even baking. Remove them from the oven and let them cool. (They'll get crispy as they rest.)

6. While the pecans are cooking, *make the Peach Topping*: In a small pan over medium heat, cook the peaches until slightly golden, stirring occasionally, for about 2 to 3 minutes. Stir in the maple syrup and cinnamon, stirring and cooking until fragrant, about 1 to 2 minutes. Set aside.

7. Divide the grains and yogurt between two bowls. Stir to combine and top with the peaches and 2 to 3 tablespoons of the pecan topping.

Calcium: 224 mg	Iron: 3 mg	Magnesium: 171 mg	Omega-3s: .3 g	Zinc: 3 mg

Calories: 532 | Protein: 12 g | Carbohydrate: 77 g | Fiber: 12 g | Fat: 20 g | Sodium: 183 mg

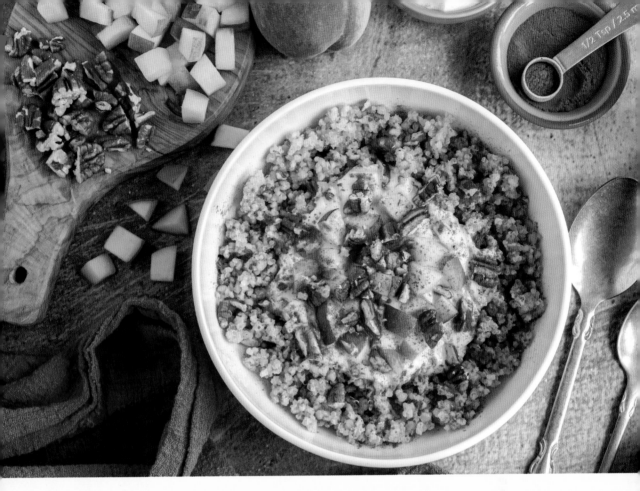

CHEF'S NOTES

Time-Saving Tips

Cook the grains ahead of time and store them in an airtight container in the refrigerator for up to 3 days.

Prepare the Sweet and Savory Pecan Topping and store it at room temperature for up to 2 weeks or in the refrigerator for up to 1 month before using.

Substitutions

Substitute rolled oats or your favorite grain of choice for the quinoa, millet, or buckwheat.

Substitute raw pecans, walnuts, almonds, hazelnuts, or macadamia nuts for the Sweet and Savory Pecan Topping.

Substitute nectarines, plums, apricots, or your favorite stone fruits for the peaches.

Storage

Store leftover cooked whole grains in an airtight container in the refrigerator for up to 3 days. Store leftover peaches in an airtight container in the refrigerator for up to 3 days. Store pecans in an airtight container at room temperature for up to 2 weeks, in the refrigerator for up to one month, or in the freezer for up to 3 months.

BERRYLICIOUS POPPY SEED PANCAKES

Buckwheat flour is a game changer in the nutrient department. It's a source of essential nutrients such as fiber, protein, B vitamins (niacin, folate, and vitamin B$_6$), and essential minerals (magnesium, manganese, and iron). These soft and hearty pancakes are bursting with sweet berry flavor and rich nuttiness. They're also brimming with omega-3 fats from the flaxseed meal, calcium from the poppy seeds, and plenty of notable nutrients that can keep you full and cheerful throughout the morning. Bonus: they also pack well as a snack during a long hike!

Serves: 4   **Prep time:** 10 minutes   **Cooking time:** 10 minutes

2 tablespoons flaxseed meal

1½ cups buckwheat flour

1 cup dry rolled oats

2 teaspoons baking powder

1 tablespoon poppy seeds

1 tablespoon lemon zest, optional

¼ teaspoon salt, optional

1¾ cups plain, unsweetened plant-based milk

2 tablespoons lemon juice

2 tablespoons maple syrup

1 cup fresh or frozen blueberries

CHEF'S NOTES

Substitutions

Instead of buckwheat flour, use whole wheat flour or oat flour.

Try a chia egg instead of the flax egg. (Add 2 tablespoons of chia seeds to 6 tablespoons of water and let rest 5 minutes before use.)

Substitute orange zest and orange juice for the lemon zest and juice.

Instead of blueberries, use another berry of choice.

Storage

Store leftover pancakes in an airtight container in the refrigerator for up to 5 days or freeze for up to 1 month.

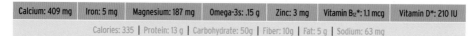

Calcium: 409 mg	Iron: 5 mg	Magnesium: 187 mg	Omega-3s: .15 g	Zinc: 3 mg	Vitamin B₁₂*: 1.1 mcg	Vitamin D*: 210 IU

Calories: 335 | Protein: 13 g | Carbohydrate: 50g | Fiber: 10g | Fat: 5 g | Sodium: 63 mg

*If using fortified plant-based milk.

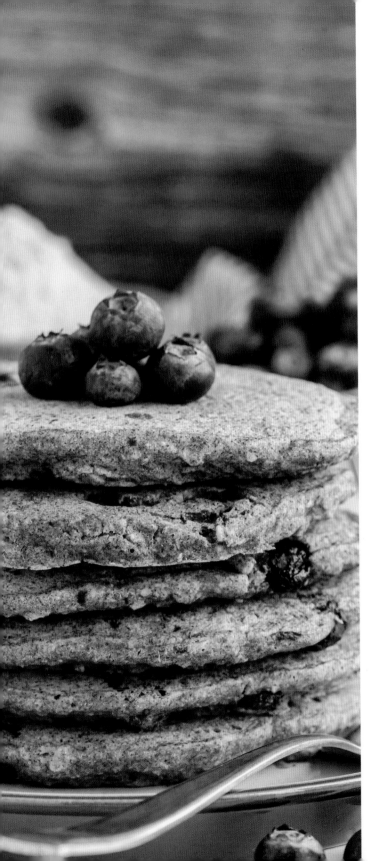

1. Preheat the oven to 200°F (unless you're serving the pancakes immediately from the griddle).

2. Prepare the flax egg: In a medium bowl, whisk together the flaxseed meal and ¼ cup water. Set the mixture aside to rest for a few minutes before using.

3. In a large bowl, combine the flour, oats, baking powder, poppy seeds, lemon zest, and salt and set aside.

4. In a second medium bowl, whisk together the plant-based milk, lemon juice, and maple syrup.

5. Add the wet ingredients to the dry ingredients and stir until just combined. Don't overmix; lumps and dry spots are okay. Note that the batter may be thicker than traditional pancake batter.

6. Fold in the flax egg and the blueberries.

7. Heat a stovetop griddle over medium heat. Grease it with ½ teaspoon or a little spray of oil to prevent the pancakes from sticking.

8. Add approximately ½ cup or a ladle-size of pancake batter to the griddle. You should be able to fit four pancakes on the griddle at a time. Cook until the sides start to brown, about 2 to 3 minutes; then flip to the other side, cooking for another minute or until fully cooked.

9. Transfer the pancakes to an oven-safe plate and warm them in the oven until ready to serve.

10. Serve warm, topped with your favorite fruit such as berries, bananas, or peaches; spread a nut or seed butter over top; or add a handful of nuts for a little crunch!

BANANA BLISS CHOCOLATE CHIP MILLET MUFFINS

Magnesium is one of the most under-consumed nutrients in our modern society. Luckily, nearly every ingredient in these delightful muffins, from the dark chocolate to the millet to the banana, contains magnesium. Make them early in the week and enjoy them all week long as a way to increase your nutrient intake, especially if you find yourself in a pinch between meals.

Serves: 6　**Prep time:** 15 minutes **Cooking time:** 15 minutes

2 tablespoons chia seeds

2 cups oat flour

½ cup dry millet, rinsed, soaked, and drained (see page 242)

2 teaspoons baking powder

2 teaspoons ground cinnamon

¼ teaspoon salt, optional

¾ cup plain, unsweetened plant-based milk

2 tablespoons tahini

¾ cup mashed ripe banana (approximately 1 large)

½ cup unsweetened applesauce

⅓ cup maple syrup

2 teaspoons vanilla extract

¾ cup chopped walnuts, optional

½ cup fair or direct trade vegan dark chocolate chips

1. Preheat the oven to 400°F. Set aside a silicone muffin mold or lined muffin tray (this recipe will make 16 to 18 regular-sized muffins or 30 to 36 mini muffins).

2. Prepare the chia egg: In a small bowl, mix the chia seeds and 6 tablespoons of water. Set the chia egg aside to rest for a few minutes before using.

3. In a large bowl, combine the flour, millet, baking powder, cinnamon, and salt and set aside. If the millet is still damp from soaking, make sure to mix all the ingredients well to evenly disperse the millet.

4. In a medium bowl, whisk together the milk, tahini, banana, applesauce, maple syrup, and vanilla. (Small pieces of banana in this mixture are okay.)

5. Add the wet ingredients to the flour mixture and stir until just combined; don't overmix.

6. Stir the chia egg, then fold it into the batter.

7. Fold in the walnuts and chocolate chips.

8. Spoon batter into muffin cups, filling about three-quarters full.

9. Bake for 15 to 17 minutes or until golden. Let the muffins cool for 5 minutes before enjoying.

Calcium: 128 mg	Iron: 6 mg	Magnesium: 128 mg	Omega-3s: 2 g	Selenium: 17 mcg	Zinc: 3 mg	Vitamin B₁₂*: 1 mcg	Vitamin D*: 10 IU

Calories: 538 | Protein: 12 g | Carbohydrate: 59 g | Fiber: 11g | Fat: 23 g | Sodium: 35 mg

*If using fortified plant-based milk.

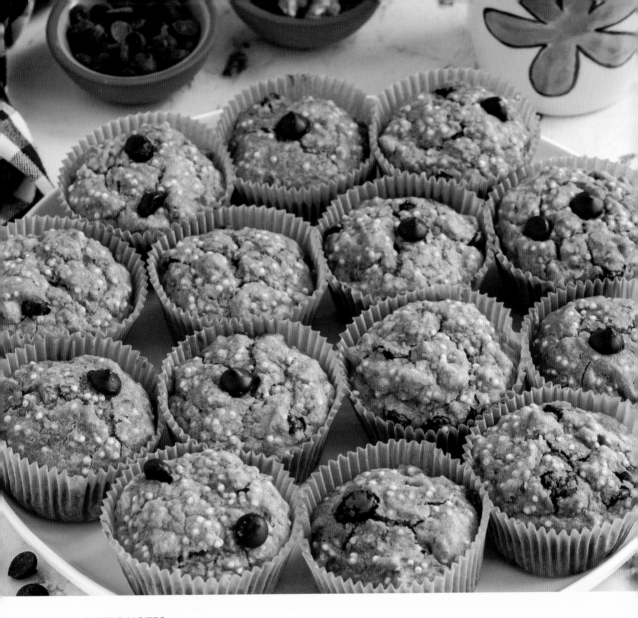

CHEF'S NOTES

Substitutions

Try flax egg instead of chia egg (page 85).

Instead of oat flour, use whole wheat, buckwheat, another flour of choice, or a blend of flours.

Use almond butter in place of tahini.

Storage

Store leftover muffins in an airtight container in the refrigerator for up to 7 days. Reheat them in the oven at 375°F for 10 minutes.

SIMPLY SAVORY POLENTA AND GREENS BREAKFAST BOWL

Filled with cheesy, umami flavor and balanced with notable nutrients like protein, fiber, iron, selenium, and calcium, this savory and nourishing meal is the perfect example of what happens when plants work together to give you the nutrients you need to tackle the day.

Serves: 2 **Prep time:** 15 minutes **Cooking time:** 12 minutes

½ cup polenta, uncooked

1½ cups plain, unsweetened plant-based milk

1 cup low-sodium vegetable broth

8 ounces sliced button mushrooms (approximately 2 cups)

1 tablespoon coconut aminos or reduced-sodium tamari

1 tablespoon sherry or red wine vinegar

½ teaspoon ground turmeric

¼ teaspoon smoked or sweet paprika

2 tablespoons nutritional yeast

½ cup chopped arugula

1 large avocado, cubed

1 jalapeño, diced, optional

Salt to taste, optional

Ground black pepper to taste, optional

Hot sauce to taste, optional

1. In a medium bowl, mix together the polenta and plant-based milk. Set aside.

2. In a medium pot, bring the vegetable broth to a boil over medium-high heat.

3. Slowly stir in the polenta and milk mixture. Bring the mixture back to a boil and then reduce the heat to low. Simmer for 10 to 12 minutes, stirring often to prevent clumping and sticking to the bottom.

4. Meanwhile, heat a large pan over medium-high heat. Add the mushrooms and ½ cup of water, cooking for 2 minutes, stirring occasionally.

5. Stir in the coconut aminos and sherry vinegar and cook until all the liquid has evaporated, about 2 to 3 minutes.

6. Once the polenta has thickened, stir in the turmeric, paprika, and nutritional yeast.

7. Divide the polenta between two bowls and top with the mushrooms, arugula, avocado, and jalapeño. Season with salt, pepper, and hot sauce.

Calcium: 358 mg	Iron: 5 mg	Magnesium: 89 mg	Omega-3s: 1 g	Selenium: 9 mcg	Vitamin B₁₂*: 4 mcg	Vitamin D*: 185 IU

Calories: 277 | Protein: 15 g | Carbohydrate: 28 g | Fiber: 9 g | Fat: 10 g | Sodium: 540 mg

*If using fortified plant-based milk.

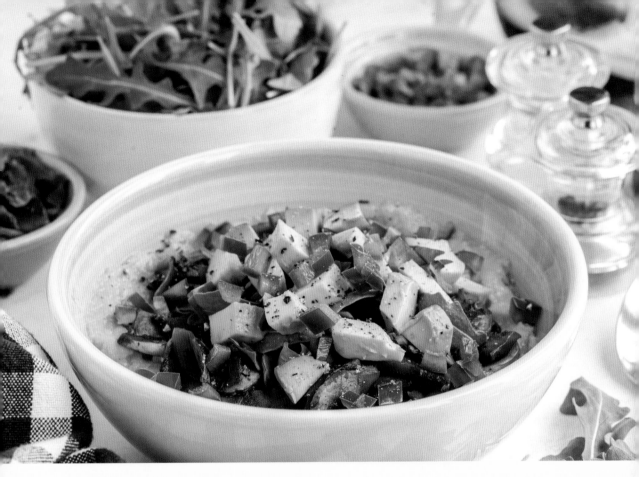

CHEF'S NOTES

Time-Saving Tips

Prepare the mushrooms ahead of time and store them in an airtight container in the refrigerator for up to 2 days.

Use frozen cubed avocado in place of fresh.

Skip chopping the arugula, or use baby arugula or arugula microgreens.

Other Tips

Omit the nutritional yeast if you're unable to tolerate it or can't find it. Or, if you like extra cheesiness, add another tablespoon!

Substitutions

Substitute water for the vegetable broth.

For the mushrooms, use cremini, portobello, or other mushrooms of your choice.

Substitute microgreens for the arugula.

Instead of jalapeño, top the polenta with 1 to 2 tablespoons of diced red bell pepper.

Storage

This dish is best consumed immediately since polenta can get clumpy very quickly! Therefore, make what you think you'll consume in a sitting.

RISE 'N' SHINE BREAKFAST HASH

Lentils are one of the most concentrated and readily available sources of nonheme iron in the plant kingdom. This dish makes for a simple and tasty way to get a diverse range of notable nutrients including fiber, protein, vitamin A, and more! Its Plant-Based Aioli is made from tofu—another good source of iron, as well as calcium.

Serves: 2 **Prep time:** 20 minutes **Cooking time:** 10 minutes

1 cup chopped onion

1 cup diced red bell pepper

4 ounces sliced mushrooms (approximately 1 cup)

2 cups diced sweet potato (approximately 1 large potato)

1 teaspoon ground cumin

1 teaspoon chili powder

1 teaspoon smoked paprika

1 teaspoon garlic powder

¼ teaspoon salt, plus more to taste, optional

1 cup home-cooked or 8 ounces canned lentils, drained

2 cups destemmed and chopped kale

Ground black pepper, to taste, optional

1 to 2 tablespoons chopped cilantro, optional

Plant-Based Aioli

8 ounces firm or extra-firm tofu, drained but not pressed

½ teaspoon mustard powder

2 teaspoons Dijon mustard

1 to 2 tablespoons lemon juice

Kala namak or salt to taste, optional (see page 85)

1. In a large pan over medium-high heat, add the onions, bell peppers, mushrooms, and sweet potatoes. Stir often for 5 minutes, or until the mushrooms start to sweat, releasing their water content. The mushrooms should naturally deglaze the pan as they sweat, but you can add 1 to 2 tablespoons of water if needed.

2. As the veggie mixture is cooking, in a small bowl, combine the cumin, chili powder, smoked paprika, garlic powder, and salt.

3. Once the mushrooms have released their water, add the spices. Stir, reduce the heat to medium, and then cover the pan with a lid three-quarters of the way to steam the potatoes for 3 to 4 minutes or until they are fork-tender.

4. Add the lentils and kale to the pan, tossing until the kale is tender, about 1 minute.

5. Add the salt and pepper to taste, and the cilantro. Set the potato mixture aside and allow it to cool slightly.

6. In a blender or food processor, blend all the Plant-Based Aioli ingredients until creamy. (If you're using a food processor, you'll want to blend it for longer, periodically pausing to scrape the aioli from the sides.) Add 1 to 2 tablespoons of water at a time to reach the desired consistency, which can range from hummus-style (great for dipping or serving on the side of the hash dish) to sauce consistency (to drizzle over the hash).

7. Divide the hash between plates and serve with the Plant-Based Aioli.

Calcium: 303 mg	Iron: 7 mg	Magnesium: 148 mg	Selenium: 9 mcg	Zinc: 3 mg

Calories: 496 | Protein: 20 g | Carbohydrate: 75 g | Fiber: 18 g | Fat: 5 g | Sodium: 292 mg

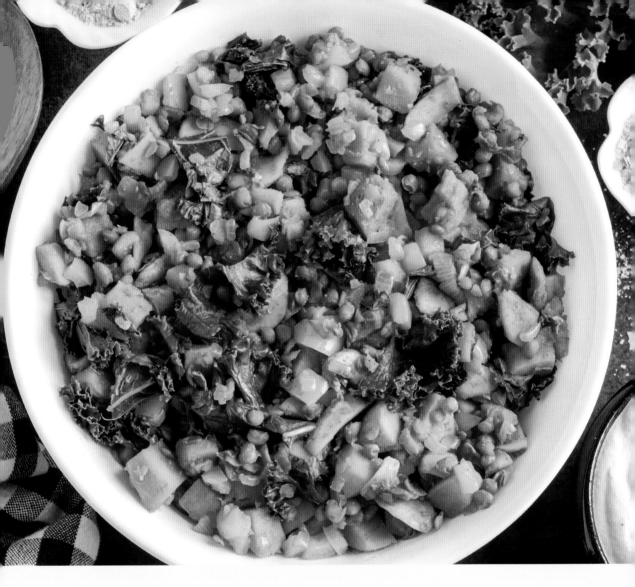

CHEF'S NOTES

Time-Saving Tips

Prepare the Plant-Based Aioli ahead of time. You can also eliminate the aioli altogether and serve the hash with a sprinkle of nutritional yeast.

Substitutions

Substitute white potatoes for the sweet potatoes, or butternut squash cubes, beets, or your favorite root vegetable of choice.

Substitute spinach, arugula, chard, or your favorite dark leafy green of choice for the kale.

Storage

Store the hash in an airtight container in the refrigerator for up to 5 days and the aioli in an airtight container in the refrigerator for up to 3 days.

WRAPPED IN WELLNESS TOFU SCRAMBLE

The term "eat the rainbow" may be familiar to you, and for good reason. Aside from the bright and cheery hues that look enticing on any plate, it's actually one of the easiest ways to ensure you are getting enough of the nutrients you need. This colorful, nutritious breakfast wrap is packed with fiber, protein, iron, calcium, zinc, and magnesium. For a culinary *je ne sais quoi*, give it a try with kala namak to give this wrap an egg-like flavor that ties it all together!

Serves: 2 **Prep time:** 20 minutes **Cooking time:** 10 minutes

8 ounces firm or extra-firm tofu, drained and crumbled (see page 81)

½ cup chopped red onion

½ cup chopped red bell pepper

½ cup seeded and chopped tomatoes

1 to 2 tablespoons minced jalapeño, optional

1 cup spinach

2 to 4 tablespoons chopped cilantro, optional

2 8-inch whole-grain tortillas

½ avocado, sliced

Salsa to taste, optional

Hot sauce to taste, optional

Cashew Sour Cream

1 cup raw cashews, soaked in hot water for 30 minutes or room-temperature water for 2 hours, drained

1 tablespoon lemon juice

1 teaspoon apple cider vinegar

¼ teaspoon salt, optional

Tahini Sauce

1 tablespoon tahini

¼ cup plain, unsweetened plant-based milk

¼ teaspoon ground turmeric

1 teaspoon chili powder

1 teaspoon ground cumin

1 teaspoon garlic powder

¼ teaspoon kala namak or salt, optional (see page 85)

2 dashes ground black pepper, optional

| Calcium: 58 mg | Iron: 10 mg | Magnesium: 312 mg | Selenium: 27 mcg | Zinc: 7 mg |

Calories: 501 | Protein: 33 g | Carbohydrate: 20 g | Fiber: 15 g | Fat: 31 g | Sodium: 591 mg

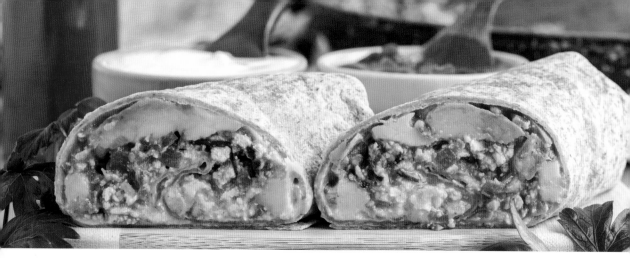

1. Prepare the Cashew Sour Cream: Rinse the soaked cashews. Transfer the cashews, ½ cup of water, lemon juice, apple cider vinegar, and salt to a blender or food processor. Blend on high until smooth. You might need to stop to scrape down the blender now and then, or add 1 to 2 tablespoons of water if it's too thick. Set aside.

2. Make the Tahini Sauce: In a medium bowl, whisk together the tahini, plant-based milk, turmeric, chili powder, cumin, garlic powder, kala namak, and black pepper until blended. Set aside.

3. In a large pan over medium-high heat, add the tofu, onion, and red bell pepper. Stir occasionally until the onion is translucent and the tofu starts to brown just a bit, about 5 minutes.

4. Reduce the heat to medium and stir in the tomatoes and jalapeños, cooking for another minute.

5. Pour the tahini sauce over the tofu and stir. Cook for another minute until fully combined.

6. Fold in the spinach and cilantro until the spinach is wilted, about 30 seconds, and remove the scramble from the heat.

7. Warm the tortillas in the microwave for 30 seconds or heat on a griddle on the stovetop for 1 to 2 minutes.

8. Divide the tofu mixture and avocado between the tortillas and then top each with salsa, Cashew Sour Cream, and your desired amount of hot sauce.

CHEF'S NOTES

Time-Saving Tips

Make the Cashew Sour Cream ahead of time and store it in an airtight container in the refrigerator for up to 5 days or freeze for up to 3 months.

Other Tips

For this dish, you don't need to press the tofu. Drain the water from the tofu and crumble it into small pieces into a bowl in preparation for adding it to the pan. However, if you want the tofu to have a firmer texture, see page 87 for recommendations.

Substitutions

Substitute crumbled, cooked tempeh for the tofu.

Substitute green bell pepper for the jalapeño.

Substitute baby kale or arugula for the spinach.

Substitute parsley or dill for the cilantro.

Use almond butter in place of tahini.

Use corn tortillas or collard wraps in place of whole-grain tortillas.

Soy-Free: Instead of tofu, try crumbled chickpeas or your favorite plant-based protein of choice.

Storage

Store the scramble in an airtight container in the refrigerator for up to 4 days.

MORNING ZEN BUCKWHEAT MUESLI

Muesli is a versatile breakfast cereal or snack that typically consists of rolled oats, nuts, seeds, dried fruits, and spices. Using buckwheat in place of oats and combining a rich medley of nuts and seeds adds extra plant-powered protein and anti-inflammatory omega-3s. These all-star ingredients are also packed with calcium, magnesium, and iron, making it a recipe you'll want to keep in your breakfast cereal archives.

Serves: 2   **Prep time:** 5 minutes   **Cooking time:** 5 minutes

½ cup dry buckwheat, rinsed, soaked, and drained (see page 241)

2 tablespoons slivered almonds

2 tablespoons raw pumpkin seeds

1 tablespoon flaxseed meal

1 tablespoon chia seeds

1 tablespoon hemp seeds

2 tablespoons unsweetened or naturally sweetened dried cranberries

1 teaspoon ground cinnamon

1 cup plain, unsweetened plant-based milk, plus more as desired

Suggested toppings (see Chef's Notes)

1. In a medium pan over medium heat, toast the buckwheat for 5 minutes, tossing or stirring often until fragrant and lightly golden brown. Set aside.

2. To a 16-ounce mason jar or storage container, add the buckwheat, almonds, pumpkin seeds, flaxseed meal, chia seeds, hemp seeds, dried cranberries, and cinnamon. Place a lid on top and shake to combine.

3. Add the plant-based milk. Stir and store in the refrigerator overnight.

4. Enjoy it cold or heat it on the stovetop the next morning. Add more plant-based milk, depending on the consistency you'd like. Add toppings of your choice.

| Calcium: 290 mg | Iron: 4 mg | Magnesium: 197 mg | Omega-3s: 1.8 g | Selenium: 8 mcg | Zinc: 2 mg | Vitamin B₁₂*: 1 mcg | Vitamin D*: 120 IU |

Calories: 365 | Protein: 15 g | Carbohydrate: 36 g | Fiber: 9 g | Fat: 15 g | Sodium: 69 mg

*If using fortified plant-based milk.

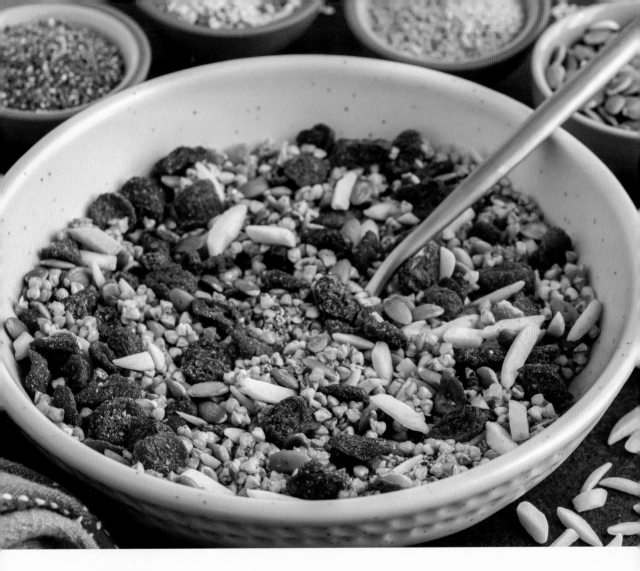

CHEF'S NOTES

Other Tips

Topping Ideas: Berries are always a great choice, but feel free to add any chopped fruit that you enjoy most, or try unsweetened shredded coconut or cacao nibs.

Substitutions

Substitute rolled oats for the buckwheat.

Substitute raisins, currants, or your favorite dried fruit of choice for the cranberries.

For a sweet vanilla flavor, add 1 teaspoon of vanilla extract and any sweetener of your choice to taste to the milk.

Storage

Store the muesli in an airtight container in the refrigerator for up to 2 days. Alternatively, you can mix all the ingredients except the plant-based milk and toppings and store them in an airtight container in the refrigerator for up to 1 week.

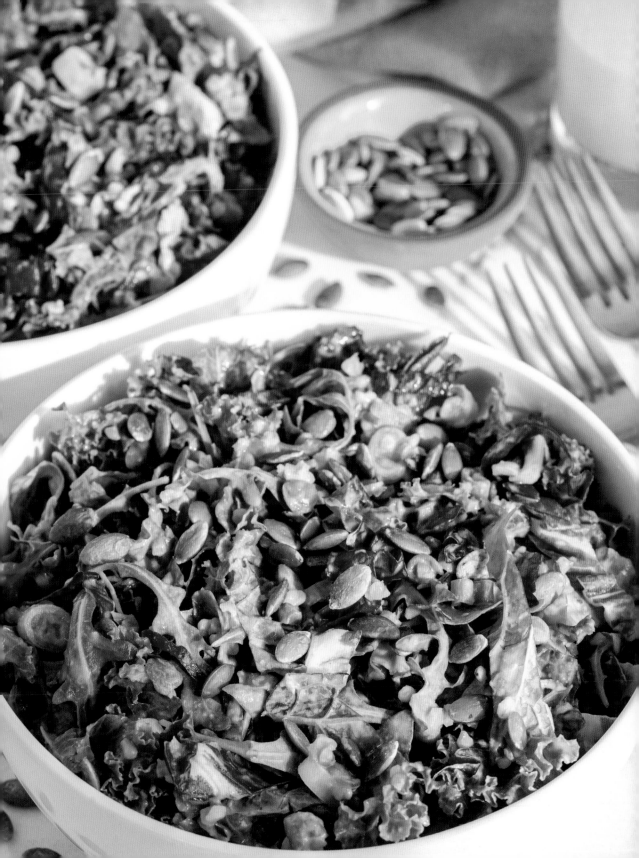

SALADS

BRIGHT AND LIVELY CITRUS SALAD

Bursting with summer flavor, this salad is a powerhouse of eye-catching color and nutrition. Citrus fruit and blackberries brighten this dish, making getting your daily dose of essential nutrients just as much fun as a day in the summer sun!

Serves: 2 **Prep time:** 15 minutes **Cooking time:** none

¼ cup dry quinoa, rinsed

4 cups chopped spinach

1 cup segmented and chopped citrus fruit pieces of your choice

½ cup halved blackberries

¼ cup chopped red onion

1 medium avocado, cubed

2 tablespoons slivered almonds or hemp seeds

1 to 2 teaspoons extra virgin olive oil, optional

2 tablespoons lemon juice

Salt to taste, optional

Ground black pepper to taste, optional

Macadamia Nut Ricotta

½ cup macadamia nuts

2 dashes nutmeg

2 teaspoons lemon juice

⅛ teaspoon salt, optional

1. In a small pot over medium-high heat, bring the quinoa and ½ cup water to a boil. Reduce the heat to low, cover, and simmer for 15 minutes. Remove from the heat and let it sit for 10 minutes with the lid on.

2. Meanwhile, make the Macadamia Nut Ricotta: In a food processor, blend the macadamia nuts, ¼ cup of water, nutmeg, lemon juice, and salt until smooth. Set aside.

3. In a large bowl, toss to combine the spinach, citrus, blackberries, red onion, avocado, almonds, and quinoa.

4. Drizzle the olive oil and lemon juice over the top. Toss to combine once more. Add salt and pepper to taste.

5. Divide between salad plates or bowls and top with 1 to 2 dollops of Macadamia Nut Ricotta.

Magnesium: 219 mg	Selenium: 6.5 mcg	Zinc: 2.9 mg

Calories: 485 | Protein: 12 g | Carbohydrate: 28 g | Fiber: 13 g | Fat: 33 g | Sodium: 56 mg

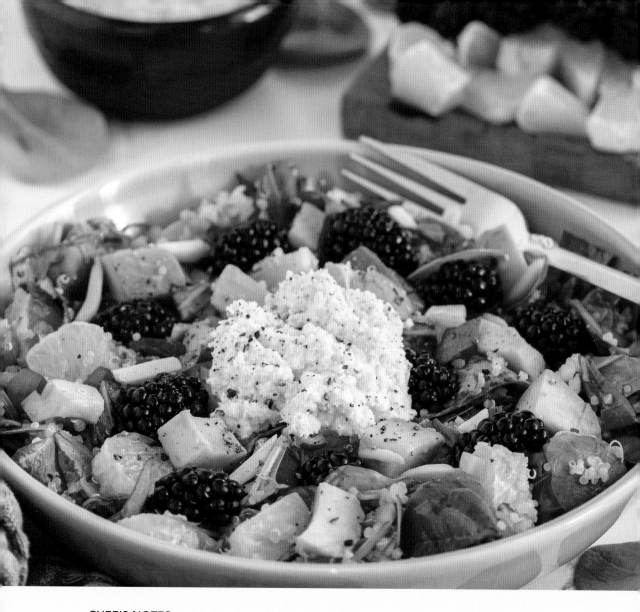

CHEF'S NOTES

Citrus Tips

For the citrus, choose seedless varieties such as navel, Cara Cara, mandarin, or Valencia. (Try to avoid using the white pith as it can create more bitter and less sweet flavors.)

Substitutions

Substitute arugula or your favorite leafy greens of choice for the spinach.

Substitute strawberries, blueberries, or raspberries for the blackberries.

In place of red onion, use shallots.

Storage

Store in an airtight container in the refrigerator for up to 3 days.

DELIGHTFULLY CREAMY AVOCADO SALAD WITH MAPLE TAHINI DRESSING

The combination of creamy avocado, chewy buckwheat, and cool cucumbers makes this salad a refreshing feast for the senses! It's a nice balance of smooth and crunchy, and the addition of tomatoes and red onion delivers exceptional flavor and nutrition, all in less than 30 minutes. Enjoy it solo, as a side dish, or in a hearty vegetable wrap.

Serves: 4   **Prep time:** 15 minutes   **Cooking time:** 8 minutes

½ cup dry buckwheat, rinsed, soaked, and drained (see page 241)

2 large avocados, cubed

1 cup diced unwaxed cucumbers

½ cup diced red onion

1 cup chopped tomatoes

1 cup chopped arugula

Salt to taste, optional

Ground black pepper to taste, optional

Maple Tahini Dressing

1 tablespoon tahini

1½ tablespoons lime juice

1½ tablespoons red wine vinegar

2 teaspoons maple syrup

½ teaspoon garlic powder

½ teaspoon dried oregano

1. In a small pan over medium heat, toast the buckwheat for 5 minutes, tossing or stirring often until fragrant and lightly golden brown. Set aside.

2. Make the Maple Tahini Dressing: In a small bowl, whisk together the tahini, lime juice, red wine vinegar, maple syrup, garlic powder, and oregano. Add 1 to 2 tablespoons of water as needed to reach your desired drizzling consistency. Set the dressing aside.

3. In a large bowl, gently toss together the avocados, cucumbers, red onion, tomatoes, arugula, and buckwheat.

4. Pour the dressing over the top and gently mix together. Add salt and pepper to taste.

Calcium: 53 mg	Iron: 2 mg	Magnesium: 83 mg	Selenium: 3 mcg	Zinc: 1.4 mg

Calories: 241 | Protein: 5 g | Carbohydrate: 21 g | Fiber: 8 g | Fat: 13 g | Sodium: 18 mg

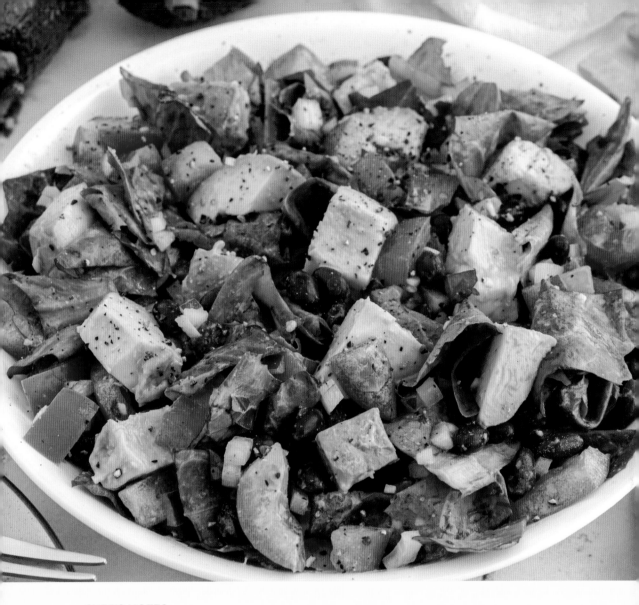

CHEF'S NOTES

Other Tips

Add chopped mango for a little sweetness. Add diced jalapeño for a little spice.

Substitutions

Instead of red onion use yellow, white, or green onion.

In place of arugula use red leaf lettuce, romaine, or kale.

Storage

Store leftovers in an airtight container in the refrigerator for up to 2 days. Note that the arugula may get soggy, so if you expect to have leftovers, add arugula to only the portion you plan to eat immediately to keep it crisp.

UNDER THE ITALIAN SUN-DRIED TOMATO, CANNELLINI, AND SPINACH SALAD

The robust flavors of Italy make getting this daily dose of leafy greens that much more enjoyable. Moreover, the ingredients in this hearty salad combine to provide a concentrated source of iron, boasting a whopping 10 milligrams per serving. Depending on your dietary needs, you may come pretty close to consuming your recommended daily requirement with this meal alone. You can enjoy this salad on a bed of leafy greens, in a whole-grain wrap, or as a warm side dish.

Serves: 2 **Prep time:** 15 minutes **Cooking time:** 15 minutes

¼ cup low-sodium vegetable broth

2 tablespoons minced shallots

4 cloves garlic, minced

¼ cup chopped sulfite-free sun-dried tomatoes

¼ cup chopped artichokes, frozen or jarred in water

2 tablespoons chopped kalamata or green olives

1½ cups home-cooked or 1 15-ounce can cannellini beans, drained

1 cup cooked quinoa (see page 242)

2 cups chopped spinach

2 tablespoons lemon juice

½ teaspoon dried oregano

¼ teaspoon ground black pepper, optional

¼ teaspoon crushed red pepper flakes, optional

2 tablespoons nutritional yeast, optional

2 tablespoons chopped basil

1. In a medium pan over medium heat, cook the vegetable broth, shallots, and garlic for 1 to 2 minutes.

2. Stir in the sun-dried tomatoes, artichokes, and olives and cook for another 30 to 60 seconds.

3. Stir in the cannellini beans and quinoa. Add more vegetable broth, if needed, to prevent sticking to the pan. Cook for another 30 to 60 seconds.

4. Stir in the spinach until wilted. Remove the pan from the heat.

5. Add the lemon juice, oregano, ground black pepper, and crushed red pepper flakes. Stir well.

6. Divide between two dishes as a side or on top of spring greens. Top with the nutritional yeast and basil.

Calcium: 133 mg	Iron: 6 mg	Magnesium: 186 mg	Selenium: 11 mcg	Zinc: 4 mg	Vitamin B$_{12}$*: 2.4 mcg

Calories: 350 | Protein: 18 g | Carbohydrate: 101 g | Fiber: 13 g | Fat: 5 g | Sodium: 261 mg

*If using fortified nutritional yeast.

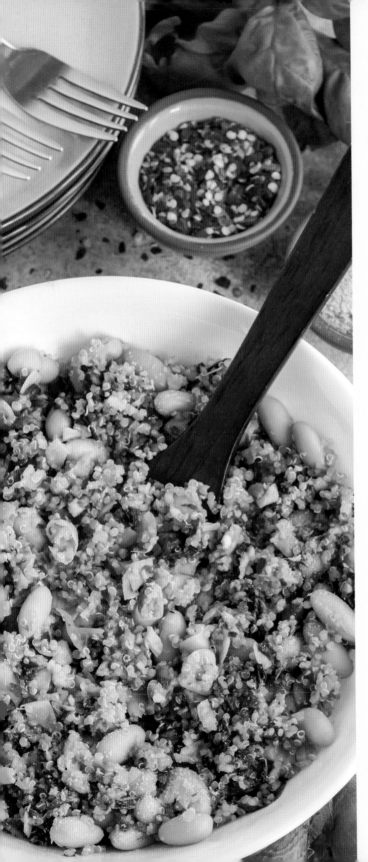

CHEF'S NOTES

Time-Saving Tips

Make the quinoa ahead of time by placing ⅓ cup thoroughly rinsed quinoa and ⅔ cup water in a medium pot. Bring to a boil and then reduce the heat to low and simmer for 10 to 15 minutes. Turn off the heat and allow the quinoa to sit, covered, for 5 minutes. Fluff with a fork before adding it to the remaining salad ingredients.

Substitutions

In place of shallots, use chopped red, yellow, or white onion.

In place of fresh garlic, use ½ teaspoon of garlic powder.

In place of cannellini beans, use chickpeas, great northern beans, fava beans, or any other beans you have on hand.

Substitute fresh tomatoes for sundried. Fresh tomatoes may call for a little salt or additional seasoning (lemon, oregano, or nutritional yeast).

Instead of quinoa, try a grain such as farro, brown rice, or Kamut.

Instead of basil, use parsley or chives.

Storage

Store leftovers in an airtight container in the refrigerator for up to 5 days or freeze for up to 1 month.

SUPER GREENS AND BEANS DETOX SALAD

Vibrantly colored and nutritious, this salad combines crisp leafy greens, hearty lentils, and fluffy bulgur to give you a heaping serving of a bunch of notable nutrients. Packed with fiber, iron, plant-based protein, magnesium, and zinc, this salad is a delicious way to support your health and relish the joy of a satisfying and tasty meal.

Serves: 2 **Prep time:** 15 minutes **Cooking time:** none

½ cup dry brown or green lentils, rinsed

½ cup dry bulgur, rinsed

2 cups destemmed and thinly sliced kale

1 cup thinly sliced radicchio (approximately 1 small head or ½ medium head)

2 cups thinly sliced arugula

⅔ cup thinly sliced radishes

⅔ cup thinly sliced unwaxed cucumbers

½ cup diced red onion

¼ cup raw walnuts or raw pistachios

Salt and pepper to taste, optional

Creamy Ginger Dressing

½ cup plain, unsweetened plant-based yogurt

1 tablespoon tahini

2 tablespoons unsweetened rice vinegar

1 tablespoon lime juice

2 teaspoons coconut aminos or reduced-sodium tamari

1 tablespoon maple syrup

2 teaspoons Dijon mustard

1 tablespoon minced ginger

1. In a medium pot over high heat, bring the lentils, bulgur, and 2⅓ cups water to a boil. Reduce the heat to low, cover, and simmer for 25 minutes.

2. Make the Creamy Ginger Dressing: In a blender, blend all the dressing ingredients along with 2 tablespoons of water until smooth. Set it aside.

3. In a large bowl, combine the kale, radicchio, arugula, radishes, cucumbers, and onion with the cooked bulgur and lentils. (Be sure to drain any excess water from the cooked bulgur and lentils before adding.)

4. Divide the salad between two bowls for a main meal or between four bowls if it's being served as a side.

5. Pour the dressing over the top and toss well. (If you're planning to save any salad for later, serve the dressing alongside the salad to avoid it getting soggy in storage.)

6. Sprinkle with walnuts and add salt and pepper to taste.

Calcium: 184 mg	Iron: 5 mg	Magnesium: 119 mg	Selenium: 4 mcg	Zinc: 2 mg

Calories: 559 | Protein: 21 g | Carbohydrate: 65 g | Fiber: 14 g | Fat: 17 g | Sodium: 325 mg

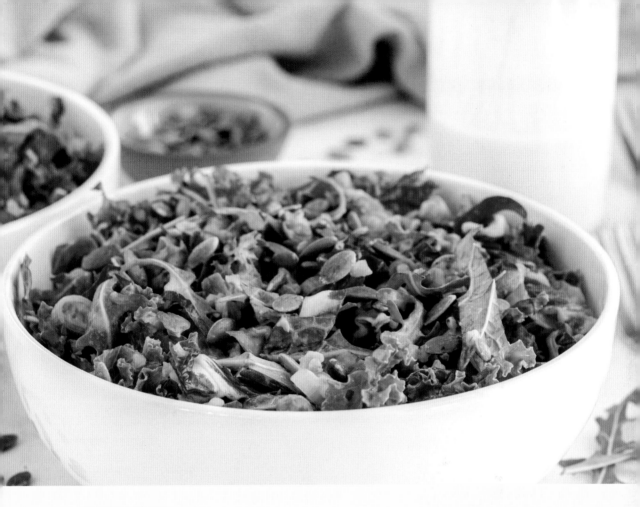

CHEF'S NOTES

Time-Saving Tips

Cook the bulgur (or another substituted grain) and lentils ahead of time and store them in an airtight container in the refrigerator for up to 5 days, or in the freezer for up to 1 month.

Substitutions

For the kale, use curly, lacinato, baby kale, or other leafy greens.

For the lentils, you can also use black or French varieties.

Instead of red onion, use green, yellow, or white onion.

Instead of walnuts or pistachios, try sunflower seeds or pumpkin seeds.

Gluten-Free:

Substitute quinoa, millet, amaranth, or buckwheat for the bulgur.

Substitute cooked and cubed sweet potatoes in place of the bulgur.

Storage

Store leftovers in airtight containers in the refrigerator for up to 3 days. Store the dressing separately from the salad ingredients to keep the vegetables crisp.

PERFECTLY BALANCED 15-MINUTE PASTA SALAD

This recipe is a great example of how you can increase your protein intake simply by choosing a legume-based pasta over a grain-based one. Depending on the serving size, you can obtain nearly 30 grams of protein—all from plants! Persian cucumbers have less water than English varieties, which keeps the dish from getting watered down (especially if you have leftovers for the next day). Mix in dark leafy greens and a few other wholesome vegetables to up your intake of iron and fiber too.

Serves: 2 **Prep time:** 15 minutes **Cooking time:** 10 minutes

8 ounces dry whole-grain or legume pasta

½ cup cherry tomatoes, halved

⅓ cup diced red onion

⅓ cup pitted and diced green or black olives

½ Persian cucumber, diced (see Chef's Notes)

1 cup arugula

¼ cup chopped basil

2 teaspoons extra virgin olive oil, optional

2 tablespoons lemon juice

½ teaspoon dried oregano

½ teaspoon garlic powder

¼ teaspoon salt, optional

Salt and pepper to taste, optional

Crushed red pepper flakes to taste, optional

2 lemon wedges

Vegan Walnut Parmesan

¾ cup raw chopped walnuts

¼ cup raw sunflower seeds

¼ teaspoon garlic powder

¼ teaspoon onion powder

2 tablespoons nutritional yeast

¼ teaspoon salt, optional

1. Prepare your pasta according to the directions on the packaging.

2. While the pasta is cooking, in a large bowl, combine the tomatoes, onion, olives, cucumber, arugula, and basil. Set aside.

3. In a small bowl, whisk together the olive oil, lemon juice, oregano, garlic powder, and salt until thoroughly combined. Set aside.

4. In a food processor, blend all the Vegan Walnut Parmesan ingredients until the walnuts and sunflower seeds are mealy. Set aside.

5. Once the pasta is finished cooking, drain and add it to the bowl containing the veggies. Toss to combine.

6. Drizzle the dressing over the top and toss again until the veggies and pasta are evenly coated.

7. Sprinkle ¼ cup Vegan Walnut Parmesan over the top and toss once again.

8. Divide the salad between bowls and add salt, pepper, and crushed red pepper flakes to taste. Serve with the lemon wedges.

Calcium: 69 mg	Iron: 2 mg	Magnesium: 48 mg	Omega-3s: 1 g	Selenium: 3.75 mcg	Zinc: 1 mg	Vitamin B₁₂*: 8 mcg

Calories: 348 | Protein: 27 g | Carbohydrate: 29 g | Fiber: 7 g | Fat: 26 g | Sodium: 422 mg

*If using fortified nutritional yeast.

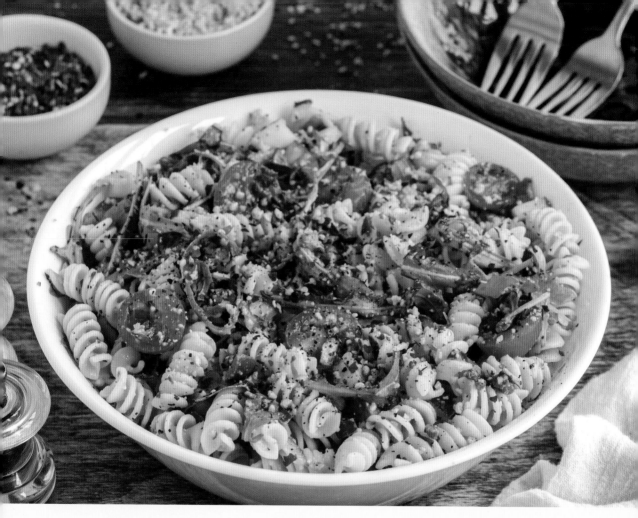

CHEF'S NOTES

Time-Saving Tips
Make the Vegan Walnut Parmesan ahead of time and store it in an airtight container in the refrigerator for up to 2 weeks.

Substitutions
Substitute shallots for the red onion.

Substitute parsley for the basil.

Substitute spinach or baby kale for the arugula.

Substitute red wine vinegar for the lemon juice.

Substitute bell peppers, celery, or radishes for the cucumber.

Nut-Free: Sprinkle nutritional yeast on top instead of the Vegan Walnut Parmesan.

Storage
Store the pasta salad in an airtight container in the refrigerator for up to 5 days.

CREAMY ALMOND MEETS CRUNCHY SLAW

Prepare your taste buds for this combination of zesty and bright napa cabbage, colorful julienned vegetables, protein-packed edamame, and a creamy almond butter–based sauce. This slaw not only incorporates delicious Asian fusion flavors but also provides you with a significant source of plant-based calcium (approximately 190 milligrams per serving to be exact!).

Serves: 4 **Prep time:** 20 minutes (while rice is cooking) **Cooking time:** 35 minutes

⅓ cup dry black rice, rinsed

4 cups thinly sliced napa cabbage

1 cup thinly sliced red bell pepper

1 cup shredded carrots

½ cup sliced green onion

1 cup shelled frozen and thawed edamame

3 tablespoons coconut aminos or reduced-sodium tamari

1 tablespoon unsweetened almond butter

2 tablespoons unsweetened rice vinegar

2 teaspoons gochujang or chili paste

2 teaspoons maple syrup

½ teaspoon garlic powder

½ teaspoon ground ginger

½ cup slivered almonds

1. In a medium pot over medium-high heat, bring the rice and 1 cup of water to a boil; then reduce the heat to low, cover, and simmer for 30 to 35 minutes.

2. Meanwhile, in a large bowl, combine the cabbage, bell pepper, carrots, green onion, and edamame. Set aside.

3. In a small bowl, whisk together the coconut aminos, almond butter, rice vinegar, gochujang, maple syrup, garlic powder, and ginger until well combined. Alternatively, place the ingredients in a mason jar, put the lid on, and shake until well combined. Or you can blend the dressing ingredients in a blender until smooth.

4. Once the rice is finished cooking, drain any remaining liquid and add the rice to the bowl with the vegetables. (It's fine to add the rice while it's hot as it will help soften up the veggies a bit.)

5. Pour the dressing over the slaw ingredients and mix until well coated.

6. Top with the almond slivers and enjoy the salad at room temperature or refrigerate for an hour to chill.

Calcium: 164 mg	Iron: 1.7 mg	Magnesium: 106 mg	Selenium: 1.8 mcg	Zinc: 2 mg

Calories: 294 | Protein: 13 g | Carbohydrate: 27 g | Fiber: 8 g | Fat: 13 g | Sodium: 589 mg

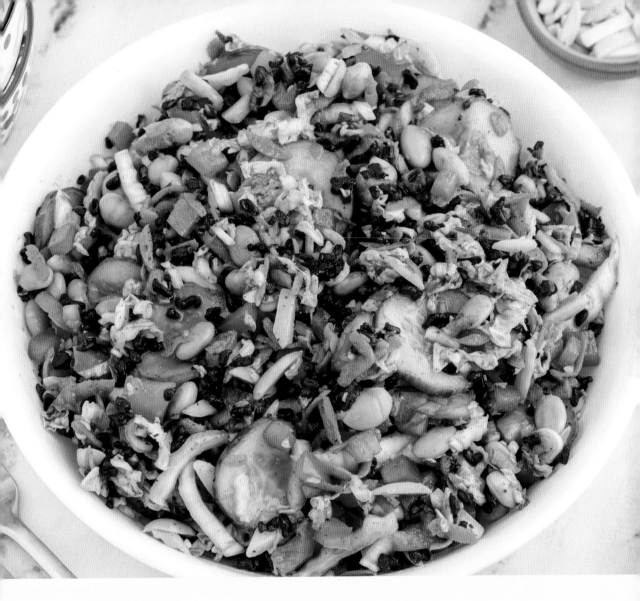

CHEF'S NOTES

Substitutions

In place of black rice, use red or brown rice.

Use another grain in place of rice, such as quinoa, farro, or millet.

Use green or red cabbage in place of napa cabbage. (Note that this will change the flavor profile.)

Use orange, yellow, or green pepper in place of the red pepper.

In place of edamame, use chickpeas or another legume of choice.

Storage

Store leftovers in an airtight container in the refrigerator for up to 5 days.

LETTUCE GO TO THE FARMERS MARKET SALAD

Farmers markets are a treasure trove of fresh, locally grown fruits, vegetables, and other goodies to delight your inner foodie. The market picks below create a salad rich in fiber, protein, iron, zinc, and magnesium, but feel free to get creative and swap in any local and seasonal produce you can get your hands on. You can also make this a heartier meal by adding a cup of cooked whole grains or beans.

Serves: 2 **Prep time:** 20 minutes **Cooking time:** none

Miso Peanut Dressing

1 tablespoon mellow white or chickpea miso

¼ cup smooth or crunchy unsweetened peanut butter

2 tablespoons coconut aminos or reduced-sodium tamari

1 tablespoon unsweetened rice vinegar

1 tablespoon maple syrup

1 tablespoon lime juice

1 to 2 teaspoons gochujang or chili paste

2 teaspoons roughly minced ginger

1 teaspoon roughly minced garlic

Salad

2 cups destemmed and chopped kale

2 cups shredded red cabbage

2 cups shredded carrots

2 cups chopped bell pepper

1½ cups home-cooked or 1 15-ounce can chickpeas, drained

1 cup cooked grain of choice, optional

½ cup sliced green onion

½ cup chopped cilantro, optional

1. Make the Miso Peanut Dressing: In a blender, blend all the dressing ingredients with ¼ cup water (plus more as needed) until smooth. Alternatively, add the ingredients to a bowl and use an immersion blender or whisk to combine. (Be sure to finely mince or grate your ginger and garlic if they won't be blended.) Set the dressing aside.

2. Place the kale in a large salad bowl. Add 2 to 3 tablespoons of the dressing and massage the kale until tender, about 30 seconds.

3. Add the cabbage, carrots, bell pepper, chickpeas, and cooked grains and toss. Drizzle three-quarters of the dressing over the top and toss to combine. Add more dressing to taste.

4. Add the green onion and the cilantro and toss once more.

5. Divide the salad between serving bowls or plates.

CHEF'S NOTES

Substitutions

Swap the kale, red cabbage, carrots, or peppers for your favorite farmers market finds. You can use broccoli, spinach, arugula, radishes, green cabbage, or any of your other favorite vegetables.

Storage

Store this salad in an airtight container in the refrigerator for up to 5 days.

Calcium: 242 mg	Iron: 5 mg	Magnesium: 185 mg	Selenium: 8 mcg	Zinc: 3 mg

Calories: 669 | Protein: 23 g | Carbohydrate: 79 g | Fiber: 22 g | Fat: 11 g | Sodium: 728 mg

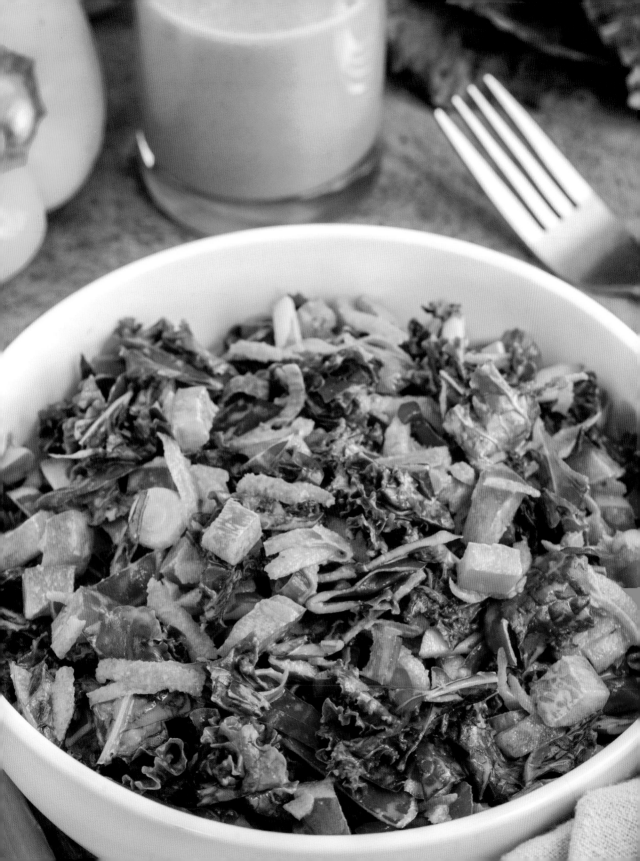

CRUNCHY SOUTHWEST SALAD WITH ZINGY LIME DRESSING

This salad hits a home run with some of our favorite notable nutrients. It scores high with fiber, iron, protein, calcium, magnesium, zinc, and selenium, making this a go-to, nutrition-packed meal for days. These plant-powered ingredients are bundled into a zesty, creamy, and crunchy salad you're sure to love.

Serves: 2   **Prep time:** 20 minutes   **Cooking time:** 10 minutes

Crunchy Tortilla Strips

1 8-inch whole-grain or gluten-free tortilla
1 tablespoon lime juice
Pinch salt, optional

Zingy Lime Dressing

2 tablespoons tahini
2 tablespoons lime juice
1 small clove garlic
1½ teaspoons Dijon or brown mustard
1½ teaspoons maple syrup
¼ teaspoon salt, optional
⅛ teaspoon ground black pepper, optional

Salad

2 cups destemmed and chopped kale
2 cups chopped romaine lettuce
1½ cups home-cooked or 1 15-ounce can black beans, drained
1 cup frozen and thawed or freshly cooked corn
1 cup halved cherry tomatoes
¼ cup sliced black olives
½ cup diced red onion
½ cup chopped cilantro, optional
¼ cup diced jalapeño, optional

1. Make the Crunchy Tortilla Strips: Preheat the oven to 350°F and line a baking sheet with parchment paper. Brush both sides of the tortilla with lime juice using a pastry brush and cut into ¼-inch by 1-inch strips. Then cut the strips across to make even pieces. Evenly space the pieces on the baking sheet and sprinkle with the salt. Bake for 5 to 7 minutes (depending on the thickness of the tortilla) or until crispy. Keep an eye on them as they can burn quickly! Remove them from the oven and set them aside.

2. Make the Zingy Lime Dressing: In a blender, blend all the dressing ingredients (or add to a bowl and use an immersion blender) until creamy and smooth. Add 1 to 2 tablespoons of water at a time to reach the desired consistency. Set the dressing aside.

3. Add the kale to a large salad bowl. Drizzle 1 to 2 tablespoons of dressing over the top and massage the dressing gently into the leaves for about 15 to 30 seconds.

4. Add the lettuce, beans, corn, tomatoes, olives, onion, cilantro, and jalapeño. Drizzle the remaining dressing over the top. Toss to combine.

5. Divide between serving bowls and top with tortilla strips.

Calcium: 281 mg	Iron: 7 mg	Magnesium: 147 mg	Selenium: 12 mcg	Zinc: 3.3 mg

Calories: 471 | Protein: 19 g | Carbohydrate: 47 g | Fiber: 25 g | Fat: 14 g | Sodium: 416 mg

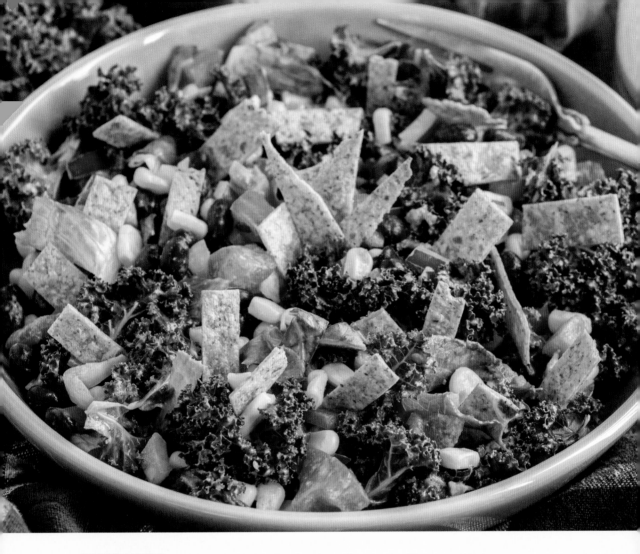

CHEF'S NOTES

Time-Saving Tips

Prepare the tortilla strips ahead of time and store them in an airtight container at room temperature for up to 3 days.

Substitutions

Instead of tahini, use sunflower butter or plant-based yogurt for the creamy base.

Substitute lemon juice for the lime juice.

Substitute ⅛ to ¼ teaspoon of garlic powder for the garlic clove.

Instead of using cherry tomatoes, consider grape tomatoes or other tomato varieties, chopped or diced.

Storage

Store the salad in an airtight container in the refrigerator for up to 3 days. Store the Crunchy Tortilla Strips separately.

PEA-NUTS ABOUT YOU THAI MILLET SALAD

Enjoy the rich, wholesome flavors of Thai cuisine with this peanut lover's dream come true. Savor the nutty flavors from the millet and peanuts along with the powerful notes of the ginger, purple cabbage, and crushed red pepper flakes. Make extra dressing if you are preparing this dish for later in the week, as the veggies soak up what's recommended below.

Serves: 4   **Prep time:** 15 minutes   **Cooking time:** 15 minutes

1 cup dry millet, rinsed, soaked, and drained (see page 242)

Sauce

¼ cup smooth or crunchy unsweetened peanut butter

3 tablespoons coconut aminos or reduced-sodium tamari

1 tablespoon unsweetened rice vinegar

1 to 2 tablespoons minced ginger

2 tablespoons lime juice

1 tablespoon maple syrup, optional

1 teaspoon sesame oil, optional

Slaw

2 cups shredded purple cabbage

1 cup shredded carrots

1 cup frozen and thawed green peas

½ cup chopped cilantro

½ cup sliced green onions

¼ cup raw or roasted unsalted chopped peanuts

½ teaspoon crushed red pepper flakes, optional

1. In a medium pot over high heat, bring the millet and 1½ cups water (or vegetable broth) to a boil. Then reduce heat to medium-low, cover, and simmer until the millet has absorbed all the water (about 15 minutes). Remove the millet from the heat and let it rest for 5 minutes, covered.

2. Meanwhile, make the sauce: Whisk together the peanut butter and coconut aminos until smooth. Whisk in the rice vinegar, ginger, lime juice, and optional maple syrup and sesame oil until smooth. If the mixture seems too thick, loosen it up with 1 to 2 tablespoons of water at a time. Alternatively, blend all the ingredients together in a blender until smooth.

3. In a large serving bowl, toss to combine the cabbage, carrots, peas, cilantro, and green onions.

4. Add the cooked and cooled millet to the vegetables. Toss to combine.

5. Drizzle the peanut sauce over the top and toss until everything is lightly coated.

6. Garnish with peanuts and crushed red pepper flakes.

Calcium: 75 mg	Iron: 2 mg	Magnesium: 135 mg	Selenium: 4 mcg	Zinc: 2.1 mg

Calories: 434 | Protein: 16 g | Carbohydrate: 49 g | Fiber: 10 g | Fat: 16 g | Sodium: 595 mg

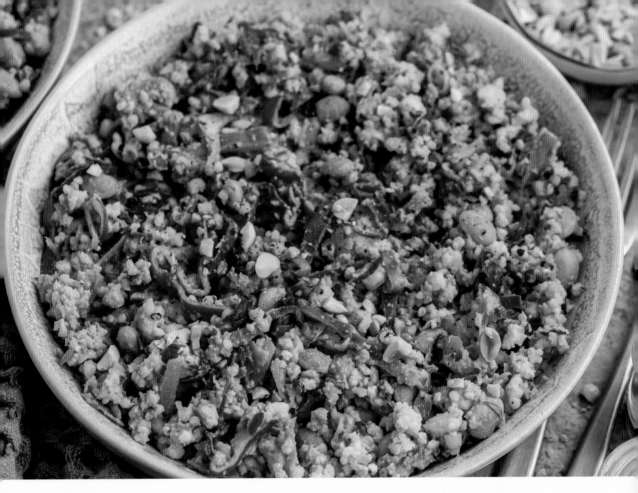

CHEF'S NOTES

Time-Saving Tips

If you don't have time to soak the millet, cook it in 2 cups of water instead of 1½ cups. Drain any excess water after cooking if needed.

Other Tips

Add more nutrients: Add steamed or raw broccoli, sliced radishes, or your veggies of choice. Toss in some fermented kimchi or kraut to add some probiotic goodness. Add grilled tofu or tempeh.

Make it a wrap: Serve in a collard leaf to make a green wrap.

Substitutions

Substitute quinoa for the millet.

In place of peas, try chickpeas, white beans, or kidney beans.

Instead of cilantro, use chopped parsley or basil.

Storage

Store leftovers in an airtight container in the refrigerator for up to 5 days or in the freezer for up to 1 month.

YUMMY TABBOULEH SALAD

Tabbouleh is a traditional Lebanese salad full of fresh vegetables, herbs, and grains. While it is typically made with cracked bulgur, parsley, mint, tomato, and green onion, this version adds another boost of protein with the addition of hemp seeds. You can also add a cup of cooked chickpeas to make this a heartier meal. Tabbouleh is a cultural symbol of hospitality and is often a mainstay at family gatherings, celebrations, and feasts in the Middle East. Keeping with tradition, we hope you decide to share this dish with family and friends!

Serves: 4   **Prep time:** 15 minutes   **Cooking time:** 10 minutes

½ cup dry bulgur, rinsed

Dash of salt, optional

¼ cup hemp seeds

¼ cup lemon juice

¼ teaspoon salt, optional

Ground black pepper to taste, optional

2 cups seeded and diced tomatoes

1 cup diced cucumbers

¾ cup chopped parsley or a parsley/
   cilantro blend (see Chef's Notes)

2 tablespoons minced mint

¾ cup sliced green onion

1. In a small pot over high heat, bring the bulgur, 1½ cups water, and salt to a boil. Reduce the heat to low, cover, and simmer for 10 minutes or until the water is absorbed. Remove from the heat and keep the lid on for another 10 minutes. Remove the lid and fluff with a fork. Drain any excess water and set aside.

2. While the bulgur simmers, in a blender, blend the hemp seeds, lemon juice, salt, and pepper until combined. (It's okay if you can't get all the hemp seeds to blend!) Set the mixture aside.

3. In a large mixing bowl, combine the bulgur, tomatoes, cucumbers, parsley, mint, and green onion. Pour the dressing over the top. Mix well and add salt and pepper to taste.

Calcium: 55 mg	Iron: 2.6 mg	Magnesium: 123 mg	Omega-3s: .95 g	Selenium: 3.6 mcg	Zinc: 1.7 mg

Calories: 148 | Protein: 7 g | Carbohydrate: 16 g | Fiber: 5 g | Fat: 5 g | Sodium: 17 mg

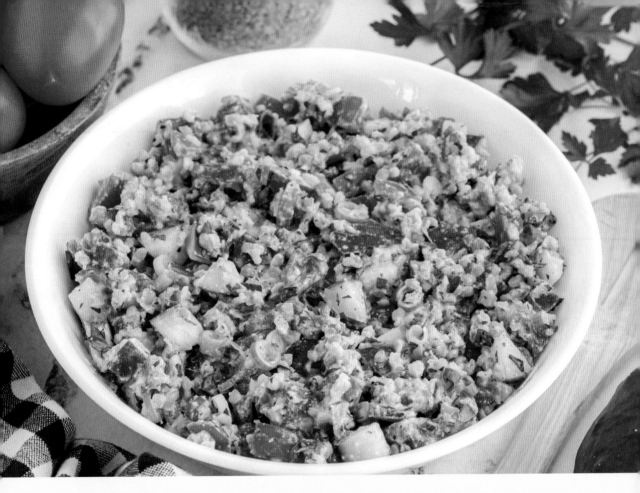

CHEF'S NOTES

Time-Saving Tips

Make the bulgur ahead of time and store it in an airtight container in the refrigerator for up to 5 days or in the freezer for up to 3 months.

Chop your vegetables ahead of time and store them in an airtight container in the refrigerator for up to 2 days. Note that the cucumbers will release some water; drain them before use.

Substitutions

We recommend a half parsley and half cilantro blend to make up the ¾ cup, but you can use all parsley, all cilantro, or substitute other herbs like oregano, thyme, chives, or basil.

Replace the mint with basil, dill, or chives.

Use sesame seeds in place of hemp seeds.

Use diced sweet or red onions in place of green onions.

Gluten-Free: Make the tabbouleh gluten-free by substituting quinoa or millet for the bulgur.

Storage

Store leftovers in an airtight container in the refrigerator for up to 5 days or freeze for up to 1 month.

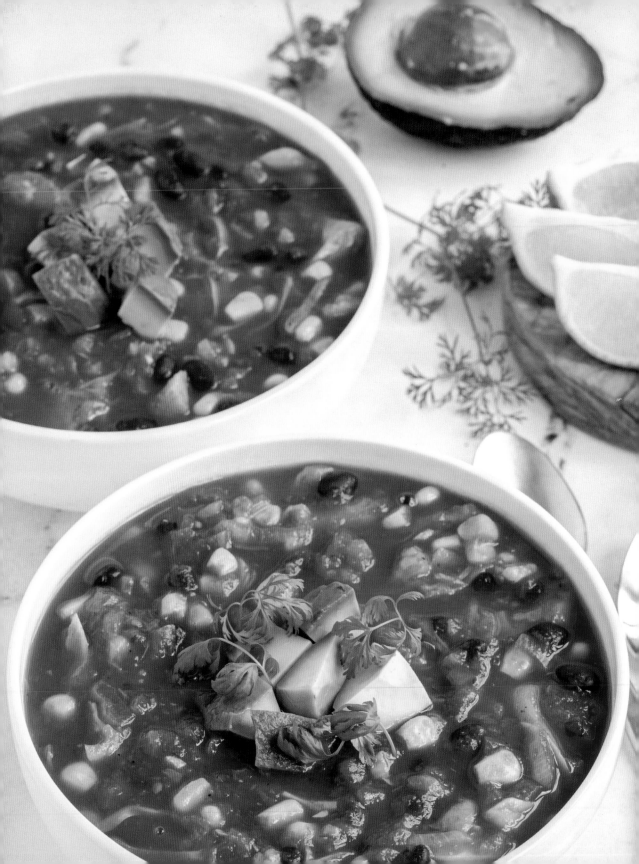

SOUPS AND STEWS

SIMPLE AND SAVORY BUCKWHEAT SOUP

The perfect bowl of soup should have a quick preparation time, uncomplicated ingredients, and rich, savory flavors (you can thank the aromatics for that). There is a certain magic that happens when beans, buckwheat, and leafy greens come together, including the healing combination of nutrients you'll get in every bite.

Serves: 4 **Prep time:** 15 minutes **Cooking time:** 15 minutes

1 large leek, sliced (white and light green parts only, approximately 2 cups)

2 medium carrots, sliced (about 1 cup)

2 large stalks celery, sliced (about 1 cup)

8 ounces mushrooms, sliced (approximately 2 cups)

4 cloves garlic, minced

2 teaspoons minced fresh sage

2 teaspoons dried oregano

½ cup dry buckwheat, rinsed, soaked, and drained (see page 241)

4 cups low-sodium vegetable broth

1½ cups home-cooked or 1 15-ounce can white beans, drained

2 cups destemmed and thinly sliced collard greens or other leafy greens of choice

¼ to ½ teaspoon salt, optional but highly recommended to bring out the flavors

¼ teaspoon ground black pepper, optional

Crushed red pepper flakes to taste, optional

4 lemon wedges

1. In a large pot over medium-high heat, cook the leek, carrots, celery, and mushrooms for 5 minutes, stirring often. The mushrooms should naturally deglaze the pan as they release moisture, but you can add 1 to 2 tablespoons of water if needed.

2. Stir in the garlic, sage, oregano, and buckwheat. Add the vegetable broth and 2 cups of water, turn the heat to high, and bring the soup to a boil. Reduce the heat to low, use a lid to cover three-quarters of the pot, and simmer for 10 minutes.

3. Remove the lid and stir in the beans and collard greens.

4. Add salt, pepper, and red pepper flakes. Serve with lemon wedges on the side.

CHEF'S NOTES

Substitutions

Substitute white or yellow onion for the leek.

Substitute quinoa, wild rice, or brown rice for the buckwheat. See the Whole Grains Cooking Guide on page 241.

Storage

Store the soup in an airtight container in the refrigerator for up to 5 days or let it cool before freezing for up to 3 months.

| Calcium: 175 mg | Iron: 5.7 mg | Magnesium: 137 mg | Selenium: 9 mcg | Zinc: 2 mg |

Calories: 250 | Protein: 16 g | Carbohydrate: 39 g | Fiber: 10 g | Fat: 1.5 g | Sodium: 525 mg

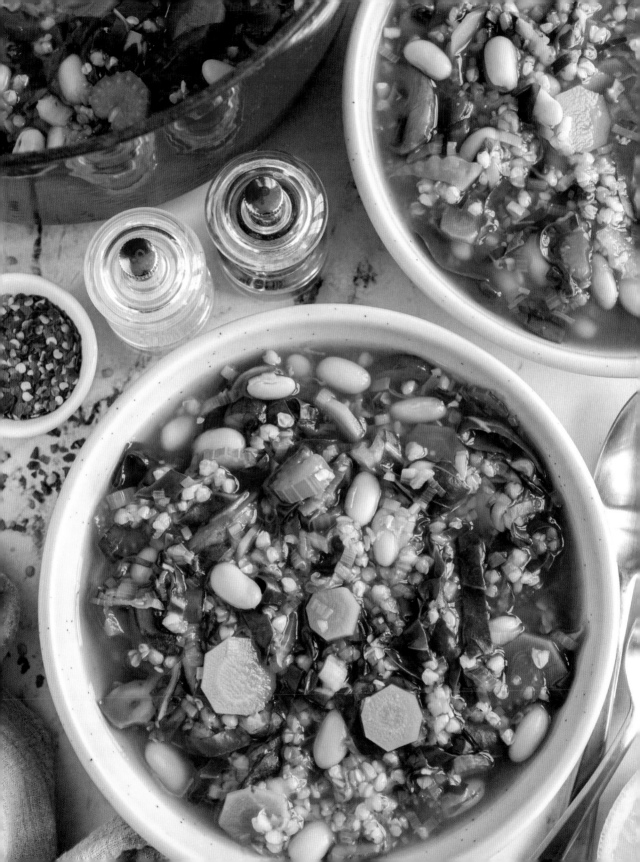

A BOWL OF GOODNESS TORTILLA SOUP

Tortilla soup, or "sopa de tortilla," is a beloved Mexican dish known for its rich, flavorful broth and crunchy tortilla strips. This hearty and comforting plant-based version is a celebration of delectable flavors and revitalizing nutrients.

Serves: 6   **Prep time:** 15 minutes   **Cooking time:** 25 minutes

1 medium yellow or white onion, chopped

3 cloves garlic, minced

1 jalapeño, minced, optional

12 ounces young green jackfruit, pulled from fresh or canned

1 14.5-ounce can crushed tomatoes

1 14.5-ounce can diced tomatoes

1 cup corn, frozen and thawed or fresh

1½ cups home-cooked or 1 15-ounce can red kidney beans, drained

2 teaspoons ground cumin

1 teaspoon chili powder

¼ teaspoon salt, optional

¼ teaspoon ground black pepper, optional

2 cups low-sodium vegetable broth

1 tablespoon lime juice

1 medium avocado, cubed

Crunchy Tortilla Strips (page 120)

¼ cup chopped cilantro, optional

1. In a large pot over medium-high heat, cook the onion, garlic, and jalapeño for 2 minutes, stirring often. Deglaze with 1 to 2 tablespoons of water or vegetable broth as needed.

2. Add the jackfruit, tomatoes, corn, beans, ground cumin, chili powder, salt, and pepper. Stir to combine and cook for an additional minute.

3. Add the vegetable broth, bring it to a boil, reduce the heat, and simmer for 15 minutes.

4. Remove the mixture from the heat, add the lime juice, and stir. Taste and add additional flavors of choice.

5. Divide into serving bowls and top with the avocado, tortilla strips, and cilantro.

| Calcium: 84 mg | Iron: 1.5 mg | Magnesium: 69 mg | Selenium: 1.7 mcg | Zinc: .73 mg |

Calories: 247 | Protein: 6 g | Carbohydrate: 37 g | Fiber: 9 g | Fat: 5 g | Sodium: 431 mg

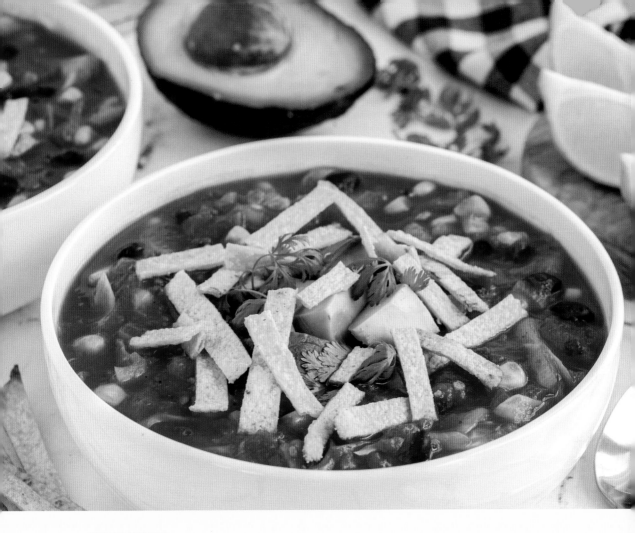

CHEF'S NOTES

Time-Saving Tips

Make the tortilla strips ahead of time and store them in an airtight container at room temperature for up to 3 days.

Substitutions

Use serrano pepper in place of jalapeño pepper.

Instead of cilantro, use another herb of choice, like parsley or chives.

In place of kidney beans, use black beans, pinto beans, or other bean of choice.

Instead of whole grain for the Crunchy Tortilla Strips, use corn tortillas.

If you prefer not to use tortillas but still want some crunch, add crispy chickpeas, kale chips, or tofu.

Storage

Store the leftover soup in an airtight container in the refrigerator for up to 5 days or freeze for up to 3 months.

CREAMY AND COZY VEGGIE RAMEN

Creamy, comforting, savory, and satisfying are just a few of the words that may come to mind when enjoying this veggie-riffic ramen! This flavorful coconut-based broth is filled with brown rice noodles, colorful vegetables, and umami mushrooms that not only are a feast for the eyes but also feed your mind, body, and soul.

Serves: 4 **Prep time:** 15 minutes **Cooking time:** 15 minutes

8 ounces chopped button mushrooms (approximately 2 cups)

1 cup chopped white or yellow onion

1 cup chopped red bell pepper

1 tablespoon grated garlic cloves

1 tablespoon grated fresh ginger

1 tablespoon finely minced fresh lemongrass, outer leaves removed

4 cups low-sodium vegetable broth

8 ounces dry brown rice noodles

2 tablespoons mellow white or chickpea miso

1 cup canned light coconut milk

2 tablespoons coconut aminos or reduced-sodium tamari

2 to 3 teaspoons gochujang or chili paste

2 cups chopped bok choy

1 cup shelled frozen and thawed edamame

2 tablespoons lime juice

3 stalks green onion, thinly sliced

¼ cup chopped cilantro

Sriracha or hot sauce of your choice to taste, optional

1. To a large stockpot over medium-high heat, add the mushrooms, onion, and red bell pepper. Stir occasionally until the onions are translucent, about 2 to 3 minutes.

2. Stir in the garlic, ginger, and lemongrass. Cook for another minute.

3. Add the vegetable broth and 2 cups of water. Bring the mixture to a boil and then add the noodles. Cook for 10 minutes or until the noodles are tender.

4. Meanwhile, in a medium bowl, whisk together the miso, coconut milk, coconut aminos, and gochujang until the miso is completely dissolved.

5. Once the noodles are tender, turn off the heat and stir in the coconut milk mixture.

6. Add the bok choy and edamame, stirring until the bok choy is slightly wilted. Add the lime juice.

7. Divide the ramen between four bowls and garnish with a generous amount of green onion, cilantro, and sriracha.

| Calcium: 109 mg | Iron: 4 mg | Magnesium: 62 mg | Selenium: 5 mcg | Zinc: 1.5 mg |

Calories: 366 | Protein: 18 g | Carbohydrate: 53 | Fiber: 7 g | Fat: 7 g | Sodium: 883 mg

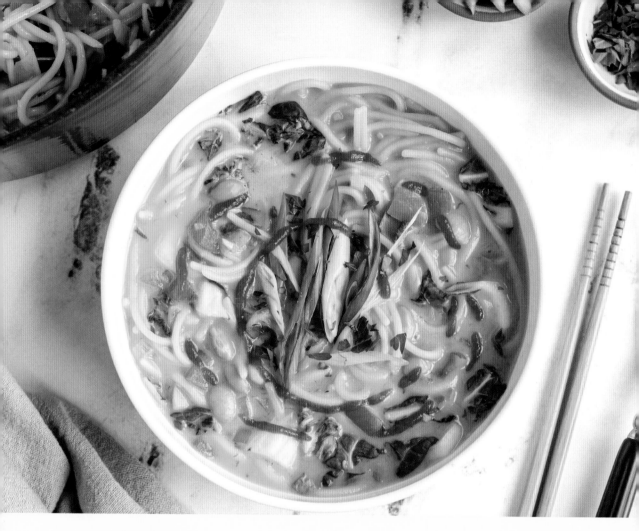

CHEF'S NOTES

Time-Saving Tips

Prepare the coconut miso mixture ahead of time and store it in an airtight container in the refrigerator for up to 48 hours.

Substitutions

For the mushrooms, anything goes! Use shiitake, cremini, or any mushroom of your choice. They're all delicious and healing.

Substitute red onion or shallots for the white or yellow onion.

Substitute green, yellow, or orange bell pepper for red bell pepper.

Instead of bok choy, use spinach or kale.

Add chickpeas in place of edamame.

Storage

Store leftovers in an airtight container in the refrigerator for up to 5 days. Note that the noodles will continue to absorb the broth and may get a bit soggy.

NOURISH AND THRIVE IMMUNE SUPPORT SOUP

Loaded with fiber, protein, iron, and magnesium, this soup harnesses the natural power of plants in a deliciously wholesome way to help support your immune system through seasonal transitions. Fiber supports the health of the gut, where 70 to 80 percent of immune cells live; selenium has been shown to lower the risk of infections; and phytonutrient-rich veggies and spices fight inflammation. We've even heard some describe this soup as a "delicious bowl of lovin'," and we couldn't agree more.

Serves: 4   **Prep time:** 10 minutes   **Cooking time:** 15 minutes

¾ cup thinly sliced leeks (white and light green parts only)

2 teaspoons mustard seeds

2 cloves garlic, minced

1-inch piece of ginger, peeled and minced

1 small head cauliflower, leaves removed and cut into 1-inch florets

2 teaspoons ground turmeric

1 tablespoon ground cumin

½ teaspoon salt, optional

Ground black pepper to taste, optional

3 cups low-sodium vegetable broth

1 cup canned light coconut milk

1½ cups home-cooked or 1 15-ounce can chickpeas, drained

2 cups destemmed and chopped kale

¼ cup chopped cilantro, optional

1 to 2 dashes cayenne pepper, optional

1 to 2 dashes smoked paprika, optional

1. In a large stockpot over high heat, add the leeks and mustard seeds. Stir for 2 to 3 minutes, until the leeks are translucent.

2. Reduce the heat to medium and add the garlic, ginger, cauliflower, turmeric, cumin, salt, and pepper. Sauté for 1 to 2 minutes, or until the spices are lightly toasted. Deglaze the pan with 2 to 3 tablespoons of water or vegetable broth as needed.

3. Add the vegetable broth, raise the heat to bring the soup to a boil, and then reduce the heat to a simmer. Cook until the cauliflower is tender, about 10 minutes.

4. Stir in the coconut milk, chickpeas, and kale. Heat through until the kale is slightly wilted.

5. Add more salt and pepper to taste.

6. Divide between bowls and serve with the cilantro, cayenne pepper, and smoked paprika.

Calcium: 134 mg	Iron: 4 mg	Magnesium: 65 mg	Selenium: 6.7 mcg	Zinc: 1.2 mg

Calories: 250 | Protein: 10 g | Carbohydrate: 49 g | Fiber: 10 g | Fat: 7 g | Sodium: 380 g

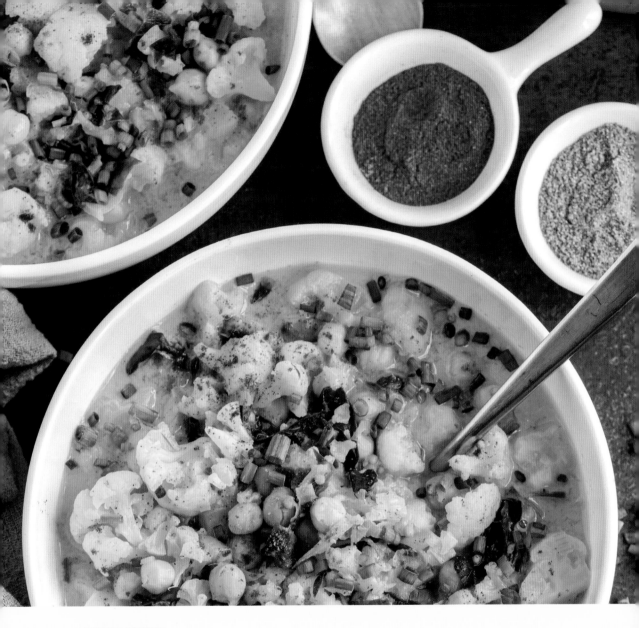

CHEF'S NOTES

Substitutions

In place of leek, use onion or shallot.

Use white beans or another legume of choice instead of chickpeas.

Use your favorite leafy green in place of kale, such as spinach, mustard greens, or bok choy.

Instead of cilantro use parsley or chives.

Storage

Store in an airtight container in the refrigerator for up to 5 days or freeze for up to 1 month.

CREAMY DREAMY MUSHROOMS, GREENS, AND BEANS SOUP

One of the things we love most about this soup is the high concentration of selenium per serving, thanks, in part, to mushrooms! This is all the more reason to cozy up to this hearty bowl of nourishing plants. This dish is a simple and tasty way to include a wide variety of nutrient-dense, plant-based ingredients in your weekly routine.

Serves: 4   **Prep time:** 20 minutes   **Cooking time:** 10 minutes

2 cups diced white onion

1 pound button mushrooms sliced (approximately 4 cups)

3 large cloves garlic, minced

1 tablespoon minced fresh sage

2 tablespoons sherry vinegar or red wine vinegar

¾ cup cashews, soaked in hot water for 30 minutes or room-temperature water for 2 hours, drained

1 tablespoon mellow white or chickpea miso

3 tablespoons nutritional yeast

3 cups low-sodium vegetable broth

2 cups destemmed and chopped kale

1½ cups home-cooked or 1 15-ounce can chickpeas, drained

Salt to taste, optional

Ground black pepper to taste, optional

4 lemon wedges

Crushed red pepper flakes to taste, optional

1. To a large pot over medium-high heat, add the onion and mushrooms, stirring often until the onions are translucent and the mushrooms have released their liquid, about 5 minutes.

2. Stir in the garlic, sage, and vinegar, and cook for another 2 minutes.

3. Reduce the heat to low. Transfer half the mushroom mixture to a high-speed blender and blend until creamy (if using a regular or immersion blender, blend longer to reach a creamy consistency).

4. Add the drained cashews, miso, nutritional yeast, and vegetable broth to the blender and blend until smooth and creamy.

5. Transfer the sauce back to the pot and raise the heat to medium.

6. Add the kale and chickpeas, stirring to combine and until the kale is tender, about one minute. Add salt and pepper to taste.

7. Serve topped with lemon wedges and crushed red pepper flakes.

Calcium: 96 mg	Iron: 3 mg	Magnesium: 108 mg	Selenium: 18.5 mcg	Zinc: 3 mg

Calories: 306 | Protein: 15 g | Carbohydrate: 29 g | Fiber: 8 g | Fat: 13 g | Sodium: 405 mg

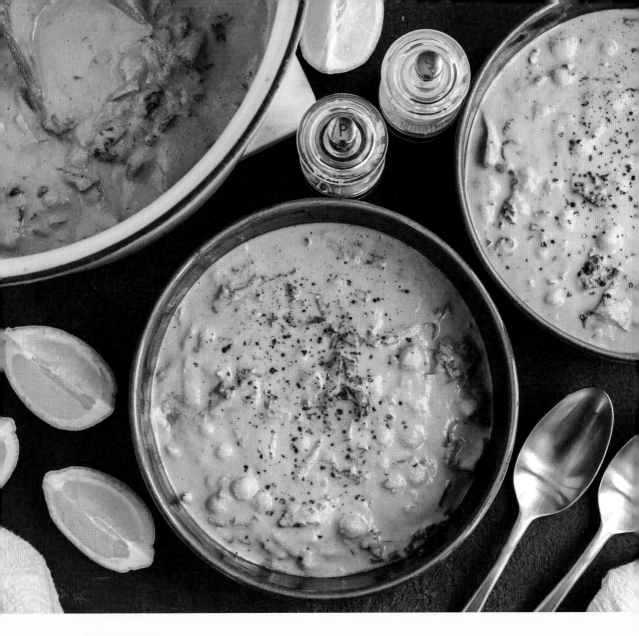

CHEF'S NOTES

Substitutions

Substitute cremini, oyster, or any mushroom you'd like for the button mushrooms.

Substitute fresh thyme or rosemary for the sage.

Substitute spinach, chard, or your favorite dark leafy greens of choice for the kale.

Substitute white beans, lentils, tofu, or your favorite plant protein of choice for the chickpeas.

Storage

Store in an airtight container in the refrigerator for up to 5 days.

BUTTERY VEGAN CORN CHOWDER

Traditional corn chowder is full of heavy butter and cream, but our plant-based alternative gets its richness from creamy coconut milk, satisfying sweet potatoes, and fiber-packed corn. Enjoy it as a main course with a slice of crusty whole-grain bread, as an appetizer, or as a cozy afternoon snack.

Serves: 4   **Prep time:** 15 minutes   **Cooking time:** 20 minutes

1 cup chopped yellow or white onion

1 cup chopped celery

1 cup chopped red bell pepper

1 tablespoon fresh thyme, minced

2 teaspoons ground cumin

1 teaspoon ground turmeric

1 teaspoon onion powder

½ teaspoon salt, optional

¼ teaspoon ground black pepper, optional

2 cups frozen or fresh corn

2 cups sweet potato, cut into ½-inch pieces (approximately 1 large potato)

4 cups low-sodium vegetable broth

2 tablespoons arrowroot powder or cornstarch

1 13.5-ounce can light coconut milk

2 to 3 tablespoons sliced green onions

¼ cup chopped parsley or cilantro

Crushed red pepper flakes to taste, optional

1. To a large stockpot over medium-high heat, add the onion, celery, and bell pepper. Stir continuously until the onion is translucent, about 2 to 3 minutes.

2. Stir in the thyme, cumin, turmeric, onion powder, and salt and pepper. Cook for another minute.

3. Add the corn, sweet potatoes, and vegetable broth. Bring the mixture to a boil and then reduce heat to low and simmer until the potatoes are tender, about 10 minutes.

4. Meanwhile, in a small bowl, whisk the arrowroot powder with 2 tablespoons of water until the powder is dissolved.

5. Once the sweet potatoes are tender, slowly pour the arrowroot mixture into the pot, stirring constantly.

6. Once the chowder thickens slightly, remove it from the heat and stir in the coconut milk (slowly to keep it from curdling).

7. Taste and adjust for more seasoning with another dash of salt, cumin, or onion powder.

8. Divide into bowls and top with sliced green onions and parsley or cilantro, as well as crushed red pepper flakes (or minced jalapeño).

Calcium: 75 mg	Iron: 1.8 mg	Magnesium: 59 mg	Zinc: 1 mg

Calories: 292 | Protein: 6 g | Carbohydrate: 48 g | Fiber: 8 g | Fat: 6 g | Sodium: 434 mg

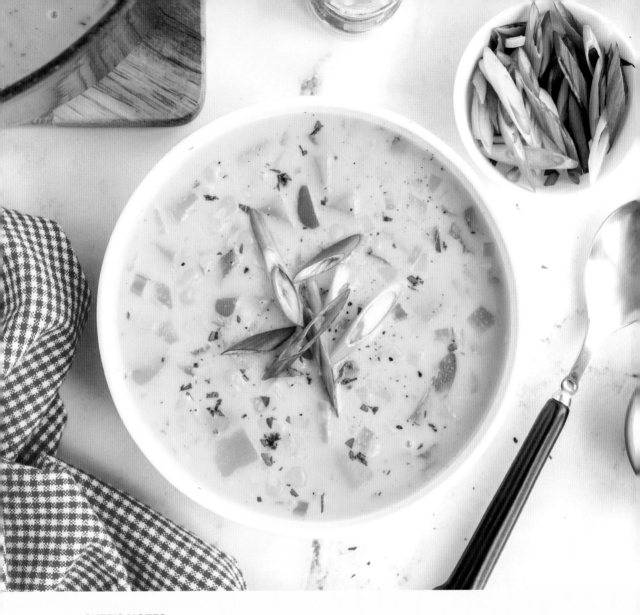

CHEF'S NOTES

Substitutions

Shallots can be used in place of onion.

For the bell pepper, use orange, yellow, or green bell pepper in place of red bell pepper.

Use fresh oregano in place of fresh thyme. Or use 1 teaspoon of dried thyme in place of the fresh (however, we do recommend fresh over dried for the best flavor).

Instead of sweet potato, use red, purple, or golden potato.

Storage

Store in an airtight container in the refrigerator for up to 5 days or in the freezer for up to 1 month.

SIP AND SHINE ASPARAGUS SOUP

Who knew that humble asparagus and simple silken tofu could come together to create the most velvety, dreamy, and flavorful soup with only a handful of ingredients? You can eat this soup as is; drizzle it over a baked potato; mix it with zucchini, whole-grain, or legume noodles; or use it as a creamy base in a casserole dish.

Serves: 2 **Prep time:** 15 minutes **Cooking time:** 15 minutes

½ cup roughly chopped shallots

4 cloves garlic, roughly minced

2 pounds asparagus, cut into 1-inch pieces

1 teaspoon ground cumin

¼ teaspoon salt, optional

¼ teaspoon ground black pepper, optional

2 cups low-sodium vegetable broth

½ cup silken tofu

Minced chives to taste

Minced dill to taste

1. In a large stockpot over medium heat, cook the shallots and garlic until fragrant, about 1 minute.

2. Add the asparagus and cumin, season with salt and pepper, and cook until slightly charred, about 5 minutes.

3. Add the veggie broth and bring the mixture to a boil. Lower the heat, cover, and simmer for 7 minutes, until the asparagus is very tender but still green.

4. After the veggies have cooled just a bit, transfer the mixture to a blender (or use an immersion blender). Add the tofu and blend until creamy.

5. Season with salt and pepper to taste. Garnish with the chives and dill.

CHEF'S NOTES

Substitutions

Substitute white or yellow onion for the shallots.

Use a teaspoon of garlic powder in place of garlic cloves.

Instead of dill or chives, try shaved vegetables, sautéed shallots, or Garlic Cashew Cream (page 186) drizzled on top.

Storage

Store in an airtight container in the refrigerator for up to 5 days or in the freezer for up to 3 months.

Calcium: 170 mg	Iron: 11 mg	Magnesium: 83 mg	Selenium: 16 mcg	Zinc: 3 mg

Calories: 170 | Protein: 17 g | Carbohydrate: 18 g | Fiber: 10 g | Fat: 1.4 g | Sodium: 110 g

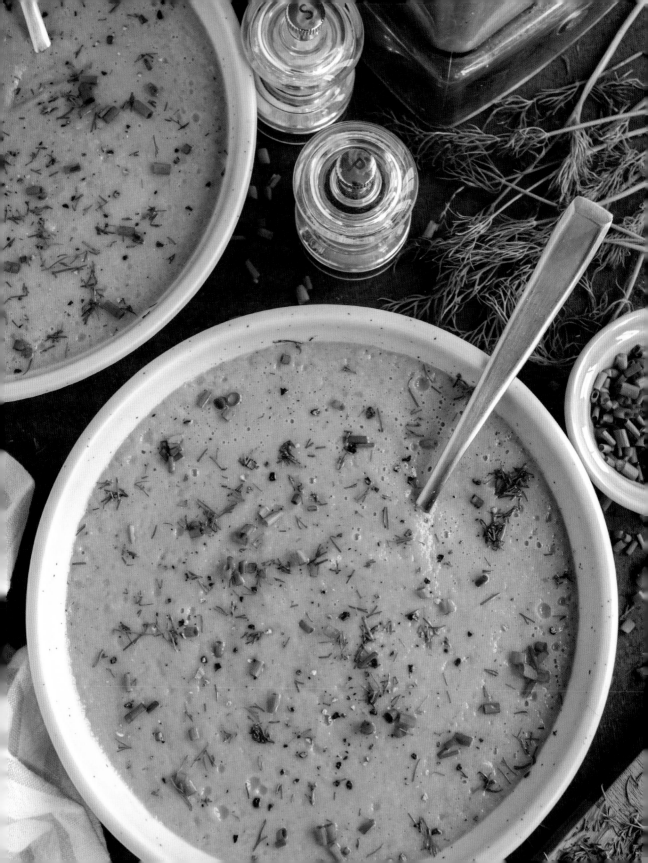

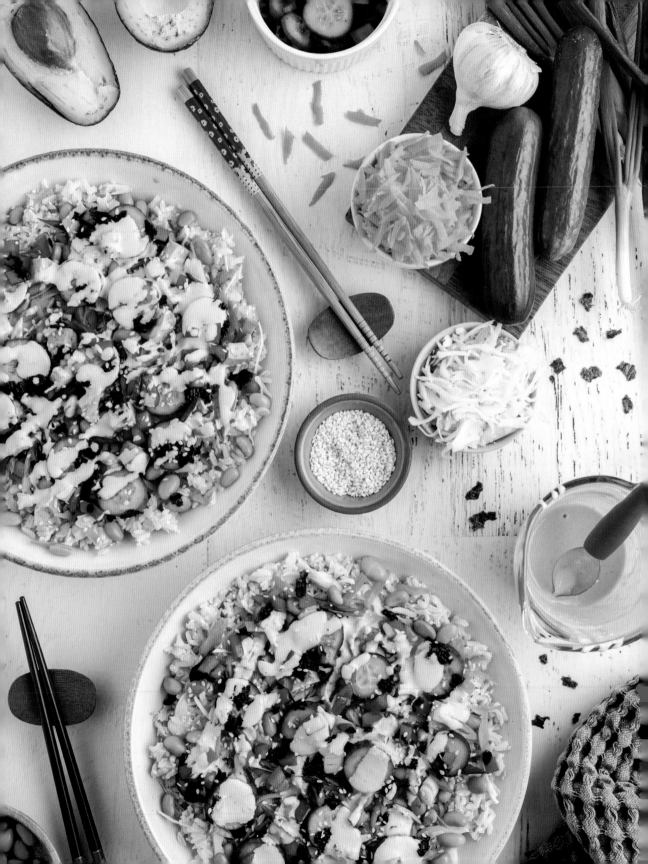

BOWLS

PURPLE PARADISE POWER BOWL

Purple to the fifth power feels like the best way to describe this remarkably colorful bowl. Purple sweet potatoes, red beets, red cabbage, red onion, and juicy blueberries are teeming with fiber, iron, and antioxidant power. Not to mention the heavenly balance of sweet and savory in this meal! The purple coloring comes from anthocyanins, a powerful family of antioxidants that does wonders for your brain, heart, immune system, and more.

Serves: 2 **Prep time:** 20 minutes **Cooking time:** 20 minutes

1½ cups home-cooked or 1 15-ounce can chickpeas, drained

2 cups diced purple sweet potato or orange sweet potato (approximately 1 large potato)

1 tablespoon, plus 1 to 2 teaspoons extra virgin olive oil (divided), optional

Salt, optional

¼ teaspoon ground black pepper, optional

1 bunch kale, destemmed and chopped (approximately 4 cups)

1 medium beet, shredded (approximately 1 cup)

¼ medium red onion, thinly sliced (approximately ¼ cup)

1 cup shredded red cabbage

2 tablespoons raw pumpkin seeds or sunflower seeds

Tangy Blueberry Dressing

1 cup blueberries, frozen and thawed or fresh

2 tablespoons tahini

2 tablespoons balsamic vinegar

2 to 3 tablespoons maple syrup

1½ teaspoons Dijon mustard

2 tablespoons lime juice

1. Preheat the oven to 425°F. Line a baking sheet with parchment paper.

2. In a large bowl, combine the chickpeas and sweet potatoes. If using olive oil, drizzle it over the top and toss to coat.

3. Spread the chickpeas and potatoes evenly onto the parchment-lined baking sheet. Sprinkle with salt and pepper. Bake for 20 minutes. If you have more time and want the chickpeas crispy, bake for 30 to 40 minutes.

4. While the chickpeas and potatoes are baking, prepare the other bowl ingredients: In a large bowl, drizzle the kale with 1 to 2 teaspoons olive oil. With clean hands, massage the kale until tender, about 30 seconds. Sprinkle with salt.

5. Divide the kale between two bowls and top with beet, onions, and cabbage.

6. Make the Tangy Blueberry Dressing: In a blender or food processor, blend all the dressing ingredients plus ¼ cup water until smooth. Add 1 to 2 tablespoons more water as needed. Set aside.

7. When the potatoes and chickpeas are finished cooking, divide them between the two bowls. Drizzle as much Tangy Blueberry Dressing as you'd like over each bowl and top with freshly ground pepper. Sprinkle with pumpkin or sunflower seeds.

Calcium: 331 mg	Iron: 6 mg	Magnesium: 155 mg	Selenium: 11.5 mcg	Zinc: 3 mg

Calories: 646 | Protein: 19 g | Carbohydrate: 74 g | Fiber: 20 g | Fat: 25 g | Sodium: 449 mg

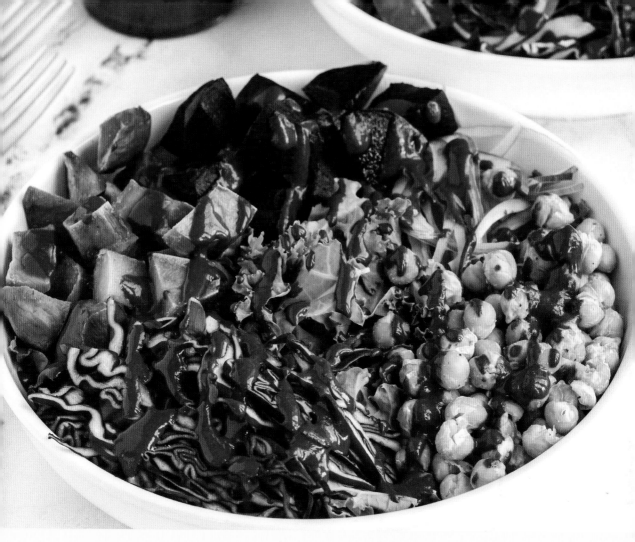

CHEF'S NOTES

Time-Saving Tips

Make the crispy chickpeas and potatoes ahead of time. Store them in an airtight container in the refrigerator for up to 5 days.

Substitutions

Instead of purple sweet potato, use any other type of potato.

If you prefer pickled beets to fresh, they taste delicious in this dish.

Instead of raw onion, use Pickled Red Onions (page 166).

In place of kale, use your favorite leafy greens.

If you prefer to forgo the dressing, add a squeeze of lemon or lime juice to the bowl.

Storage

Store bowl leftovers and leftover dressing in separate airtight containers in the refrigerator for up to 5 days.

THE ULTIMATE LOADED MASHED POTATO BOWL

Loaded (literally) with lots of protein-rich black beans, tender massaged kale, naturally sweet corn, and crunchy red onion, and topped with a few dashes of hot sauce, this veggie-rich bowl has every notable nutrient packed into one wholesome serving. This is the indulgent loaded potato you've been longing for!

Serves: 2 **Prep time:** 20 minutes **Cooking time:** 10 minutes

5-Minute Cheesy Sauce

1 cup cashews, soaked in hot water for 30 minutes or room-temperature water for 2 hours, drained

4 tablespoons nutritional yeast

2 tablespoons lemon juice

1 teaspoon garlic powder

¼ to ½ teaspoon salt, optional

Bowl Ingredients

2 cups russet potato, cut into ¾-inch cubes (approximately 1 large potato)

¼ cup plain, unsweetened plant-based milk, plus 1 to 2 tablespoons

¼ teaspoon garlic powder

½ teaspoon onion powder

¼ to ½ teaspoon salt, optional

¼ teaspoon ground black pepper, optional

¼ teaspoon cayenne pepper, optional

1 tablespoon tahini

2 tablespoons lemon juice

1 tablespoon nutritional yeast

½ teaspoon smoked or sweet paprika

¼ teaspoon ground turmeric

¼ teaspoon salt, optional

¼ teaspoon ground black pepper, optional

2 cups destemmed and thinly sliced kale

1½ cups cooked fresh or frozen corn

1½ cups home-cooked or 1 15-ounce can black beans, drained

½ cup chopped red onion

¼ cup chopped cilantro, optional

Hot sauce to taste, optional

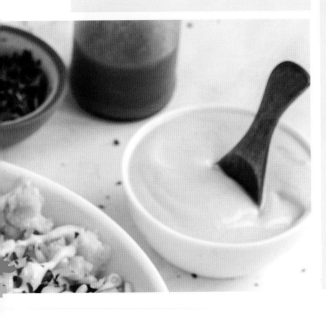

Calcium: 378 mg	Iron: 11 mg	Magnesium: 366 mg	Selenium: 25 mcg	Zinc: 7 mg	Vitamin B₁₂*: 1.5 mcg	Vitamin D*: 45 IU

Calories: 837 | Protein: 35 g | Carbohydrate: 97 g | Fiber: 26 g | Fat: 29 g | Sodium: 570 mg

*If using fortified plant-based milk.

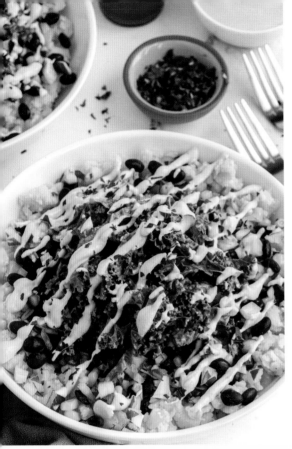

1. Make the 5-Minute Cheesy Sauce: In a high-speed blender or food processor, blend all the sauce ingredients along with ½ cup of water (plus more if needed) until smooth. Set the sauce aside.

2. To a large pot, add enough water to cover the potatoes and heat on high until boiling. Boil the potatoes until tender, about 10 minutes, then drain.

3. In a large bowl, mash together the potatoes, plant-based milk, garlic powder, onion powder, salt, pepper, and cayenne with a potato masher or fork until mostly mashed (lumpy mashed potatoes are okay if you like!). Taste for additional seasoning of choice.

4. In a medium bowl, mix the tahini, lemon juice, nutritional yeast, paprika, turmeric, salt, and pepper until the tahini is completely blended. Add the kale and stir until the leaves are coated. To make coating easier, you can massage the kale with clean hands for about 30 seconds. Set this mixture aside.

5. Divide the mashed potatoes, corn, black beans, red onion, and kale between two bowls. Drizzle the Cheesy Sauce on top. Sprinkle with chopped cilantro and hot sauce.

CHEF'S NOTES

Time-Saving Tips

Make the potatoes ahead of time and store them in an airtight container in the refrigerator for up to 5 days.

Make the kale ahead of time and store it in an airtight container in the refrigerator for up to 3 days.

Make the 5-Minute Cheesy Sauce ahead of time and store it in an airtight container in the refrigerator for up to 5 days or in the freezer for up to 1 month.

Make the corn and beans ahead of time and store them in an airtight container in the refrigerator for up to 5 days.

Substitutions

Substitute red, purple, or golden potatoes for the russet potatoes.

Use sweet potato in place of regular potato.

Substitute spinach, romaine, or spring greens for the kale.

In place of black beans, use chickpeas, edamame, or white beans of choice.

Substitute sliced green onion, chives, or shallots for the red onion.

Storage

Store leftovers in an airtight container in the refrigerator for up to 5 days. Store leftover 5-Minute Cheesy Sauce in an airtight container in the refrigerator for up to 5 days.

BOUNTIFUL BULGUR BOWL WITH SAVORY ORANGE VINAIGRETTE

You know you have a near-perfect, delicious bowl when you can't quite decide which element of this recipe deserves the spotlight. Could it be the toasty Moroccan-inspired chickpeas? Or maybe the creamy and wonderfully savory orange vinaigrette? What we do know for sure is that this meal is a culinary must-have.

Serves: 2 **Prep time:** 20 minutes **Cooking time:** 10 minutes

Moroccan Baked Chickpeas

½ teaspoon ground cumin
¼ teaspoon ground cinnamon
¼ teaspoon garlic powder
¼ teaspoon ground ginger
¼ teaspoon ground turmeric
¼ teaspoon smoked or sweet paprika
¼ teaspoon salt, optional
1½ cups home-cooked or 1 15-ounce can chickpeas, drained

Bulgur

1 cup dry bulgur (fine or medium grind), rinsed
2½ cups low-sodium vegetable broth
1 teaspoon ground cumin
1 dash ground cinnamon
½ teaspoon onion powder
¼ teaspoon salt, optional
1 teaspoon lemon zest
1 tablespoon lemon juice

Savory Orange Vinaigrette

1 medium orange, peeled (preferably sweet and seedless)
1 tablespoon tahini
1 tablespoon apple cider vinegar
¼ teaspoon salt, optional
¼ cup chopped cilantro, optional

Bowl Ingredients

1 cup chopped spinach
1 cup frozen and thawed or freshly cooked corn
¼ cup finely diced red onion
¼ cup unsweetened or naturally sweetened dried cranberries
2 tablespoons minced mint or parsley
2 to 4 tablespoons chopped raw pistachios, optional

| Calcium: 201 mg | Iron: 5 mg | Magnesium: 208 mg | Selenium: 10 mcg | Zinc: 3 mg |

Calories: 720 | Protein: 25 g | Carbohydrate: 105 g | Fiber: 24 g | Fat: 16 g | Sodium: 617 mg

1. Preheat the oven to 400°F. Line a baking sheet with parchment paper.

2. In a medium bowl, mix the chickpea spices until they are blended. Toss with the chickpeas until evenly coated.

3. Spread the chickpeas on the baking sheet and bake for 30 minutes (or until crispy), stirring halfway through.

4. Meanwhile, cook the bulgur: In a medium pot over high heat, bring the bulgur, vegetable broth, cumin, cinnamon, onion powder, salt, lemon zest, and lemon juice to a boil. Reduce the heat to low, cover, and simmer for approximately 10 minutes, until the bulgur is tender and all or most of the liquid is absorbed. Depending on the grind size of the bulgur, you may need a longer cooking time.

5. Make the Savory Orange Vinaigrette: In a food processor, combine all the dressing ingredients except the cilantro. Puree until smooth, adding water as needed. Add the cilantro to the smooth mixture, pulse a few times, and set the dressing aside.

6. If you'd like your spinach slightly cooked, add it to a colander. Once the bulgur is finished cooking, pour it over the spinach in the colander (draining any liquid left with your bulgur) and stir until the spinach is tender. If you prefer your spinach raw, skip this step and add the spinach with the other bowl ingredients in the next step.

7. Divide the bulgur and spinach between two bowls as well as the chickpeas, corn, and red onion. Drizzle the desired amount of dressing on top of each bowl. Top with cranberries, mint, and pistachios.

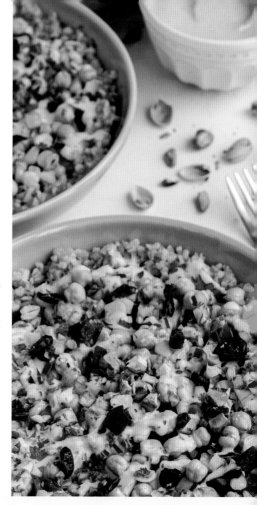

CHEF'S NOTES

Time-Saving Tips

Use canned chickpeas in place of Moroccan Baked Chickpeas.

Make the bulgur ahead of time and store in an airtight container in the refrigerator for up to 5 days.

Make the Moroccan Baked Chickpeas ahead of time and store in an airtight container in a cool, dark place for up to 3 days.

Substitutions

In place of lemon zest and juice for the bulgur, use orange zest and juice.

Substitute cilantro for mint or parsley.

Substitute raisins for cranberries.

For the red onion, use yellow or white instead.

Gluten-Free: Use quinoa or millet in place of bulgur.

Storage

Store bowl leftovers and leftover dressing in separate airtight containers in the refrigerator for up to 5 days.

ZESTY FIESTA MUSHROOM LENTIL CHORIZO TACO BOWL

Mushrooms, lentils, and walnuts transform into a meaty "chorizo" so infused with robust flavors you just might be convinced it's the real thing! Piled high on brown rice and topped with all the right elements, including a generous dollop of Cashew Sour Cream, it's a flavor-packed twist on a traditional Tex-Mex meal that will leave you savoring every bite. Try this bowl as filling in your favorite whole-grain tortilla wrap, corn taco shell, or collard green leaves.

Serves: 2   **Prep time:** 20 minutes   **Cooking time:** 5 minutes

Mushroom Lentil Chorizo

8 ounces sliced cremini mushrooms (approximately 2 cups)
1 teaspoon chili powder
1 teaspoon ancho chili powder, optional
1 teaspoon ground cumin
¾ teaspoon dried oregano
½ teaspoon ground coriander
½ teaspoon garlic powder
¼ teaspoon onion powder
1 teaspoon smoked paprika
½ teaspoon sweet paprika
⅛ teaspoon ground cinnamon
1 cup home-cooked or 8 ounces canned green or brown lentils, drained
½ cup raw walnuts
¼ teaspoon salt, optional
¼ teaspoon ground black pepper, optional

Bowl Ingredients

2 cups cooked brown rice
1 cup romaine lettuce, thinly sliced
½ cup diced Roma tomatoes
¼ cup diced red onion
1 avocado, cubed
1 to 2 tablespoons lime juice
Salt to taste, optional
Ground black pepper to taste, optional
2 to 4 tablespoons chopped cilantro
Cashew Sour Cream (page 100), optional
¼ cup salsa of your choice

1. Make the Mushroom Lentil Chorizo: In a medium pan over medium-high heat, cook the mushrooms until lightly browned, about 5 minutes. Add 1 to 2 tablespoons of water as needed to deglaze the pan. Meanwhile, in a small bowl, mix all the chorizo spices and set them aside. In a food processor, pulse the mushrooms, lentils, walnuts, and spices until a coarse meal is formed. Add salt and pepper to taste.

2. Divide the cooked rice, chorizo, lettuce, tomatoes, onion, and avocado between two bowls.

3. Drizzle the lime juice on top and sprinkle with salt, pepper, and cilantro.

4. Top with Cashew Sour Cream along with 2 tablespoons of salsa per serving.

Calcium: 104 mg	Iron: 8.7 mg	Magnesium: 297 mg	Omega-3s: 2.8 g	Selenium: 29.7 mcg	Zinc: 6.6 mg

Calories: 820 | Protein: 29 g | Carbohydrate: 78 g | Fiber: 20 g | Fat: 40 g | Sodium: 364 mg

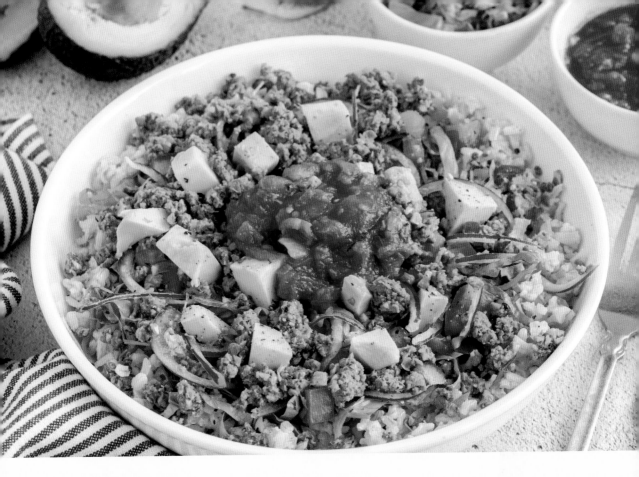

CHEF'S NOTES

Time-Saving Tips

Make the spice blend ahead of time and store it in an airtight container in a cool, dark place for up to 30 days.

Make the chorizo ahead of time and store it in an airtight container in the refrigerator for up to 3 days.

Make the Cashew Sour Cream ahead of time and store it in an airtight container in the refrigerator for up to 5 days.

Substitutions

Instead of cremini mushrooms, use button or portobello mushrooms.

Substitute any whole grain of choice for rice.

For the tomatoes, use heirloom, grape, or any other tomatoes you have on hand.

Substitute another leafy green for romaine lettuce.

Use white or yellow onion or shallots in place of red onion.

Substitute lemon juice in place of lime juice.

Storage

Store leftovers in an airtight container in the refrigerator for up to 3 days or freeze them for up to one month.

DECONSTRUCTED SUSHI BOWL

Sushi night may become as highly requested as your family's favorite taco or pizza night after you give this dish a try. Wholesome veggies like edamame, carrots, cabbage, and green onion get a flavor boost thanks to the sweet, tangy, and refreshing sunomono topping. Sunomono is a Japanese cucumber salad that takes this recipe from good to amazing. Teeming with fiber, protein, selenium, iodine, and zinc, what's not to love?

Serves: 2 **Prep time:** 25 minutes **Cooking time:** 35 minutes

1 cup dry brown or black rice, rinsed

2 cups thinly sliced cucumbers

1 sheet nori, torn into pieces or ground

⅓ cup diced red bell pepper

2 tablespoons unsweetened rice vinegar

1 tablespoon maple syrup

1 tablespoon coconut aminos or reduced-sodium tamari

¼ cup tahini

2 teaspoons sriracha or other chili sauce

1 small clove garlic, chopped

1 tablespoon lemon juice

1 large avocado, cut into 1-inch cubes

1 cup shredded cabbage

1 cup shredded carrots

½ cup shelled frozen and thawed edamame

½ cup sliced green onion

1 tablespoon sesame seeds

½ cup chopped cilantro, optional

1. In a small pot, bring the rice and 2 cups of water to a boil over medium-high heat. Reduce the heat to low, cover, and simmer for 30 to 35 minutes.

2. Meanwhile, make the sunomono: In a medium bowl, toss to combine the cucumbers, torn nori sheets (which will rehydrate and soften), and bell pepper. In a small bowl, whisk together the rice vinegar, maple syrup, and coconut aminos. Pour over the cucumber mixture, toss to combine, and set aside.

3. Make the sauce: In a blender, blend the tahini, sriracha, garlic, and lemon juice plus 2 to 4 tablespoons of water until smooth. Set aside.

4. Once the rice has finished cooking, divide the rice, avocado, cabbage, carrots, edamame, and green onion between two bowls. Top with the sunomono, drizzle with the sauce, and garnish with sesame seeds and cilantro.

| Calcium: 262 mg | Iodine: 27 mcg | Iron: 6.8 mg | Magnesium: 236 mg | Omega-3s: .4 g | Selenium: 29.4 mcg | Zinc: 5.4 mg |

Calories: 826 | Protein: 22 g | Carbohydrate: 94 g | Fiber: 18 g | Fat: 35 g | Sodium: 385 mg

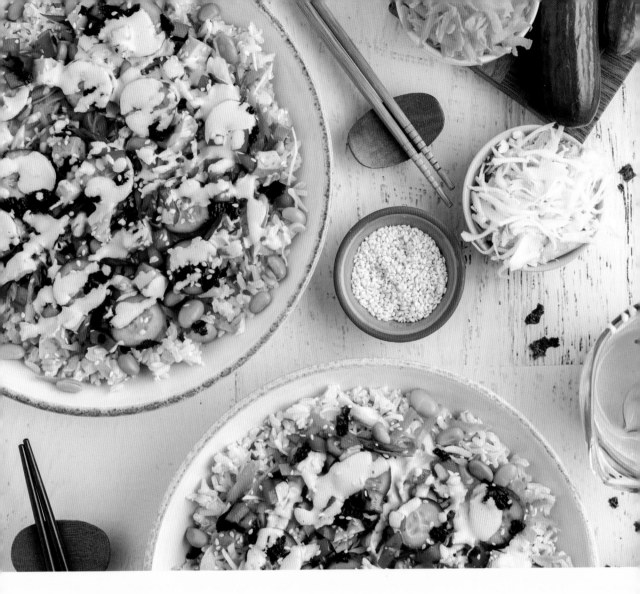

CHEF'S NOTES

Time-Saving Tips

Make the sunomono ahead of time and store it in an airtight container in the refrigerator for up to 2 days.

Make the rice ahead of time and store it in an airtight container in the refrigerator for up to 5 days.

Substitutions

Use yellow, green, or orange bell pepper in place of red bell pepper.

Substitute arame or wakame in place of nori.

Storage

Store in an airtight container in the refrigerator for up to 5 days.

FANTASTICALLY FERMENTED NATTO BLACK RICE BOWL

Meet natto! This Japanese staple hasn't yet made its way to mainstream Western cuisine, but it certainly deserves mainstream status. During its fermentation process, something magical happens: one of our favorite notable nutrients, vitamin K_2, is created . . . and a lot of it! This tangy, pungent, and umami black rice bowl is your chance to experiment with this nutrient-packed food. We know you'll love it!

Serves: 2 **Prep time:** 10 minutes **Cooking time:** 10 minutes

2 cups chopped bok choy

2 cups cooked black or brown rice

1 cup wet or dry natto

1 cup sliced radishes

1 cup sliced cucumbers

1 large avocado, cubed

¼ cup coconut aminos or reduced-sodium tamari

2 tablespoons unsweetened rice vinegar

1 tablespoon maple syrup

1 to 2 teaspoons sriracha or chili paste, optional

1 tablespoon minced ginger

1½ teaspoons minced garlic

1 tablespoon arrowroot powder or cornstarch

2 stalks sliced green onions

¼ cup chopped cilantro, optional

1 to 2 tablespoons sesame seeds

1. To a medium pan over medium-high heat, add the bok choy. Reduce the heat to medium, place a lid over the pan, and steam the bok choy for 1 to 2 minutes or until wilted. Transfer the bok choy to two bowls. (Turn off the heat, but keep the pan on the stovetop for the sauce.)

2. Split the rice, natto, radishes, cucumber, and avocado between the bowls.

3. Make the sauce: In a medium bowl, whisk together the coconut aminos, rice vinegar, maple syrup, sriracha, ginger, garlic, and arrowroot powder with ½ cup of water until the powder is dissolved. Heat the saved pan on medium-high and add this sauce, stirring until it thickens, about 1 to 2 minutes.

4. Divide the sauce between the two bowls, using as much as you prefer. Top each bowl with green onions, cilantro, and sesame seeds.

Calcium: 325 mg	Iron: 12 mg	Magnesium: 201 mg	Omega-3s: .8 g	Selenium: 12.8 mcg	Zinc: 4.5 mg

Calories: 815 | Protein: 35 g | Carbohydrate: 97 g | Fiber: 16 g | Fat: 16 g | Sodium: 830 mg

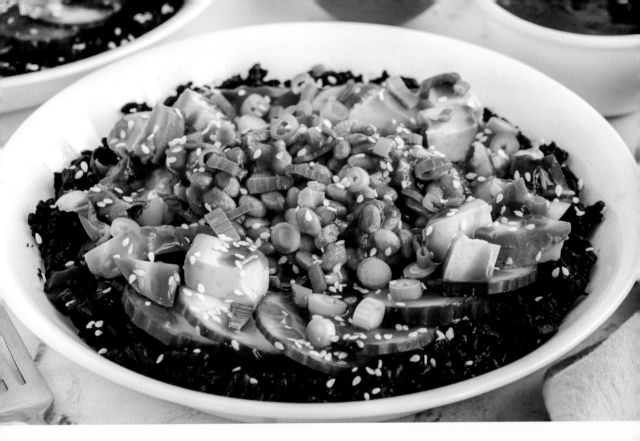

CHEF'S NOTES

Time-Saving Tips

Make the rice ahead of time so you have it ready to use.

Other Tips

Make brown or black rice by adding ¾ cup of rinsed rice to a pot with 1½ cups of water. Bring the rice to a boil over high heat, reduce heat to low, cover, and simmer for approximately 30 to 35 minutes. Prepare your bowl ingredients while the rice is cooking to save time!

If you haven't tried natto, you might prefer starting with the dry variety as it doesn't have the same sticky texture as the wet natto, and may be preferred by those with texture sensitivities. You can find natto at your local natural grocer or buy it online.

Substitutions

For the rice, use red in place of black or brown.

We used radishes, cucumbers, and avocado, but feel free to use any raw veggies you have on hand. If you prefer all raw ingredients, replace the cooked bok choy with raw baby bok choy or a raw leafy green like spinach or kale.

Instead of cilantro, try basil or chives.

Storage

Store the bowl in an airtight container in the refrigerator for up to 3 days.

Store any extra sauce in an airtight container in the refrigerator for up to 5 days.

SWEET ON YOU CHILI BROCCOLI AND TOFU BOWL

This simple-to-make yet flavorful tofu stir-fry includes a true megastar in the plant kingdom: broccoli. This dish includes lots of notable nutrients, including calcium, vitamin C, fiber, and vitamin K_1. Coating the broccoli and tofu in a sweet and sticky chili sauce makes it comforting and inviting. We added in more veggies with mushrooms (hello, selenium!), red bell pepper, and onion, but feel free to use any other veggies you like.

Serves: 2 **Prep time:** 10 minutes **Cooking time:** 20 minutes

14 ounces firm or extra-firm tofu, pressed (optional, see page 87) and cut into ½-inch cubes

2 tablespoons plus 1 teaspoon coconut aminos or reduced-sodium tamari, divided

1 tablespoon arrowroot powder or cornstarch

⅓ cup unsweetened rice vinegar

⅓ cup date paste

1 tablespoon sambal oelek or other chili paste

1 teaspoon ginger, minced

6 ounces button mushrooms, sliced (approximately 1½ cups)

1½ cups broccoli florets, chopped into 1-inch pieces

1 medium red bell pepper, chopped

1 small onion, thinly sliced

3 cups cooked brown rice

2 tablespoons raw cashews

2 tablespoons sliced green onion

Chopped cilantro to taste, optional

1. Preheat the oven to 400°F and line a baking sheet with parchment paper.

2. In a medium bowl, gently toss the tofu with 2 tablespoons of coconut aminos until the tofu is coated.

3. Spread the tofu out evenly on the baking sheet and bake it for 20 minutes, flipping halfway through.

4. Meanwhile, prepare the sauce: In a small bowl, whisk together the arrowroot powder and 1 tablespoon of water until dissolved. In a blender, blend the arrowroot slurry, rice vinegar, date paste, sambal oelek, ginger, 1 teaspoon coconut aminos, and ¼ cup of water until smooth, and set the sauce aside.

5. To a large pan over medium-high heat, add the mushrooms, broccoli, red bell pepper, and onion. Stir for 1 minute and then add ½ cup of water. Cover three-quarters of the pan with a lid, and cook for 3 to 5 minutes or until the vegetables are as tender as you like.

6. Transfer the cooked tofu and sauce to the pan with the veggies. Stir until the sauce thickens and everything is heated through, about 30 to 60 seconds.

7. Divide the stir-fry and rice between serving plates. Top with the cashews, green onion, and cilantro.

Calcium: 867 mg	Iron: 7.2 mg	Magnesium: 286 mg	Omega-3s: .9 g	Selenium: 61 mcg	Zinc: 7.2 mg

Calories: 853 | Protein: 43 g | Carbohydrate: 117 g | Fiber: 12 g | Fat: 21 g | Sodium: 509 mg

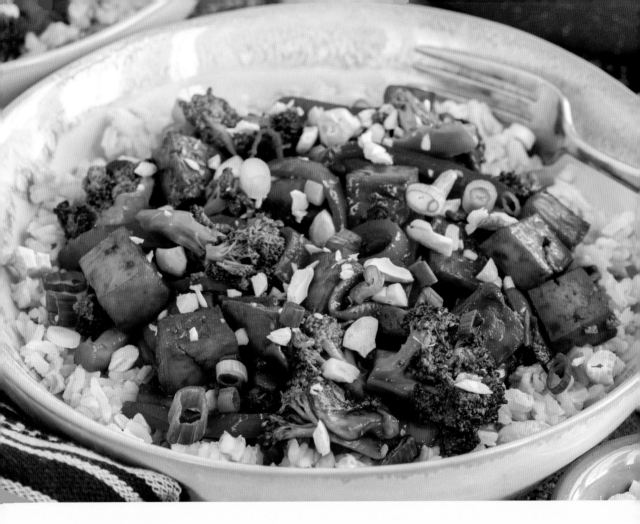

CHEF'S NOTES

Time-Saving Tips

Make the tofu ahead of time and store it in an airtight container in the refrigerator for up to 3 days.

Substitutions

If you don't want to make your own sweet chili sauce, feel free to use a store-bought brand. However, check the ingredients label to avoid unnecessary fish sauce, preservatives, and processed sugar.

Instead of red bell pepper, use yellow, orange, or green bell pepper.

Substitute another vegetable of choice in place of broccoli, such as cauliflower, carrots, or brussels sprouts.

Substitute any mushroom you love for the button mushrooms.

Substitute parsley or basil for the cilantro.

Storage

Store leftovers in an airtight container in the refrigerator for up to 5 days.

SWEET POTATO LENTIL BOWL WITH SILKY GREEN TAHINI SAUCE

If there is one thing we love about plant-based eating, it is the range of creativity you can have when crafting the perfect nourishing bowl. Blending leafy green spinach, cilantro, and jalapeño with tahini is a delicious way to sneak in a few extra veggies too. Drizzled over sweet potatoes and lentils with a sprinkle of nutty and seedy dukkah seasoning on top, this creamy, savory, and oh-so-green bowl of plants is anything but boring.

Serves: 2 **Prep time:** 15 minutes **Cooking time:** 15 minutes

½ cup dry green or brown lentils, rinsed

1½ cups sweet potato, cut into 1-inch cubes (approximately ¾ large potato)

2 cups spinach

1 cup shredded carrots

1 cup shredded beet (approximately 1 medium beet)

⅓ cup thinly sliced red onion

Herb of choice, to taste (cilantro, parsley, or mint)

Salt to taste, optional

Ground black pepper to taste, optional

Green Tahini Sauce

¼ cup tahini

2 tablespoons seeded and roughly minced jalapeño, optional

¼ cup chopped cilantro, optional

1 cup roughly chopped spinach

2 small cloves garlic, chopped

3 tablespoons lime juice

1 to 2 pinches salt, optional

Dukkah Seasoning

⅛ cup finely chopped raw almonds

⅛ cup finely chopped raw pecans

1 tablespoon sesame seeds

½ teaspoon mustard seeds

½ teaspoon coriander seeds

½ teaspoon cumin seeds

⅛ teaspoon ground ginger, optional

⅛ teaspoon salt, optional

| Calcium: 346 mg | Iron: 10 mg | Magnesium: 234 mg | Omega-3s: .35 g | Selenium: 17 mcg | Zinc: 5.5 mg |

Calories: 768 | Protein: 28 g | Carbohydrate: 83 g | Fiber: 23 g | Fat: 29 g | Sodium: 338 mg

1. To a small pot over medium-high heat, add 1½ cups water and the lentils. Bring to a boil and then reduce the heat to low. Cover the lentils, simmer them for 25 minutes, and then drain any excess water and set them aside.

2. While the lentils simmer, fill a medium pot halfway with water and bring it to a boil over medium-high heat. Add the sweet potatoes and cook until tender, about 10 minutes. Pierce the potatoes with a fork to determine doneness. Drain any excess water and set aside.

3. Make the Green Tahini Sauce: In a blender, blend all the sauce ingredients plus ¼ cup of water until smooth. Add 1 to 2 tablespoons more water as needed for desired consistency.

4. Make the Dukkah Seasoning: In a small pan over medium heat, toast the almonds and pecans for 3 minutes, tossing frequently so they don't burn. Add the sesame, mustard, coriander, and cumin seeds, tossing for an additional 2 minutes. Transfer the dukkah ingredients to a mortar and pestle (or spice grinder), allow them to cool slightly, and then crush the seeds and nuts until combined well. Stir in the ginger and salt. Set the dukkah aside.

5. Divide the spinach between the two bowls and then divide the lentils and potatoes between the two bowls. (Their warmth will soften and wilt the spinach a bit.) Divide the carrots, beet, and onion between the two bowls.

6. Divide the Green Tahini Sauce between the two bowls and toss to combine. Add 1 to 2 tablespoons of dukkah to each bowl, along with your herb of choice. Add salt and pepper to taste.

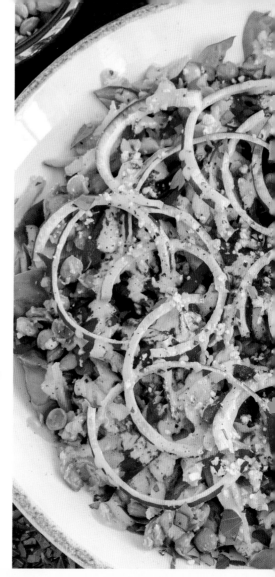

CHEF'S NOTES

Time-Saving Tips
Prepare the dukkah seasoning ahead of time and store it in an airtight container in the refrigerator for up to 1 month.

Substitutions
Substitute butternut squash or your favorite winter squash for the sweet potato.

Substitute green bell pepper for the jalapeño.

Substitute kale or your favorite dark leafy green for the spinach.

Storage
Store bowl leftovers and leftover dressing in separate airtight containers in the refrigerator for up to 5 days.

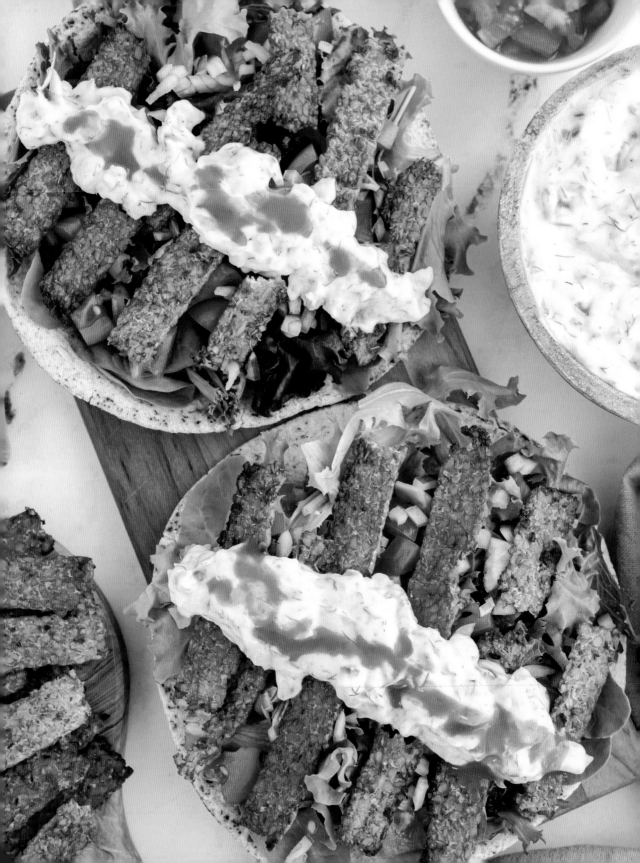

SANDWICHES, WRAPS, AND PIZZA

MEET ME IN THE MEDITERRANEAN TORTILLA PIZZA WITH TOFU RICOTTA

Made with creamy tofu "ricotta" instead of dairy cheese, this family favorite is packed with protein as well as calcium and iron. The combination of tofu and nutritional yeast creates a cheesy texture and flavor that everyone will love. Have the kiddos help out during the preparation stage to build one-of-a-kind homemade pizzas and memories together!

Serves: 4 **Prep time:** 15 minutes **Cooking time:** 15 minutes

8 ounces firm or extra-firm tofu, drained well

1 tablespoon tahini

1½ tablespoons nutritional yeast

2 tablespoons minced shallots

1 clove garlic, minced

½ teaspoon dried oregano

1 dash ground nutmeg

1 tablespoon lemon juice

¼ teaspoon salt, optional

⅛ teaspoon ground black pepper, optional

¾ cup diced red onion

1 cup halved cherry tomatoes

1 cup shaved or thinly sliced asparagus

1 tablespoon red wine vinegar

2 dashes salt, optional

4 8-inch whole-grain tortillas or flatbreads

Extra virgin olive oil, optional

¼ cup sliced green or kalamata olives

1 cup arugula

2 tablespoons chopped fresh basil

Vegan Walnut Parmesan (page 114) to taste, optional

Crushed red pepper flakes to taste, optional

1. Preheat the oven to 425°F.
2. Make the Tofu Ricotta: In a medium bowl, crumble the tofu. In a small bowl, whisk together the tahini, nutritional yeast, shallots, garlic, oregano, nutmeg, lemon juice, salt, and pepper. Add the tahini mixture to the tofu and gently mix with a fork until well combined. Note: The tofu should be a little wet and in clumps, not totally mashed.
3. In a large skillet over medium-high heat, sauté the onion, tomatoes, and asparagus for 2 minutes.
4. Add the vinegar and salt, and cook for another minute. Remove from the heat.
5. Place the tortillas or flatbread on two baking sheets, or pizza stones if you own them. Lightly brush the tortillas with olive oil and sprinkle with salt.
6. Divide the sautéed veggies and olives between the tortillas. Spread approximately 4 to 6 tablespoons of Tofu Ricotta over each tortilla, leaving about a 1-inch space around the edges. Press the tofu down to keep the veggies in place.
7. Bake for 10 minutes or until the edges are golden crispy.
8. Remove the pizzas from the oven and top them with arugula, basil, and Vegan Walnut Parmesan to taste. Sprinkle the crushed red pepper flakes over the top.

| Calcium: 313 mg | Iron: 4.4 mg | Magnesium: 61 mg | Omega-3s: .5 g | Selenium: 12 mcg | Zinc: 1.75 mg |

Calories: 308 | Protein: 18 g | Carbohydrate: 59 g | Fiber: 13 g | Fat: 15 g | Sodium: 518 mg

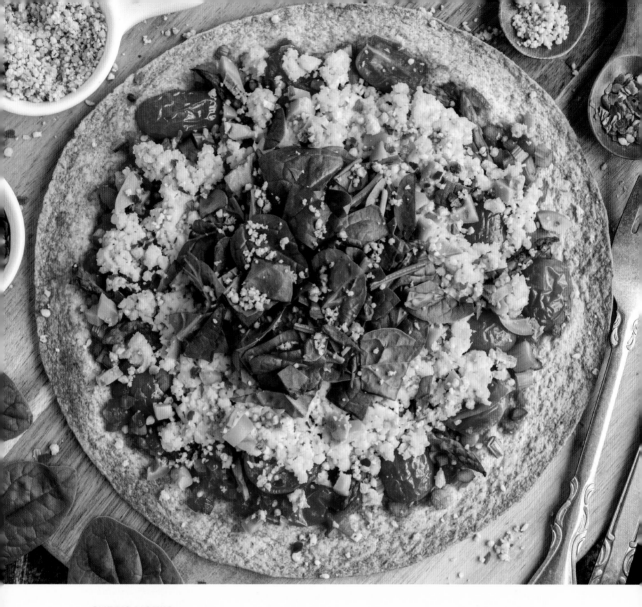

CHEF'S NOTES

Time-Saving Tips

Make the Vegan Walnut Parmesan ahead of time.

Make the Tofu Ricotta ahead of time and store it in an airtight container in the refrigerator for up to 3 days.

Substitutions

In place of nutritional yeast, use 1 tablespoon of mellow white or chickpea miso.

Storage

Store the pizzas in an airtight container in the refrigerator for up to 3 days. Reheat at 425°F for 5 to 7 minutes.

SMOTHERED IN TZATZIKI TEMPEH GYRO

Savory tempeh strips are seasoned with Mediterranean spices and generously dolloped with cool and creamy dairy-free Tzatziki Sauce, then sprinkled with fresh onion and tomato. Gyros are typically served in a warm pita or flatbread but can be just as delicious with the gluten-free vessel of your choice (see Chef's Notes). This veggie-packed, all-in-one meal has comfort, flavor, and nourishment in every bite.

Serves: 4   **Prep time:** 15 minutes   **Cooking time:** 15 minutes

8 ounces tempeh (see Chef's Notes)

1 tablespoon tahini

2 tablespoons coconut aminos or reduced-sodium tamari

2 tablespoons lemon juice

½ teaspoon garlic powder

1 teaspoon dried oregano

4 whole-grain pitas or lavash bread or leafy green wraps

2 cups leafy greens of your choice (spinach, arugula, baby kale, romaine)

½ cup diced red onion

½ cup diced tomato

Hot sauce of your choice, to taste

Tzatziki Sauce

2 cups grated cucumbers

1½ cups plain, unsweetened plant-based yogurt

¼ cup lemon juice

2 cloves garlic, finely minced

4 tablespoons minced fresh herb of choice (parsley, dill, cilantro, or mint)

¼ teaspoon salt, optional

⅛ teaspoon ground black pepper, optional

1. Boil the tempeh: In a small pan, add the tempeh and enough water to cover it by 1 inch. Bring it to a boil and cook for 10 minutes.

2. Meanwhile, in a shallow baking dish, make the marinade by combining the tahini, coconut aminos, lemon juice, garlic powder, oregano, and ¼ cup water.

3. Make the Tzatziki Sauce: Drain 1 cup of cucumbers at a time by pressing the grated cucumbers until the water stops draining from them (press about three times). In a medium bowl, mix the cucumbers with the remaining sauce ingredients until well combined.

4. Once the tempeh is done boiling, drain and transfer it to a cutting board and cut into ½-inch by 1-inch strips to make 8 strips.

5. Add the tempeh to the marinade, gently tossing until it is completely covered.

6. Heat a large pan over medium heat. Depending on your pan, you may need to lightly oil the bottom to prevent the tempeh from sticking. Once the pan is hot, add each piece of tempeh, reserving any extra marinade. Cook 1 to 2 minutes per side, until slightly golden brown. Remove the tempeh from the heat and pour any remaining marinade over the top.

7. Add a layer of greens to each pita and then add 2 tablespoons each of onion and tomato. Divide the tempeh between the four wraps. Top with 2 to 4 tablespoons of tzatziki and hot sauce.

| Calcium: 188 mg | Iron: 6.2 mg | Magnesium: 72 mg | Omega-3s: .175 g | Selenium: 1.8 mcg | Zinc: 1.1 mg |

Calories: 422 | Protein: 30 g | Carbohydrate: 40 g | Fiber: 8 g | Fat: 13 g | Sodium: 655 mg

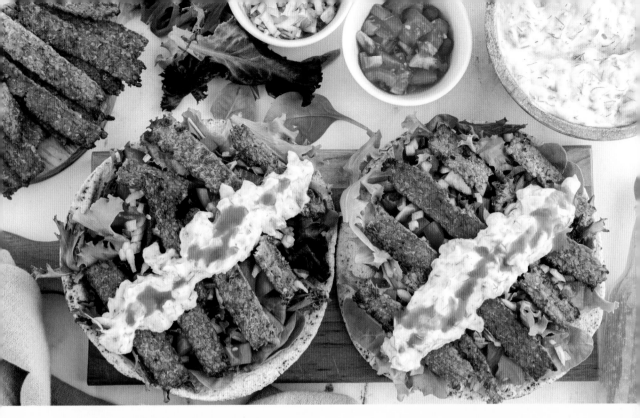

CHEF'S NOTES

Time-Saving Tips

Boil or steam the tempeh ahead of time and let it marinate overnight (or for at least 20 minutes) in the refrigerator.

Other Tips

Boiling or steaming tempeh for 10 minutes can minimize its bitterness and allow it to absorb more of the flavors paired with it. It's not a mandatory step if you don't have time.

Keep the cucumber skin intact if the cucumbers do not have a wax coating. If the cucumbers are waxed, we recommend that you peel the skins before grating them.

You can also use sprouted whole-grain tortillas. Note that if you use an 8-inch tortilla or smaller pitas, you may get more than 4 wraps. In this case, use 2 to 3 pieces of tempeh for each small wrap rather than dividing the tempeh pieces between four wraps.

Gluten-Free: Instead of pitas, use large, leafy green wraps like collard greens, Swiss chard, or romaine.

Substitutions

Substitute drained and pressed firm or extra-firm tofu in place of the tempeh (you don't need to boil or steam the tofu).

Use lime juice in place of lemon juice.

Storage

Store leftover tzatziki in an airtight container in the refrigerator for up to 3 days and leftover tempeh in an airtight container in the refrigerator for up to 5 days.

TURN UP THE BEET BURGER WITH SMASHED AVOCADO AND PICKLED ONIONS

This burger gets rave reviews, and for good reason—it's simple to make, delicious, and extremely satisfying. You'll get iron from the beet and beans, omega-3 fatty acids from the flaxseed meal, and prebiotic fiber from the oats and onions, which may help synthesize vitamin K_2 in your gut. Pile the burgers high with avocado and Pickled Red Onions to make this a meal high in vitamins C, E, and K. Try topping the burger with microgreens, sprouts, tomato slices, or leafy greens like kale or spinach for an extra nutrition boost!

Makes: 6 burgers **Prep time:** 15 minutes **Cooking time:** 10 minutes

¾ cup raw sunflower seeds

¼ cup flaxseed meal

3 cloves garlic, roughly chopped

1½ tablespoons mellow white or chickpea miso

1 tablespoon chili powder

1 tablespoon ground cumin

1 teaspoon ground turmeric

1 tablespoon onion powder

1 teaspoon dried oregano

¼ teaspoon salt, optional

⅛ teaspoon ground black pepper, optional

1 cup shredded beet (approximately 1 medium-sized beet)

1 cup rolled oats

1½ cups home-cooked or 1 15-ounce can white beans, drained

2 tablespoons plain, unsweetened plant-based yogurt

Whole-grain bread or lettuce

1 to 2 teaspoons extra virgin olive oil

1 to 2 avocados, smashed with a fork

Pickled Red Onions

1 red onion, thinly sliced

½ cup red wine vinegar

¼ teaspoon salt, optional

1. In a food processor, blend the sunflower seeds, flaxseed meal, garlic, miso, chili powder, cumin, turmeric, onion powder, oregano, salt, and pepper until a moist, coarse dough forms.

2. Add the beet, oats, beans, and yogurt. Blend until combined, using a spatula to scrape the sides and bottom of the food processor, making sure that everything is blended.

3. With clean hands, scoop out the burger mix to form 4-inch patties about ½-inch thick. You should get about 6 patties. Set aside.

4. Make the Pickled Red Onions: Add onion, red wine vinegar, and salt plus ½ cup water to a large bowl. Massage the liquids into the onions. Set them aside.

5. Heat a large skillet over medium heat. Once hot, add the patties, cooking on one side until lightly browned, about 3 to 5 minutes. Flip to cook the other side. Depending on your skillet, you may need to lightly coat it with avocado or olive oil to prevent the patties from sticking. When they are done cooking, place the burgers on a plate or clean cutting board.

6. Place the burgers between slices of whole-grain bread or in a lettuce wrap and top them with the smashed avocado and Pickled Red Onions. Add other veggies of choice and your favorite plant-based sauce or condiments.

Calcium: 151 mg	Iron: 4.9 mg	Magnesium: 93 mg	Omega-3s: .375 g	Selenium: 11 mcg	Zinc: 1.9 mg

Calories: 510 | Protein: 19 g | Carbohydrate: 49 g | Fiber: 15 g | Fat: 16 g | Sodium: 653 mg

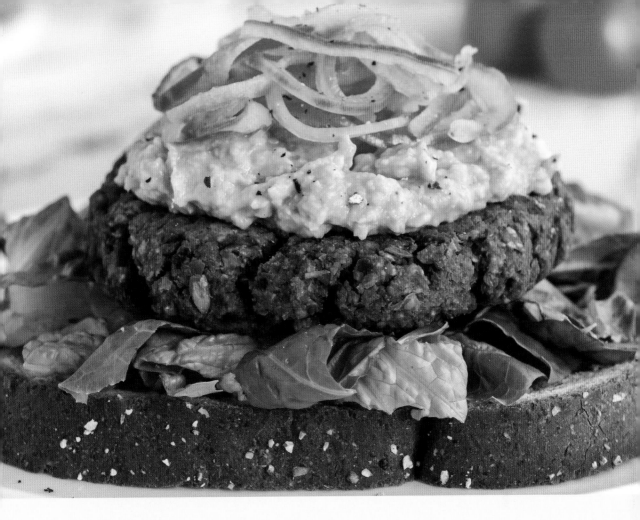

CHEF'S NOTES

Time-Saving Tips

Prepare the Pickled Red Onions ahead of time and store them in the refrigerator for up to 10 days.

Substitutions

Replace Pickled Red Onions with raw red onion, kimchi, or kraut.

In place of sunflower seeds, use walnuts or cashews.

For the white beans, use great northern, cannellini, or navy beans.

Instead of oats, try millet or quinoa.

Oven Directions

Preheat the oven to 375°F. Bake the patties on a parchment-lined baking sheet for 30 minutes, flipping halfway through.

Storage

Store leftover burger patties in an airtight container in the refrigerator for up to 7 days or freeze, separated by parchment paper, for up to 3 months.

SEOUL-FUL TLT WITH PICKLED VEGGIES AND SPICY MAYO

This is a winning TLT (in this case, tofu, lettuce, and tomato) sandwich, where you can easily substitute the tofu with tempeh if you prefer. Marinated with lots of garlic and ginger, slathered with spicy Korean-inspired mayo, and piled high with pickled veggies—all between two fiber-rich slices of whole-grain bread—this is probably one of the most satisfying ways to enjoy plant-loving nutrients in every delicious bite.

Serves: 2 **Prep time:** 20 minutes **Cooking time:** 20 minutes

2 tablespoons coconut aminos or reduced-sodium tamari

1 tablespoon sherry vinegar or red wine vinegar

¼ teaspoon garlic powder

¼ teaspoon ginger powder

½ teaspoon white or black sesame seeds

7 ounces pressed firm or extra-firm tofu, cut into 2-inch by 4-inch strips (see page 87 for pressing instructions)

4 slices whole-grain bread

2 to 4 pieces dark leafy greens of your choice

2 to 4 slices tomato

Pickled Red Onions (page 166)

2 tablespoons chopped cilantro, optional

Spicy Mayo

¼ cup tahini

1 tablespoon gochujang

1 tablespoon lime juice

1 clove garlic, roughly chopped

1. Preheat the oven to 400°F and line a baking sheet with parchment paper.

2. In a shallow dish (a pie dish works well), combine the coconut aminos, vinegar, garlic powder, ginger powder, and sesame seeds. Add the tofu to the marinade. Coat both sides of the tofu with a pastry brush and let it sit for 30 minutes. (See Chef's Notes for time-saving options.)

3. Spread the tofu out evenly on the baking sheet. Bake for 20 minutes, flipping halfway through.

4. Meanwhile, make the Spicy Mayo: In a blender, blend all the ingredients with ¼ cup water until smooth. Set the mayo aside.

5. Toast the bread; then, spread 1 to 2 tablespoons of the mayo on top of each slice.

6. Place leafy greens on two of the slices of bread. Place 2 to 4 pieces of tofu on top of the leafy greens. Add a slice of tomato and 2 to 3 tablespoons of Pickled Red Onions on top of the tofu. Sprinkle cilantro on top.

7. Place the other slice of bread on top of each sandwich, or fold in half, and enjoy!

| Calcium: 297 mg | Iron: 4.4 mg | Magnesium: 116 mg | Omega-3s: .3 g | Selenium: 13.9 mcg | Zinc: 2.65 mg |

Calories: 413 | Protein: 31 g | Carbohydrate: 73 g | Fiber: 11 g | Fat: 15 g | Sodium: 327 mg

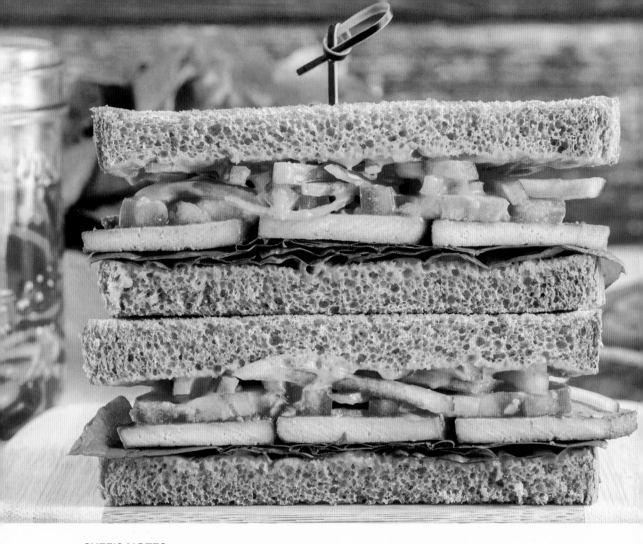

CHEF'S NOTES

Time-Saving Tips

Add the tofu marinade just before baking instead of marinating for 30 minutes. You can also marinate the tofu ahead of time and store it in an airtight container in the refrigerator overnight or for up to 48 hours.

Prepare the Pickled Red Onions ahead of time and store them in the refrigerator for up to 10 days. You can also use raw red onion.

Substitutions

Use leafy greens, like collard greens, kale, romaine, or Swiss chard, as your wrap instead of bread.

Use tempeh instead of tofu.

Storage

Store leftover tofu in an airtight container in the refrigerator for up to 5 days and leftover Spicy Mayo in an airtight container in the refrigerator for up to 7 days.

IT'S SLICE TO MEET YOU PLANT-POWERED PESTO PIZZA

Traditional pesto sauce may not be seen as versatile, but in the right hands, it can transform into something truly unique. Kale Walnut Basil Pesto is just as delicious as the classic pesto sauce you may remember, but the addition of kale, walnuts, and nutritional yeast unlocks a new layer of flavor! Feel free to slather on a generous layer if you like your pizza heavy on the sauce.

Serves: 2   **Prep time:** 20 minutes   **Cooking time:** 10 minutes

Kale Walnut Basil Pesto

2 cups destemmed kale

⅔ cup raw walnuts

1 cup packed fresh basil

2 tablespoons nutritional yeast

2 cloves garlic

½ cup cubed avocado

2 to 3 tablespoons lemon juice

¼ teaspoon salt, optional

¼ teaspoon ground black pepper, optional

¼ teaspoon crushed red pepper flakes, optional

Pizza Ingredients

2 10-inch whole-grain tortillas or flatbread

Vegan Walnut Parmesan (page 114)

1 tomato, thinly sliced

½ red onion, thinly sliced

5 to 6 rinsed and chopped artichoke hearts, canned or jarred in brine

1 handful arugula

Crushed red pepper flakes to taste, optional

1. Preheat the oven to 425°F.
2. Make the Kale Walnut Basil Pesto: In a food processor, blend all ingredients plus ¼ cup of water. Add more water, if needed, 1 tablespoon at a time until you achieve the desired consistency. Set the pesto aside.
3. Assemble your pizza: Place the tortillas on a baking sheet, or on a pizza stone if you own one.
4. Spread approximately ½ cup pesto on each tortilla, leaving about a 1-inch space around the edges.
5. Divide the tomatoes, onions, and artichokes between the tortillas.
6. Bake the tortillas for 10 minutes or until the edges are golden crispy. (Flatbread may need 5 minutes longer.)
7. Remove from the oven and top with arugula, 1 to 2 tablespoons of Vegan Walnut Parmesan, and a sprinkle of crushed red pepper flakes. Serve the leftover pesto and walnut parmesan on the side or save them for later to use in recipes throughout the week!

Calcium: 299 mg	Iron: 6 mg	Magnesium: 224 mg	Omega-3s: 4.5 g	Selenium: 16 mcg	Zinc: 4 mg	Vitamin B₁₂*: 3 mcg

Calories: 718 | Protein: 29 g | Carbohydrate: 52 g | Fiber: 30 g | Fat: 49 g | Sodium: 682 mg

*If using fortified nutritional yeast.

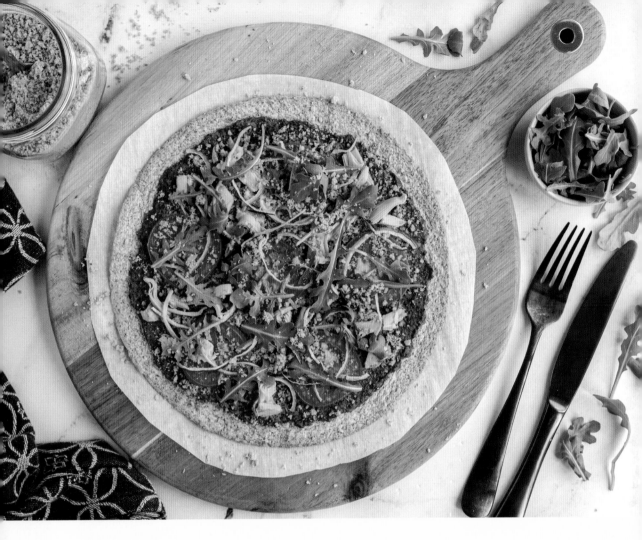

CHEF'S NOTES

Time-Saving Tips

Prepare the Kale Walnut Basil Pesto ahead of time and store it in an airtight container in the refrigerator for up to 3 days.

Prepare the Vegan Walnut Parmesan and store it in an airtight container in the refrigerator for up to 2 weeks.

Substitutions

Instead of arugula use chopped spinach, adding it with the tomatoes, onions, and artichokes, and cooking it with the pizza.

Substitute microgreens in place of the arugula, adding them after the pizza is finished cooking.

Substitute green or black olives for the onions.

Storage

Store leftover pizza in an airtight container in the refrigerator for up to 3 days.

SWEET 'N' SMOKY
BBQ TEMPEH COLLARD WRAP

Between the barbecue flavor, "meaty" tempeh, and crunchy slaw—all bundled into one tasty package—this collard leaf wrap combines the comfort of a hearty meal with the freshness of a salad, embodying a perfect harmony of taste and health.

Serves: 2 **Prep time:** 20 minutes **Cooking time:** 20 minutes

8 ounces tempeh cut into ½-inch by 3-inch strips (see Chef's Notes)

½ cup silken tofu

2 tablespoons apple cider vinegar

1 tablespoon maple syrup

2 teaspoons brown mustard

¼ teaspoon salt, optional

¼ teaspoon ground black pepper, optional

2 cups shredded red cabbage

1 cup shredded carrots

1 cup apples (Granny Smith, Pink Lady, Honeycrisp, or Envy), shaved, finely julienned, or shredded

½ cup slivered almonds

2 stalks thinly sliced green onion

¼ teaspoon ground black pepper, optional

4 collard green leaves

2 to 3 tablespoons Pickled Red Onions (page 166)

1 sliced avocado

BBQ Sauce

3 tablespoons tomato paste

4 tablespoons vegan Worcestershire sauce

1 tablespoon apple cider vinegar

1 tablespoon maple syrup

½ teaspoon garlic powder

½ teaspoon smoked paprika

¼ teaspoon onion powder

1. Preheat the oven to 375°F. Line a baking sheet with parchment.

2. Make the BBQ Sauce: In a small bowl, combine all the sauce ingredients. Add more maple syrup for sweetness, apple cider vinegar for tang, or spices for more garlic or onion flavor, to taste.

3. With a pastry brush, brush each side of the tempeh with BBQ Sauce so it's lightly coated. Place the tempeh on the baking sheet and bake it for 20 minutes, flipping halfway through. Set aside the leftover BBQ Sauce to use for assembling the wrap.

4. Make the dressing: In a food processor or blender, blend the tofu, apple cider vinegar, maple syrup, mustard, salt, and pepper until smooth and creamy. Taste and adjust the ingredients as needed (more salt, apple cider vinegar, or mustard).

5. Make the slaw: In a large bowl, combine the cabbage, carrots, and apples and pour the dressing over the top. Stir well. Stir in the almonds, green onion, and black pepper.

6. On a cutting board, lay out the collard green leaves vertically. Add 2 strips of tempeh to each collard. Add 1 to 2 teaspoons of BBQ Sauce to each wrap, spreading it out evenly. Add 2 to 3 tablespoons of slaw to each wrap. Add 2 tablespoons of Pickled Red Onions and sliced avocado.

7. Roll the wrap by first tucking in the bottom and then folding over the left side of the leafy green, and then the right side.

Calcium: 263 mg	Iron: 4.8 mg	Magnesium: 96 mg	Omega-3s: .27 g	Selenium: 6 mcg	Zinc: 1.7 mg

Calories: 776 | Protein: 20 g | Carbohydrate: 51 g | Fiber: 19 g | Fat: 43 g | Sodium: 626 mg

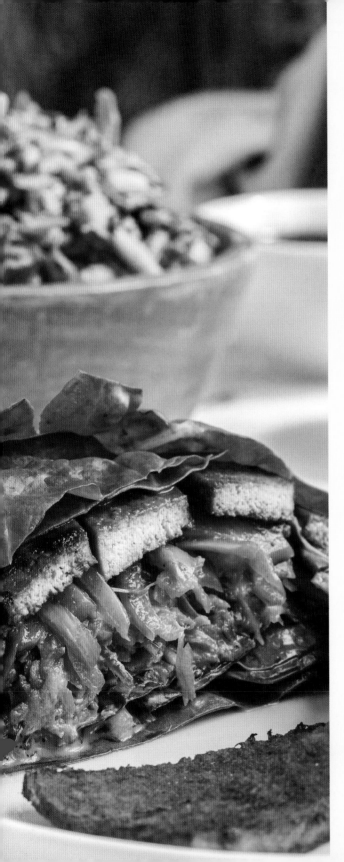

CHEF'S NOTES

Time-Saving Tips

Prepare your tempeh ahead of time and store in an airtight container in the refrigerator for up to 5 days.

Make the dressing and slaw while the tempeh is cooking.

Prepare the Pickled Red Onions ahead of time and store it in the refrigerator for up to 10 days. Or use raw red onion in place of Pickled Red Onions.

Make the slaw ahead of time and store it in an airtight container in the refrigerator for up to 5 days.

Make your BBQ Sauce ahead of time and store it in the refrigerator for up to 1 week, or use store-bought sauce.

Other Tips

Boil the tempeh for 10 minutes in a medium saucepan filled with enough water to cover the tempeh. Alternatively, you can steam the tempeh in a steamer basket for 10 minutes. This reduces the bitterness and will help the tempeh absorb the marinade better. Once it's done, drain and pat it dry. Set it aside.

Add 1 to 2 teaspoons of your favorite hot sauce or a dash of cayenne pepper.

Substitutions

Instead of carrots and cabbage, try radishes, cucumbers, shaved brussels sprouts, or other crunchy veggies.

Substitute Swiss chard or kale leaves for collard leaves.

In place of brown mustard, use Dijon.

In place of tempeh, use firm or extra-firm tofu.

Storage

Store leftover barbecue sauce in an airtight container in the refrigerator for up to 7 days. Store leftover slaw in an airtight container in the refrigerator for up to 5 days.

SMASHED AVOCADO CHICKPEA SALAD WRAP

In this rich and creamy wrap, tantalizing chickpeas, crunchy veggies, and lush smashed avocado are reminiscent of the flavors of chicken salad but with so many more plant-based nutrients to offer. While we opted to make this recipe gluten-free by using collard wraps, you can still enjoy this wholesome chickpea salad between two slices of crusty whole-grain bread.

Serves: 2 **Prep time:** 15 minutes **Cooking time:** none

1½ cups home-cooked or 1 15-ounce can chickpeas, drained

1 avocado

¼ teaspoon ground black pepper

½ teaspoon ground turmeric

½ teaspoon smoked or sweet paprika

½ teaspoon garlic powder

1 teaspoon ground cumin

2 to 3 tablespoons lime juice

1 tablespoon apple cider vinegar

¼ cup chopped green onion

¼ cup chopped celery

¼ cup chopped cilantro

¼ teaspoon salt, optional

2 collard green leaves

1. In a medium bowl, combine the chickpeas, avocado, black pepper, turmeric, paprika, garlic powder, cumin, lime juice, and apple cider vinegar.

2. Smash the avocado and chickpeas with a fork or potato masher until most chickpeas are fully smashed (to keep the mixture together when adding to a wrap or sandwich).

3. Mix in the green onion, celery, and cilantro. Taste and season with salt and more pepper as needed. Sprinkle with more paprika.

4. Scoop a generous amount into each collard wrap and serve.

Calcium: 125 mg	Iron: 3.25 mg	Magnesium: 75 mg	Selenium: 4.5 mcg	Zinc: 1.6 mg

Calories: 305 | Protein: 11 g | Carbohydrate: 22 g | Fiber: 15 g | Fat: 14 g | Sodium: 272 mg

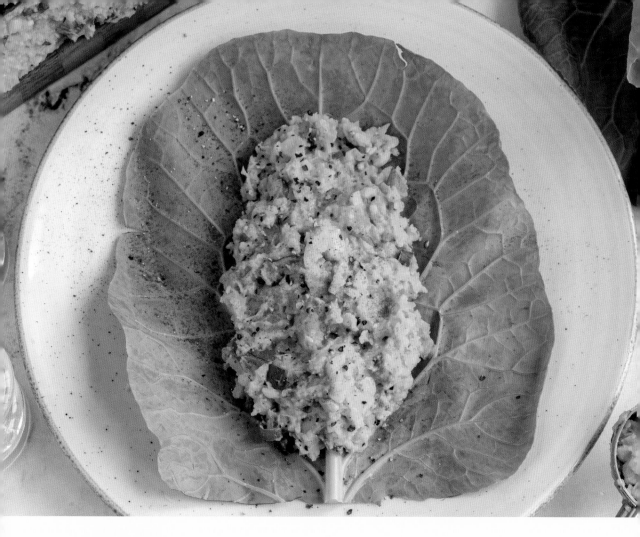

CHEF'S NOTES

Other Tips

Add microgreens, radish, kimchi, or kraut, and sprinkle with sliced almonds or hemp seeds.

If you love heat, add 1 to 2 tablespoons diced jalapeño and ½ teaspoon chipotle chili powder (or regular chili powder if you like less spice). Or you can simply add crushed red pepper flakes.

Substitutions

Use a coconut wrap, whole-grain lavash or bread, or romaine leaves instead of collard greens.

Omit the cilantro or replace it with dill.

Don't have celery on hand? This dish is still delicious without it.

Storage

Store leftover Smashed Avocado Chickpea Salad in an airtight container in the refrigerator for up to 7 days.

PILE 'EM HIGH PAD THAI TOFU BURGERS

The vibrant, nutty, and sweet-and-sour flavors of Pad Thai are even better as a juicy plant-based burger! Not only is this burger extraordinarily delicious but it's also fun to make and stack high with colorful veggie slaw and vibrant arugula that ties it all together. The other reason this recipe is so special is thanks to the high concentration of protein, iron, calcium, and omega-3 fatty acids in every saucy bite.

Serves: 4   **Prep time:** 25 minutes   **Cooking time:** 20 minutes

1½ tablespoons tomato paste

4 tablespoons coconut aminos or reduced-sodium tamari, divided

1½ tablespoons maple syrup

2 tablespoons lime juice

1½ teaspoons chili paste, optional

1 tablespoon mellow white or chickpea miso

14 ounces pressed firm or extra-firm tofu (page 87)

¼ cup smooth or crunchy unsweetened peanut butter

2 tablespoons unsweetened rice vinegar

2 tablespoons lime juice

1 tablespoon maple syrup

1 tablespoon minced ginger

2 cloves garlic, minced

2 cups shredded carrots

2 cups shredded cabbage

½ cup sliced green onion

½ cup chopped cilantro, optional

1 tablespoon white or black sesame seeds

2 teaspoons chili flakes, optional

8 slices whole-grain bread or 4 buns

Spicy Mayo (page 168)

½ cup arugula

1. Preheat the oven to 400°F and line a baking sheet with parchment paper.

2. Make the marinade: In a medium bowl, whisk the tomato paste, 2 tablespoons of coconut aminos, maple syrup, lime juice, chili paste, and miso with 3 tablespoons of water until the miso is dissolved. Alternatively, you can use a blender. Set this marinade aside.

3. Slice the tofu block in half lengthwise and then slice it in half again so you're left with four tofu steaks.

4. Place the tofu in a shallow dish and pour the marinade over the top, gently coating the tofu. Let the tofu sit for 20 minutes. (See Chef's Notes.)

5. Place the tofu evenly on the baking sheet. Leave any remaining marinade in the dish (it'll burn if you add extra to the baking sheet), reserving it for after the tofu is baked. Bake for 20 minutes, flipping halfway through.

6. Meanwhile, prepare the carrot and cabbage slaw: In a medium bowl, mix the peanut butter, 2 tablespoons of coconut aminos, rice vinegar, lime juice, maple syrup, ginger, and garlic until the peanut butter is well blended. Add the carrots, cabbage, green onion, and cilantro and toss to combine. Top with sesame seeds and chili flakes. Set aside.

7. Toast the bread or buns, if desired. Spread Spicy Mayo on each slice of bread (about a tablespoon on each). Divide the arugula equally between the four sandwiches. Add a tofu steak and ¼ cup slaw to each and top with another slice of bread.

| Calcium: 543 mg | Iron: 6 mg | Magnesium: 112 mg | Omega-3s: .72 g | Selenium: 24 mcg | Zinc: 4 mg |

Calories: 671 | Protein: 27 g | Carbohydrate: 53 g | Fiber: 10 g | Fat: 36 g | Sodium: 660 mg

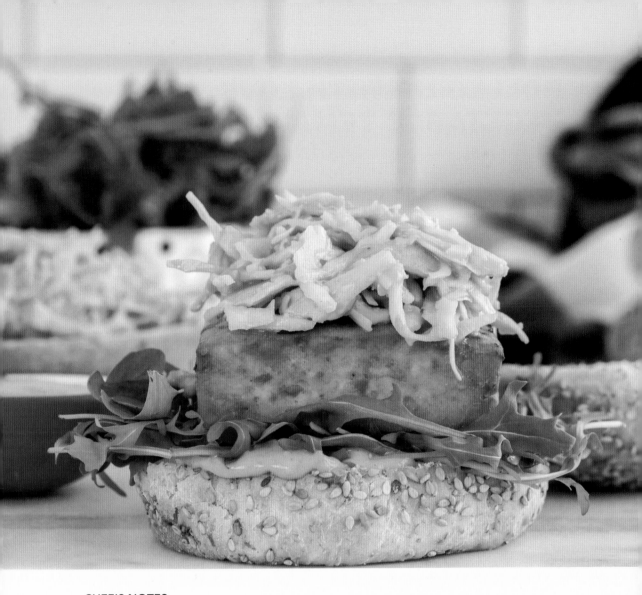

CHEF'S NOTES

Time-Saving Tips

Instead of marinating the tofu for 20 minutes, add the marinade just before baking. Or marinate the tofu ahead of time and store it in an airtight container in the refrigerator overnight or for up to 48 hours.

Prepare the carrot and cabbage slaw ahead of time and store it in an airtight container in the refrigerator for up to 7 days.

Substitutions

Substitute tempeh for the tofu.

Storage

Store the tofu in an airtight container in the refrigerator for up to 5 days.

ROLLED UP WITH LOVE VEGETABLE TEMAKI HAND ROLL

Temaki can be enjoyed like any other wrap. Add whole grains such as brown rice or quinoa, plant-based protein like tofu or tempeh, colorful vegetables—think carrots, sprouts, and cucumbers—and your favorite sauce to a nori sheet before wrapping it into a cone shape. Use iodine-rich nori to switch things up from traditional lunchtime wraps.

Serves: 2   **Prep time:** 20 minutes   **Cooking time:** 20 minutes

8 ounces pressed firm or extra-firm tofu (see page 87)

4 tablespoons coconut aminos or reduced-sodium tamari, divided

3 tablespoons white or black sesame seeds, divided

1 tablespoon unsweetened rice vinegar

2 teaspoons maple syrup

3 cups cooked short grain brown rice (see page 243)

6 nori sheets

1 cup chopped leafy green of your choice

1 cucumber, julienned

1 carrot, julienned

1 cup broccoli sprouts

1 avocado, sliced

Miso Peanut Dressing (page 118)

Wasabi to taste, optional

Pickled ginger to taste, optional

1. Preheat the oven to 400°F and line a baking sheet with parchment paper.

2. Cut the tofu into 3-inch by ⅛-inch strips. Carefully coat it in 2 tablespoons coconut aminos and then cover it with 2 tablespoons sesame seeds.

3. Place the tofu on the baking sheet and bake it for 20 minutes, flipping halfway through.

4. Meanwhile, make the sushi rice: In a medium bowl, combine 2 tablespoons coconut aminos, the rice vinegar, and the maple syrup. Add the rice and 1 tablespoon of sesame seeds. Mix well and set the rice aside.

5. Place a nori sheet on a clean surface, shiny side down. Take a handful of rice and place it on the left third of the nori sheet. Stack the greens, cucumber, carrot, sprouts, avocado, and tofu in order on top of the rice. Make sure not to overfill the nori.

6. Fold the bottom left corner of the nori over and roll it into a cone shape. You can seal the edge so it stays together by adding just a dab of water. Or use rice as "glue" by adding a small piece of rice at the bottom right corner of the cone and closing tightly.

7. Serve the hand rolls with the Miso Peanut Dressing and wasabi and pickled ginger.

Calcium: 285 mg	Iodine: 159 mcg	Iron: 5 mg	Magnesium: 163 mg	Omega-3s: .4 g	Selenium: 22 mcg	Zinc: 3.3 mg

Calories: 515 | Protein: 21 g | Carbohydrate: 50.5 | Fiber: 10.5 g | Fat: 22.5 | Sodium: 513 mg

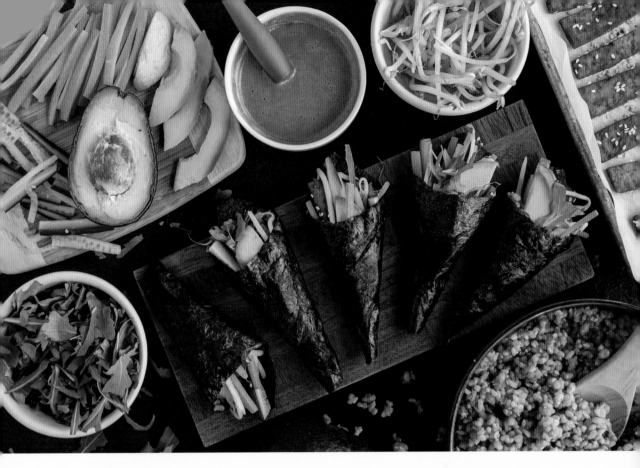

CHEF'S NOTES

Time-Saving Tips

Make the Miso Peanut Dressing ahead of time and store it in the refrigerator for 7 to 10 days.

Make the rice the day before and store it in an airtight container in the refrigerator.

Julienne the cucumber and carrot ahead of time and store them in an airtight container in the refrigerator for up to 2 days.

Other Tips

It's important to use short grain rice for this, as long grain rice will not stick together. If your rice is made several days ahead of time, it's possible that it will dry out. It's best if the rice is made as close as possible to when you plan to make the rolls.

Add nutritional yeast or herbs like cilantro, chives, or basil either inside or on top. Add wasabi and pickled ginger or other veggies to the inside of the roll.

Substitutions

Substitute any vegetables you'd like with your favorites. Just make sure they're thinly sliced so that they don't overcrowd your roll and can form a cone shape!

Use quinoa or millet in place of rice. They both stick together really well.

Storage

Store leftovers in an airtight container in the refrigerator for up to 5 days.

GARDEN OF GOODNESS SANDWICH

Incorporate an abundance of colors, including green spinach and avocado, red tomato, purple onion, orange turmeric, and white seeds, to make a texture-rich and nutrient-dense sandwich. This sandwich has some crunch from the veggies and sunflower seeds, a creaminess from the sauce and avocado, and loads of flavor! To increase the protein content of this sandwich, you can add a few slices of grilled tofu or tempeh.

Serves: 2 **Prep time:** 15 minutes **Cooking time:** none

Turmeric Tahini Sauce

¼ cup tahini

3 tablespoons lemon juice

1 teaspoon ground turmeric

¼ teaspoon ground black pepper

⅛ teaspoon garlic powder

2 dashes cayenne pepper, optional

Sandwich Ingredients

4 slices whole-grain bread

½ cup chopped spinach

6 to 8 slices cucumber

4 to 6 slices tomato

1 avocado, mashed

½ cup broccoli sprouts

Pickled Red Onions (page 166)

2 tablespoons raw sunflower seeds

2 dashes dried oregano

2 dashes ground black pepper, optional

1. Make the Turmeric Tahini Sauce: Mix all sauce ingredients plus ¼ cup water. Set the sauce aside.

2. Toast the bread in a toaster or toaster oven.

3. Evenly layer the spinach, cucumber, tomato, avocado, and sprouts on two of the slices of bread. Top with 1 to 2 tablespoons of Pickled Red Onions.

4. On the remaining two slices of bread, spread 1 to 2 tablespoons of Turmeric Tahini Sauce. Sprinkle with one tablespoon of sunflower seeds, making sure they stick to the sauce so they don't fall out of your sandwich when you're trying to eat it! Sprinkle with oregano and black pepper.

5. Place the sauce and sunflower seed bread slices on top of the layered veggie slices to form 2 sandwiches. Cut in half and enjoy!

Calcium: 167 mg	Iron: 5.5 mg	Magnesium: 145 mg	Omega-3s: 0.2 g	Selenium: 15 mcg	Zinc: 3.7 mg

Calories: 537 | Protein: 17 g | Carbohydrate: 33 g | Fiber: 16 g | Fat: 32 g | Sodium: 237 mg

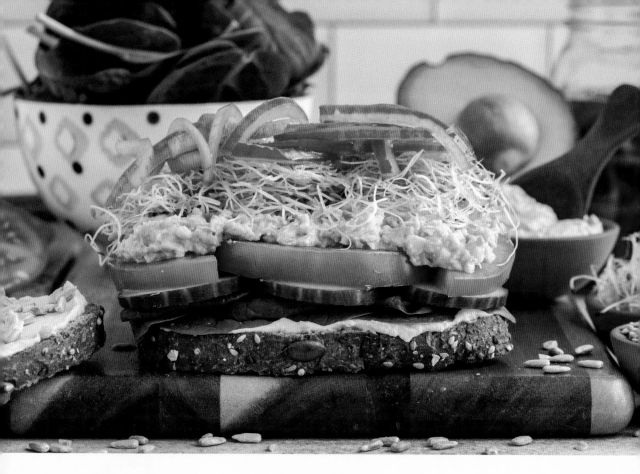

CHEF'S NOTES

Time-Saving Tips

Use store-bought hummus in place of the Turmeric Tahini Sauce.

Make the Turmeric Tahini Sauce ahead and store it in an airtight container in the refrigerator for up to 7 days.

Prepare the Pickled Red Onions ahead of time and store them in the refrigerator for up to 10 days.

Substitutions

Any greens go here! You can use kale, arugula, endive, mustard greens, or any other greens you have on hand in place of the spinach.

You can use any other sprouts you prefer in place of broccoli sprouts.

Instead of the Turmeric Tahini Sauce, use another sauce of your choice. Examples include anything creamy made with cashews or tahini, tapenade, hummus, or other bean spread.

Instead of Pickled Red Onions, use raw red onion, kimchi, or sauerkraut.

Gluten-Free: Use collards or large lettuce leaves to wrap everything up.

Storage

Store leftover Turmeric Tahini Sauce in an airtight container in the refrigerator for up to 7 days.

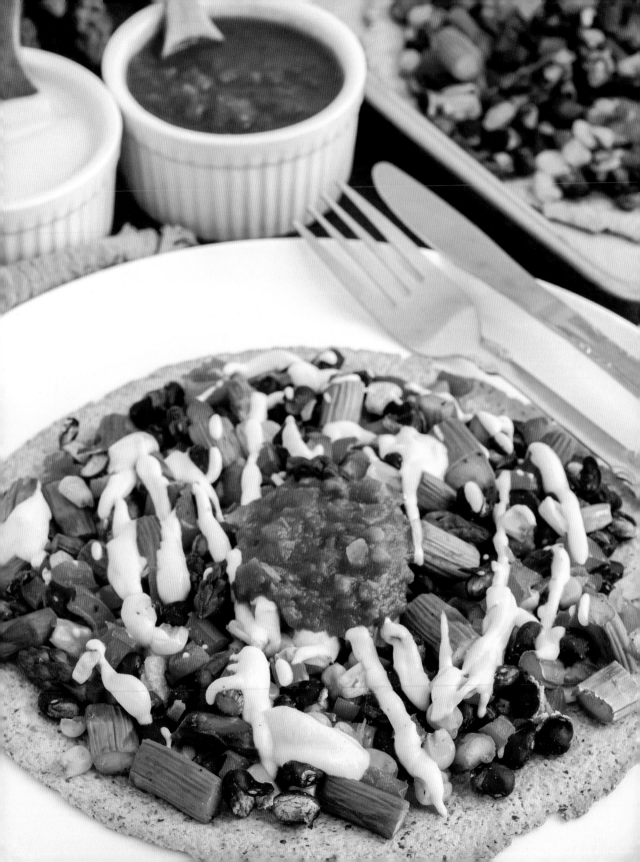

TACOS AND TOSTADAS

BANH MI OH MY VIETNAMESE-INSPIRED TACOS

This take on a classic Vietnamese sandwich reimagines it as a taco with plant-based takes on traditional elements, including tangy pickled veggies, meaty marinated mushrooms, and other fresh and vibrant fixins.

Serves: 4 **Prep time**: 10 minutes **Cooking time**: 10 minutes

1 cup thinly sliced carrots

1 cup thinly sliced red radishes

½ cup thinly sliced red onion

2 jalapeños, seeded and thinly sliced

1 cup plus 1 tablespoon unsweetened rice vinegar, divided

3 tablespoons maple syrup

½ teaspoon salt, optional

2 tablespoons coconut aminos or reduced-sodium tamari

1 tablespoon sriracha, optional

1 pound sliced mushrooms (approximately 4 cups)

8 corn tortillas

1 cup arugula

1 avocado, sliced

Spicy Mayo (page 168)

Chopped cilantro to taste, optional

1. Prepare the pickled veggies: In a large sealable container, combine the carrots, radishes, onion, jalapeños, 1 cup rice vinegar, maple syrup, salt, and 1 cup of water. Place the lid over the container and shake well. Set the veggies aside or store them in the refrigerator. The longer the storage, the better the flavors—we recommend at least 8 hours if you have the time.

2. In a large pan, whisk together the coconut aminos, 1 tablespoon rice vinegar, and sriracha. Add the mushrooms and cook over medium heat until the mushrooms caramelize and the liquid evaporates, about 10 minutes.

3. Divide the arugula, mushrooms, and avocado between the tortillas.

4. Top with the pickled veggies and drizzle with Spicy Mayo. Garnish with fresh cilantro and serve.

Calcium: 144 mg	Iron: 6 mg	Magnesium: 81 mg	Selenium: 18 mcg	Zinc: 2.3 mg

Calories: 307 | Protein: 10 g | Carbohydrate: 28 g | Fiber: 9.5 g | Fat: 15 g | Sodium: 366 mg

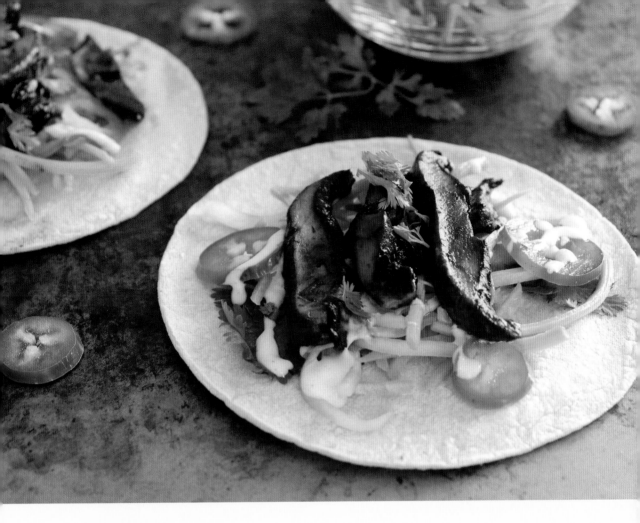

CHEF'S NOTES

Time-Saving Tips

Make the pickled veggies ahead of time and store them in an airtight container in the refrigerator for up to 2 weeks.

Other Tips

Use a mandoline slicer or a sharp kitchen knife to carefully slice the veggies into thin medallions. The thinner the slices, the more pickled, briny flavor they will absorb. They become perfectly tender and crunchy after marination.

Substitutions

Instead of corn tortillas, serve the tacos in whole-grain, cauliflower, or nut-flour tortillas; lettuce cups; or over a bed of greens.

Mushroom Alternatives: Substitute cubed tofu, chickpeas, or cauliflower for the mushrooms.

Storage

Store leftover pickled vegetables in an airtight container in the refrigerator for up to one month.

CLEAN OUT THE PANTRY EVERYDAY TACOS

Having pantry staples like canned beans, jarred salsa, and a variety of spices on hand, plus fresh produce like onions, peppers, and tomatoes, makes meals come together in minutes. Once you get the hang of how to use your plant-based pantry to the fullest, you'll be enjoying these tacos frequently!

Serves: 4   **Prep time:** 15 minutes   **Cooking time:** 10 minutes

Garlic Cashew Cream

1 cup raw cashews, soaked in hot water for 30 minutes or room-temperature water for 2 hours, drained

½ cup plain, unsweetened plant-based milk

1 teaspoon garlic powder

½ teaspoon salt, optional

Tacos

8 6-inch whole-grain or corn tortillas

½ cup salsa of your choice

1 avocado, cubed

¼ cup chopped cilantro, optional

¼ cup chopped jalapeño, optional

Hot sauce to taste, optional

8 lime wedges

Beans

1 teaspoon cumin seeds

1 cup chopped red onion

1 cup chopped red bell pepper

1 cup chopped tomatoes

1½ cups home-cooked or 1 15-ounce can black beans, drained

1 tablespoon ground cumin

½ teaspoon chili powder

½ teaspoon garlic powder

½ teaspoon onion powder

½ teaspoon sweet or smoked paprika

¼ teaspoon salt, optional

¼ teaspoon ground black pepper, optional

2 tablespoons lime juice

Calcium: 184 mg	Iron: 5.3 mg	Magnesium: 196 mg	Selenium: 12 mcg	Zinc: 3.7 mg

Calories: 347 | Protein: 17 g | Carbohydrate: 39 g | Fiber: 15 g | Fat: 11 g | Sodium: 514 mg

1. Make the Garlic Cashew Cream: In a blender, blend all the ingredients plus ¼ cup water until smooth. Add more water 1 tablespoon at a time as needed to reach desired consistency. Set the cashew cream aside.

2. Make the beans: In a large pan over medium heat, heat the cumin seeds until fragrant (about a minute), tossing often.

3. Add the onion, peppers, and tomatoes. Cook until the onion is translucent, about 3 to 4 minutes. Add 1 to 2 tablespoons of water as needed to deglaze the pan, stirring occasionally.

4. Meanwhile, add the black beans to a large bowl. Mash half the beans with a potato masher or fork.

5. Transfer the beans to the onion, pepper, and tomato mixture. Reduce the heat to medium and stir well to combine. Add the ground cumin, chili powder, garlic powder, onion powder, paprika, salt, pepper, and lime juice. Stir well once again and turn off the heat.

6. On a stovetop griddle on medium heat, warm each side of the tortillas (probably 2 at a time) for 1 to 2 minutes (just until warm, not crispy).

7. Place the tortillas on a plate and fill them with your toppings: Add 1 to 2 heaping tablespoons of the bean mixture, 1 tablespoon of salsa, 1 tablespoon of avocado, and 1 to 2 teaspoons of Garlic Cashew Cream. Add cilantro jalapeño, and hot sauce to taste. Serve with lime wedges and enjoy!

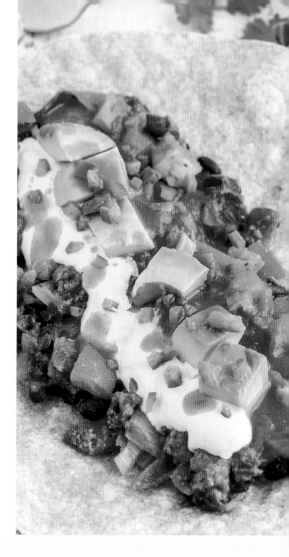

CHEF'S NOTES

Time-Saving Tips
Prepare the Garlic Cashew Cream ahead of time and store it in an airtight container in the refrigerator for up to 5 days or in the freezer for up to one month.

Alternatively, use your favorite whole-food, store-bought sour cream or plain dairy-free yogurt.

Substitutions
Instead of black beans use kidney beans, pinto beans, or other beans of choice.

Substitute white or yellow onion for red.

Gluten-Free: Use leafy green wraps (romaine, collards, or Swiss chard) instead of tortillas.

Storage
Store the leftover Garlic Cashew Cream and the beans separately in airtight containers in the refrigerator for up to 5 days.

ASPARAGUS AND BLACK BEAN TASTY TOSTADAS

Enjoying a toasty tostada is our idea of a day well spent, especially when you are craving something flavorful and exciting but are short on time. Tostadas not only function as a satisfying main meal, fun appetizer, or sustainable snack but they're also packed with vitamins and phytonutrients from the beans, corn, asparagus, and Pico de Gallo.

Serves: 4   **Prep time:** 20 minutes   **Cooking time:** 10 minutes

½ cup diced red onion

1 cup diced red bell pepper

2 cups chopped asparagus, cut into ½-inch pieces

1 cup frozen and thawed or fresh corn

1½ cups home-cooked or 1 15-ounce can black beans, drained

2 teaspoons ground cumin

1 teaspoon garlic powder

¾ teaspoon smoked paprika

¼ teaspoon salt, optional

¼ teaspoon ground black pepper, optional

8 6-inch whole-grain or corn tortillas

5-Minute Cheesy Sauce (page 146)

Pico de Gallo

1 cup diced tomatoes

½ cup diced red onion

¼ cup seeded and diced jalapeño, optional

2 tablespoons lime juice

2 to 4 tablespoons chopped cilantro, optional

Salt to taste, optional

1. Preheat oven to 350°F.

2. Make the Pico de Gallo: In a medium bowl, combine all ingredients and stir well. Set the Pico de Gallo aside.

3. In a large pan over medium-high heat, sauté the onion, bell pepper, and asparagus until the onion is translucent, about 3 minutes.

4. Stir in the corn, beans, cumin, garlic powder, paprika, salt, and pepper. Cook until the corn is warmed through, about 2 minutes.

5. Lay the tortillas on two separate baking sheets, 4 tortillas per sheet. Divide the vegetable topping between the tortillas, spreading it out to cover each tortilla.

6. Bake for 7 to 10 minutes or until the tortillas are golden brown and crispy on the outside.

7. Transfer the tostadas to plates and top them with 5-Minute Cheesy Sauce and Pico de Gallo.

Calcium: 121 mg	Iron: 6.5 mg	Magnesium: 191 mg	Selenium: 19 mcg	Zinc: 19 mg	Vitamin B₁₂*: 2.4 mcg

Calories: 455 | Protein: 20 g | Carbohydrate: 48 g | Fiber: 15 g | Fat: 16 g | Sodium: 286 mg

*If using fortified nutritional yeast.

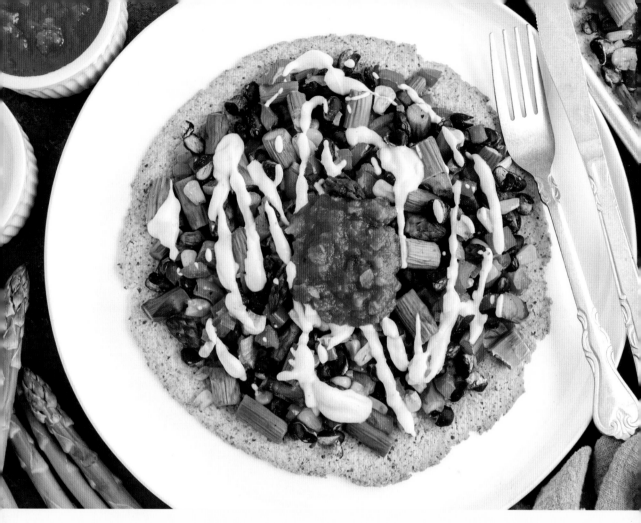

CHEF'S NOTES

Time-Saving Tips

Prepare the Pico de Gallo ahead of time or use your favorite store-bought Pico.

Make the 5-Minute Cheesy Sauce ahead of time and store it in an airtight container in the refrigerator for up to 5 days or in the freezer for up to 1 month.

Substitutions

Substitute pinto beans or your favorite legume of choice for the black beans.

Substitute broccoli, cauliflower, brussels sprouts, or green beans for the asparagus.

Substitute white or yellow onion for the red onion.

Substitute yellow, orange, or green bell pepper for red bell pepper.

Use regular paprika or chili powder in place of smoked paprika.

Storage

Store leftover Pico de Gallo and tostadas, separately, in airtight containers in the refrigerator for up to 4 days.

AIR FRYER CRUNCHY CHICKPEA AND CAULIFLOWER TACOS

Fiber-rich cauliflower and protein-packed chickpeas become crunchy nuggets of gold in an air fryer—taking a fraction of the cooking time needed for a traditional oven. Add them to your favorite whole-grain tortillas, top with vibrant Kale Salad, and drizzle with Spicy Mayo (or feel free to use your own favorite sauce). After you give this combination a try, substitute some of your favorite taco fillings for these ingredients.

Serves: 4   **Prep time:** 20 minutes   **Cooking time:** 20 minutes

2 tablespoons tahini

4 tablespoons lime juice, divided

1 teaspoon ground cumin

1 teaspoon chili powder

½ teaspoon garlic powder

½ teaspoon salt, divided, optional

3 cups cauliflower, cut into 1- to 2-inch florets

1½ cups home-cooked or 1 15-ounce can chickpeas, drained

Kale Salad

2 cups destemmed and chopped kale

½ teaspoon extra virgin olive oil, optional

¼ cup diced red onion

¼ cup diced tomato

1 jalapeño, seeded and minced, optional

6 6-inch or 4 8-inch whole-grain tortillas

Spicy Mayo (page 168)

1 avocado, sliced

Chopped cilantro to taste, optional

4 to 6 lime wedges for garnish

1. In a large bowl, combine the tahini, 3 tablespoons of the lime juice, cumin, chili powder, garlic powder, and ¼ teaspoon salt.

2. Add the cauliflower and chickpeas. Toss until well coated.

3. In an air fryer set at 380°F, cook the cauliflower and chickpeas for 20 minutes, shaking the basket or tray halfway through.

4. Make the Kale Salad: To a large bowl, add the kale, olive oil, and ¼ teaspoon salt. Massage together for about 30 seconds until the kale is tender. Add 1 tablespoon of lime juice.

5. Toss the red onion, tomato, and jalapeño with the kale. Set this salad aside.

6. Divide the cauliflower and chickpeas between the tortillas. Add 1 to 2 tablespoons of Kale Salad on top of each taco. Add the desired amount of Spicy Mayo and avocado to each taco. Top with cilantro. Serve with lime wedges.

Calcium: 274 mg	Iron: 4.8 mg	Magnesium: 65 mg	Selenium: 10.3 mcg	Zinc: 1.9 mg

Calories: 404 | Protein: 18 g | Carbohydrate: 22 g | Fiber: 18 g | Fat: 45 g | Sodium: 508 mg

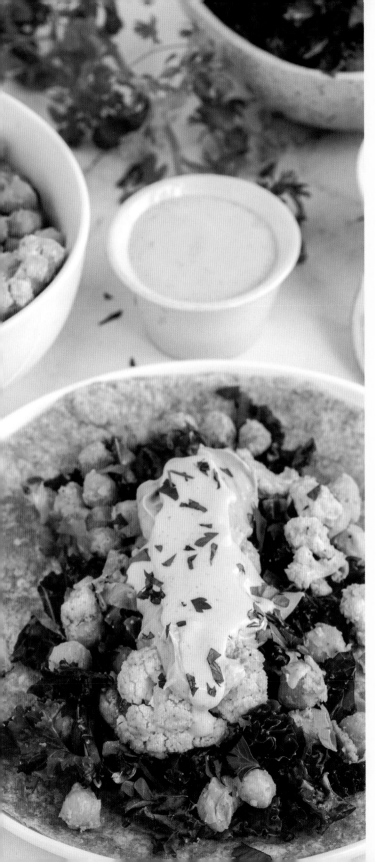

CHEF'S NOTES

Time-Saving Tips

Prepare the Kale Salad ahead of time and store in an airtight container in the refrigerator for up to 3 days.

Other Tips

Before adding the cauliflower and chickpeas to the marinade, make sure they are completely dry. This will help the marinade coat them better.

Substitutions

In place of kale, use another leafy green of your choice.

Replace the olive oil in the Kale Salad with 1 tablespoon of lime juice.

Gluten-Free: Use collard greens, Swiss chard, or romaine leaves in place of the whole-grain tortillas.

Traditional Oven Directions

Preheat the oven to 400°F. Line a baking sheet with parchment paper. Add the cauliflower and chickpeas to the baking sheet, leaving any remaining marinade behind as it'll burn. (Feel free to use excess marinade after they bake by drizzling it over the top.) Bake for 40 minutes, flipping halfway through.

Storage

Store leftovers in an airtight container in the refrigerator for up to 5 days. Store the cauliflower and chickpeas separately from the Kale Salad and tortillas until you're ready to assemble the tacos.

WARM AND SMOKY WHITE BEAN AND SPINACH FLAUTAS

Flautas are crispy little treats that are something between a burrito and a taco. Typically, they are made of a savory filling wrapped in a flour tortilla and fried. By using whole-grain tortillas and baking them instead, these fiber-rich flautas become a delicious make-ahead meal that you can freeze until you need them. Oh, and they make a tasty take-along snack too!

Serves: 4   **Prep time:** 20 minutes   **Cooking time:** 20 minutes

3 cups home-cooked or 2 15-ounce cans white beans, drained

½ cup chopped red onion

½ cup chopped orange bell pepper

½ cup frozen and thawed spinach

2 teaspoons ground cumin

1 teaspoon garlic powder

1 teaspoon onion powder

2 to 3 teaspoons smoked paprika

¼ teaspoon salt, optional

2 tablespoons lime juice

¼ cup seeded and minced jalapeño, optional

¼ cup chopped cilantro, optional

8 6-inch whole-grain tortillas

1 avocado, chopped

2 to 4 tablespoons Pico de Gallo (page 188)

2 to 4 tablespoons Cashew Sour Cream (page 100)

1. Preheat the oven to 400°F. Line a baking sheet with parchment paper.

2. In a food processor, pulse the white beans, onion, orange bell pepper, spinach, cumin, garlic powder, onion powder, paprika, salt, lime juice, jalapeño, and cilantro until it reaches your desired consistency.

3. Lay the tortillas out on the baking sheet.

4. Spoon 3 to 4 tablespoons of the bean mixture into each tortilla, forming a line in the center only. Roll each tortilla into a tight tube and place them seam side down on the baking sheet.

5. Bake for 20 minutes or until crispy and brown on the outside.

6. Divide the flautas between serving plates and top them with avocado, Pico de Gallo, and Cashew Sour Cream.

Calcium: 182 mg	Iron: 10.3 mg	Magnesium: 221 mg	Selenium: 10 mcg	Zinc: 4.5 mg

Calories: 512 | Protein: 28 g | Carbohydrate: 59 g | Fiber: 18 g | Fat: 15 g | Sodium: 458 mg

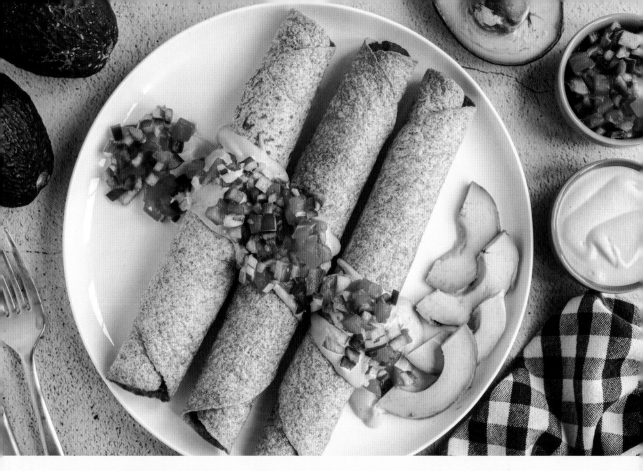

CHEF'S NOTES

Time-Saving Tips

Make the bean spread ahead of time and store it in an airtight container in the refrigerator for up to 5 days.

Prepare the Pico de Gallo ahead of time, or use your favorite store-bought Pico to save time.

Substitutions

Substitute another bean of choice, such as kidney, black, or pinto beans, in place of white beans.

Instead of red onion, use yellow or white onion, or use shallots.

Substitute yellow, red, or green bell pepper for orange bell pepper.

Substitute parsley or chives for cilantro.

Gluten-Free: Instead of whole-grain tortillas, use nut-flour tortillas, or use leafy green wraps like collards, romaine, or Swiss chard. Bypass baking if you use leafy greens.

Air Fryer Instructions

Bake in the air fryer at 400°F for 5 to 7 minutes or until crispy and brown on the outside.

Storage

Store leftover bean filling in an airtight container in the refrigerator for up to 5 days.

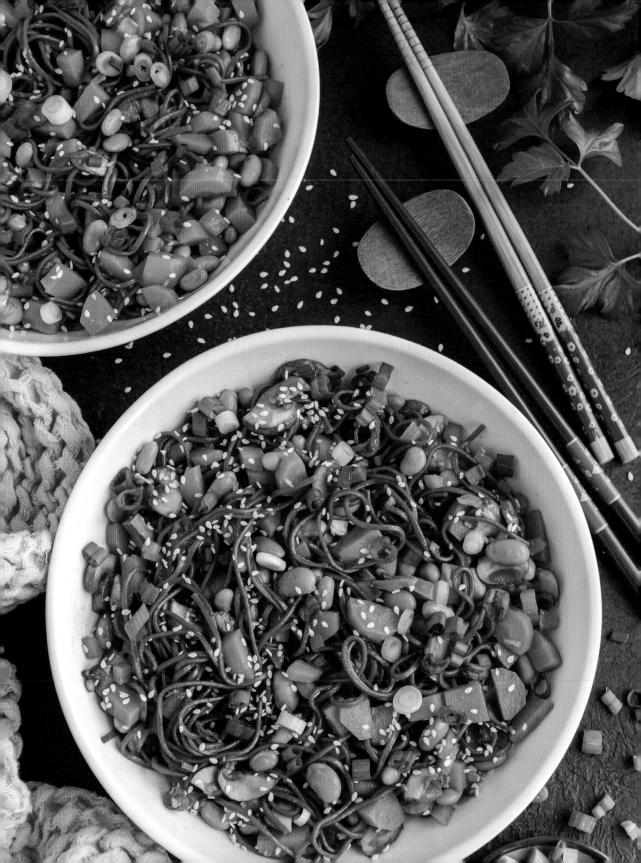

NOODLES

VEGGIELICIOUS MAC 'N' CHEESE

Soul-fulfilling and *comforting* are words that come to mind when thinking about the goodness that is Veggielicious Mac 'n' Cheese. Wholesome cauliflower, butternut squash, and just the right amount of nutritional yeast create a deliciously cheesy, creamy sauce with a remarkable umami flavor. It's the perfect complement to broccoli and nutty Vegan Walnut Parmesan. The cherry (or should we say cheese) on top is all the essential nutrients you get when you indulge in a scoop or two!

Serves: 4 **Prep time:** 15 minutes **Cooking time:** 15 minutes

8 ounces dry whole-grain or legume macaroni

1 cup chopped yellow onion

3 cups chopped cauliflower florets

1 cup cubed fresh or frozen butternut squash

3 cloves garlic, minced

1 teaspoon ground turmeric

¼ teaspoon ground black pepper, optional

1 cup low-sodium vegetable broth or water

1 cup broccoli florets, chopped into small pieces

1 tablespoon mellow white or chickpea miso

3 tablespoons nutritional yeast, plus more to taste

½ to 1 teaspoon smoked paprika

1 cup plain, unsweetened, plant-based milk

¼ to ½ teaspoon salt, optional

Vegan Walnut Parmesan (page 114), optional

Salt to taste, optional

Crushed red pepper flakes to taste, optional

1. Make the pasta according to package directions. Set it aside.

2. In a large skillet over medium-high heat, sauté the onions, cauliflower, squash, and garlic for 3 minutes.

3. Stir in the turmeric, ground black pepper, and vegetable broth. Bring to a boil and then reduce the heat to a simmer. Cover and cook for 7 minutes or until the cauliflower and squash are tender.

4. Meanwhile, steam the broccoli florets: In a large pot, bring an inch of water to a boil. Add a steamer basket to the pot. Place the broccoli florets in the steamer basket and reduce the heat to medium. Cover and steam for 3 to 5 minutes.

5. After the cauliflower is cooked, transfer it to a blender or food processor (you may need to do this in two batches). Blend it with the miso, nutritional yeast, paprika, plant-based milk, and salt until smooth.

6. In a large bowl, combine the macaroni, broccoli, and cheese sauce. Note: It will seem like a lot of sauce! The sauce gets absorbed pretty quickly by the noodles and broccoli, so you'll most likely want to use it all. However, if desired, pour three-quarters of the sauce over the top first and then add more as desired. Add a little more salt, as well as Vegan Walnut Parmesan or more nutritional yeast and crushed red pepper flakes over the top.

Calcium: 339 mg	Iron: 6 mg	Magnesium: 183 mg	Selenium: 14 mcg	Zinc: 3.2 mg	Vitamin B₁₂*: 2.4 mcg	Vitamin D*: 60 IU

Calories: 508 | Protein: 26 g | Carbohydrate: 65 g | Fiber: 24 g | Fat: 9 g | Sodium: 439 mg

*If using fortified plant-based milk and nutritional yeast.

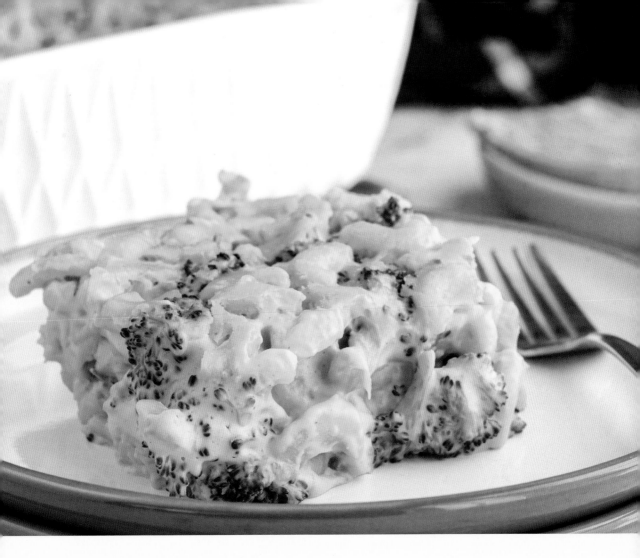

CHEF'S NOTES

Time-Saving Tips

Prepare the Vegan Walnut Parmesan ahead of time.

Substitutions

Use white onion in place of yellow.

Use sweet paprika in place of smoked paprika (but note that you'll lose the smoky flavor!).

Substitute yellow summer squash, kabocha squash, acorn squash, or sweet potato for the butternut squash.

Storage

Store leftovers in an airtight container in the refrigerator for up to 5 days or freeze for up to one month.

YUM-AMI CACIO E PEPE

In Italian, Cacio e Pepe translates to "cheese and pepper," and it's traditionally made with butter, cheese, and, depending on the chef, sometimes milk. Here we used cashews, cauliflower, garlic, and shallots to create a scrumptiously creamy sauce. Plus, we threw in chopped spinach to add even more deliciousness, nutrients (vitamin A, magnesium, and iron, to name a few), and a vibrant pop of color!

Serves: 4   **Prep time:** 15 minutes   **Cooking time:** 15 minutes

12 ounces dry whole-grain pasta

3 to 4 cups chopped spinach

4 ounces roughly chopped shiitake mushrooms (approximately 1 cup)

1 cup roughly chopped cauliflower florets

½ cup roughly chopped shallots

2 tablespoons roughly minced garlic

2 cups low-sodium vegetable broth

½ cup cashews, soaked in hot water for 30 minutes or room-temperature water for 2 hours, drained

¼ teaspoon salt, optional

Ground black pepper to taste, optional

Crushed red pepper to taste, optional

Vegan Walnut Parmesan (page 114)

1. Cook the pasta according to package directions. Meanwhile, add the spinach to the colander you plan to use to drain the noodles. Once the pasta is finished cooking, drain it in the colander to cook the spinach. Set aside.

2. Meanwhile, heat a large pan on medium-high heat. Add the mushrooms, cauliflower, shallots, and garlic, stirring often for 3 minutes.

3. Add the veggie broth and cashews, stirring to combine.

4. Cover and simmer for 7 minutes or until the cauliflower is fork-tender.

5. In a blender, blend the cashew mushroom mixture and salt until smooth.

6. Place the pasta and spinach into a large serving bowl. Pour the desired amount of shiitake cream over the top and stir to coat.

7. Divide between plates and top with ground pepper and crushed red pepper flakes. Add Vegan Walnut Parmesan.

Calcium: 85 mg	Iron: 5 mg	Magnesium: 166 mg	Selenium: 5.5 mcg	Zinc: 4.5 mg

Calories: 405 | Protein: 17 g | Carbohydrate: 59 g | Fiber: 15 g | Fat: 9 g | Sodium: 105 mg

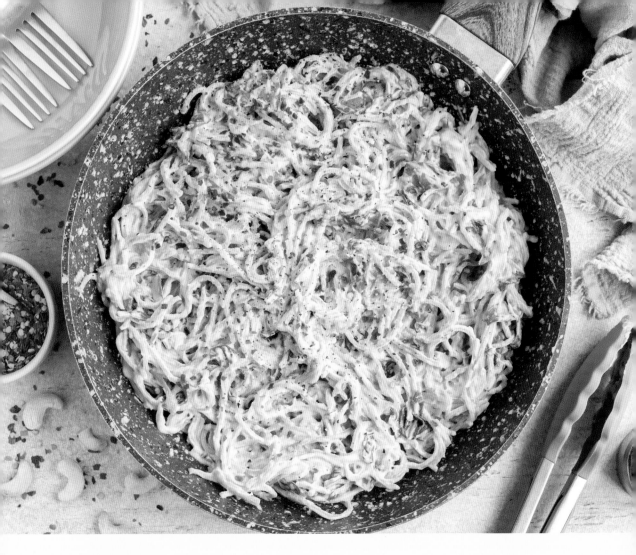

CHEF'S NOTES

Time-Saving Tips

Make the Vegan Walnut Parmesan ahead of time and store it in an airtight container in the refrigerator for up to 2 weeks.

Substitutions

Use another mushroom of choice for the shiitake mushrooms, such as cremini, chanterelle, portobello, or porcini.

Instead of shallots, use white or yellow onion.

Substitute another leafy green of choice in place of spinach.

For the pasta, use linguine, spaghetti, shells, or any pasta you love.

Gluten-Free: Substitute zucchini noodles or legume pasta for whole-grain pasta.

Storage

Store leftovers in an airtight container in the refrigerator for up to 5 days.

MISO ZEN SPICY NOODLE BOWL

Protein-packed, plant-based noodles are one of life's simple pleasures. Bright and slightly sweet edamame paired with crunchy, carotenoid-containing carrots and savory, mineral-dense cremini mushrooms make for a restaurant-worthy meal that can be whipped up in minutes!

Serves: 4 **Prep time:** 15 minutes **Cooking time:** 10 to 12 minutes

6 ounces dry brown or purple rice noodles

Sauce

¼ cup coconut aminos or reduced-sodium tamari

2 tablespoons lime juice

2 tablespoons maple syrup

2 tablespoons mellow white or chickpea miso

1 to 2 tablespoons roughly minced ginger

1 teaspoon sesame oil, optional

1 to 2 tablespoons sriracha, optional

1 cup sliced carrots

1 cup chopped orange bell pepper

8 ounces sliced cremini mushrooms (approximately 2 cups)

2 cups shelled frozen and thawed edamame

½ cup chopped green onion

2 to 3 tablespoons black or white sesame seeds

½ cup chopped cilantro, optional

1. Cook the noodles according to package instructions.

2. Meanwhile, make the sauce: In a blender, blend the coconut aminos, lime juice, maple syrup, miso, ginger, and sesame oil and sriracha until smooth. Set the sauce aside.

3. Once the noodles are finished cooking, drain them and run them under cold water to prevent them from sticking. Set them aside.

4. In a large pan or wok over medium-high heat, sauté the carrots, pepper, and mushrooms, stirring every couple of minutes until the mushrooms and carrots are fully cooked and tender, about 5 to 7 minutes. If needed, add 1 to 2 tablespoons of water to deglaze the pan.

5. Reduce the heat to medium and add the edamame, cooking until warmed through, about a minute.

6. Add the noodles and pour the sauce over the top. Mix until combined.

7. Turn off the heat and stir in the green onion, sesame seeds, and cilantro.

Calcium: 148 mg	Iron: 3.4 mg	Magnesium: 92 mg	Omega-3s: .4 g	Selenium: 6.9 mcg	Zinc: 2.3 mg

Calories: 357 | Protein: 15 g | Carbohydrate: 46 g | Fiber: 8 g | Fat: 10 g | Sodium: 456 mg

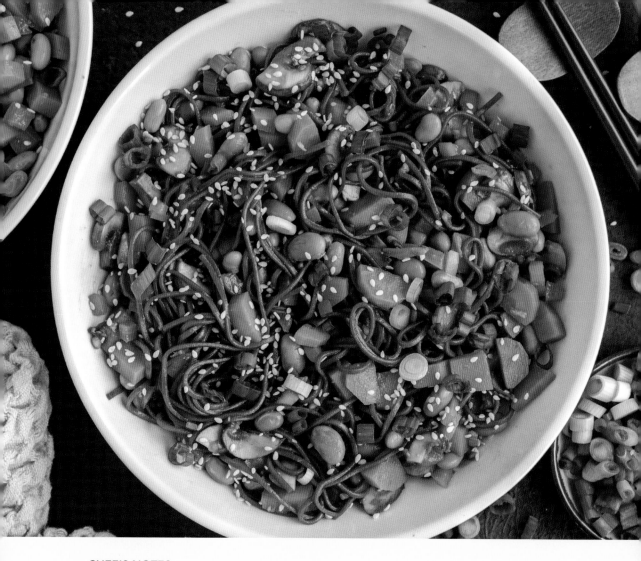

CHEF'S NOTES

Tips

Add a handful of peanuts or cashews before serving for a plant-based protein crunch.

Add an extra squeeze of citrus with more lime juice or orange juice before serving.

Substitutions

Use any noodle you love here—zucchini noodles, spiralized sweet potato, udon, whole wheat, rice, or legume.

Feel free to use any of your favorite vegetables that you have on hand instead of those listed here.

Lima beans, kidney beans, or chickpeas would be great substitutes for edamame.

Storage

Store leftovers in an airtight container in the refrigerator for up to 5 days.

LIVING AND THRIVING ZUCCHINI NOODLES WITH RAW MARINARA SAUCE

Zucchini noodles are a delicious, grain-free alternative to pasta, and are absolutely divine when paired with savory marinara sauce. Juicy ripe tomatoes blended with fragrant garlic, sweet red peppers, and fresh herbs bring new life to the classic spaghetti and red sauce pairing. You can keep the noodles raw or lightly sauté them for a softer, more pasta-like texture. Enjoy this incredible dish knowing that you're getting lots of fiber and carotenoids from the zucchini.

Serves: 2 **Prep time:** 30 minutes **Cooking time:** none

2 to 3 green or yellow zucchini

2 cups thinly sliced asparagus

Raw Marinara Sauce

¼ cup sun-dried tomatoes

2 cloves garlic, roughly chopped

1 tablespoon roughly chopped shallot

½ tablespoon tahini

1 red bell pepper, roughly chopped

1 cup seeded and roughly chopped tomatoes (Roma or heirloom)

1 teaspoon maple syrup

1 teaspoon dried oregano

¼ teaspoon salt, optional

¼ teaspoon ground black pepper, optional

¼ teaspoon crushed red pepper flakes, optional

¼ cup chopped basil

Vegan Walnut Parmesan to taste (page 114)

1. Boil 1 cup of water and pour it over the sun-dried tomatoes in a small bowl. Set the tomatoes aside to soak for 20 minutes.

2. Spiralize your zucchini. Or you can peel the zucchini into 1½-inch wide noodles using a vegetable peeler or mandoline.

3. Remove the excess water from the zucchini: Place the zucchini in the center of a tea towel, piece of cheesecloth, or nut milk bag. Bring the corners together to make a pouch, and twist. Use both hands to twist and squeeze out as much liquid as possible. Place the drained zucchini in a large bowl and add the asparagus.

4. Make the Raw Marinara Sauce: Once the sun-dried tomatoes finish soaking, drain them, reserving the liquid. In a high-speed blender, blend the sun-dried tomatoes, garlic, shallot, tahini, and ¼ cup reserved liquid into a smooth paste.

5. Add the red bell pepper, tomatoes, maple syrup, oregano, salt, pepper, and red pepper flakes. Blend the sauce until smooth. Add up to ¾ cup more reserved liquid to thin the sauce, depending on the consistency you desire. Add the basil and pulse to combine.

6. Pour the marinara sauce on top of the zucchini noodles and asparagus.

7. Top with optional Vegan Walnut Parmesan or nutritional yeast and crushed red pepper flakes.

Calcium: 128 mg	Iron: 5.6 mg	Magnesium: 109 mg	Selenium: 5.9 mcg	Zinc: 2.3 mg

Calories: 187 | Protein*: 9.9 g | Carbohydrate: 23 g | Fiber: 10 g | Fat: 4 | Sodium: 49 mg

*If using the Vegan Walnut Parmesan.

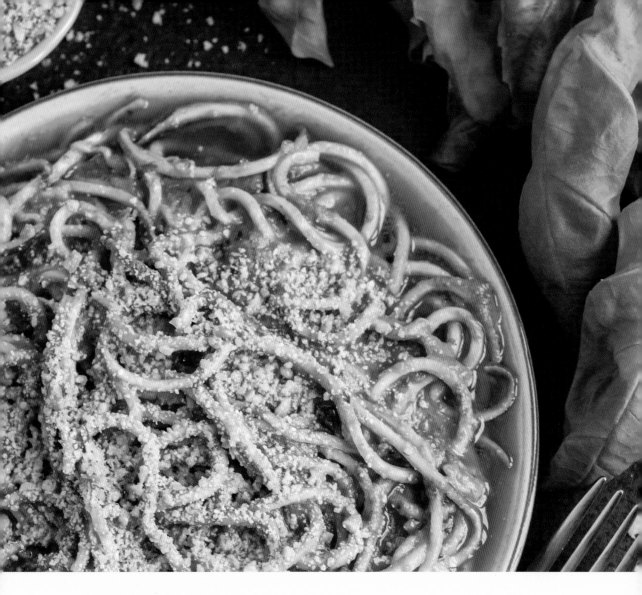

CHEF'S NOTES

Substitutions

Instead of Roma or heirloom tomatoes, use other tomatoes on hand or from your own garden.

In place of chopped shallots, use yellow or white onion.

Instead of basil, use parsley.

In place of sun-dried tomatoes, use olives (start with half the portion and then add more as desired).

Storage

Store leftovers in an airtight container in the refrigerator for up to 3 days or freeze for up to 1 month.

PRESTO PESTO PASTA

The winning combination of kale, avocado, basil, garlic, and nutritional yeast makes this vibrant green pesto super nourishing. Add omega-3-rich walnuts, mineral-dense mushrooms, and sweet green peas to your favorite legume or whole-grain pasta and you'll have a high-fiber and delightfully fresh dish ready in a jiffy!

Serves: 2   **Prep time:** 15 minutes   **Cooking time:** 10 minutes

8 ounces dry legume or whole-grain angel hair

8 ounces sliced mushrooms (approximately 2 cups)

1 large sliced zucchini

1 cup frozen and thawed peas

1 teaspoon garlic powder

Salt to taste, optional

¼ cup diced olives

Kale Walnut Basil Pesto (page 170)

Crushed red pepper flakes to taste, optional

2 lemon wedges

2 teaspoons extra virgin olive oil, optional

1. Make your pasta according to the package instructions.

2. Heat a large pan over medium-high heat until hot. Sauté the mushrooms, zucchini, and peas until tender, about 5 minutes, stirring continuously. Add 1 to 2 tablespoons of water as needed to deglaze the pan. Stir in the garlic powder and salt.

3. Add the cooked and drained pasta, olives, and Kale Walnut Basil Pesto to the pan. Stir until combined and warmed through.

4. Divide between plates, top with crushed red pepper flakes, and serve with lemon wedges. Drizzle with olive oil.

CHEF'S NOTES

Time-Saving Tips

Prepare the Kale Walnut Basil Pesto ahead of time. Store it in an airtight container in the refrigerator for up to 5 days.

Substitutions

Substitute broccoli, spinach, or another veggie of your choice for the zucchini.

Substitute capers, sun-dried tomatoes, or artichoke hearts packed in water for the olives for a similar umami bite.

Gluten-Free: Skip the pasta entirely and serve this dish as a side, or spiralize your favorite veggie to serve as your noodles.

Storage

Store leftovers in an airtight container in the refrigerator for up to 5 days.

Calcium: 245 mg	Iron: 12 mg	Magnesium: 243 mg	Selenium: 27 mcg	Zinc: 6.5 mg	Vitamin B$_{12}$*: 2.4 mcg

Calories: 842 | Protein: 40 g | Carbohydrate: 60 g | Fiber: 23 g | Fat: 42 g | Sodium: 297 mg

*If using fortified nutritional yeast.

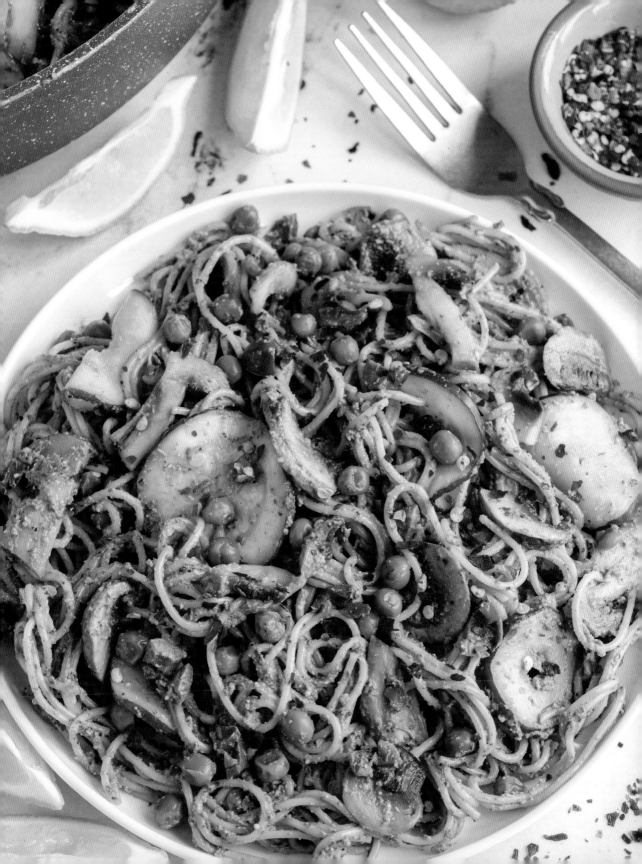

ZESTY GINGER SOBA NOODLE SALAD

Buckwheat soba noodles add a unique texture and nutty flavor that, combined with a zesty ginger dressing, make this dish a knockout! Loaded with protein and an assortment of fresh, fiber-rich vegetables, this restaurant-worthy meal can be served warm or cold. Add your favorite plant proteins on top to create a meal that is unique to you!

Serves: 2 **Prep time:** 20 minutes **Cooking time:** 10 minutes

8 ounces dry buckwheat noodles

1 cup chopped spinach

1 cup sliced radishes cut into matchsticks

1 cup julienned carrots

1 cup julienned cucumbers

2 green onions, sliced

½ cup chopped cilantro, optional

2 tablespoons white or black sesame seeds

Ginger Dressing

1 tablespoon tahini

1 tablespoon mellow white or chickpea miso

1 tablespoon coconut aminos or reduced-sodium tamari

4 tablespoons unsweetened rice vinegar

1 tablespoon maple syrup

1 tablespoon lime juice

2 tablespoons minced ginger

1 minced garlic clove

1. Bring a large pot of water to a boil. Add the noodles and cook for 5 to 7 minutes, until the noodles are just tender.

2. Meanwhile, add the spinach to the colander you plan to use to drain the noodles. Set it aside until you're ready to drain the noodles.

3. Make the Ginger Dressing: In a medium bowl, whisk all the dressing ingredients until the miso and tahini are dissolved. Set the dressing aside.

4. In a large bowl, combine the radishes, carrots, and cucumbers.

5. Once the noodles are finished cooking, drain them into the colander with the spinach to cook it. Rinse the drained noodles and cooked spinach with cold water.

6. Transfer the noodles and spinach to the bowl with the vegetables.

7. Pour the dressing over the top and stir until the noodles and veggies are coated. Note: If you think you'll have leftovers, pour the dressing over only the portion you plan to eat.

8. Top with green onion, cilantro, and sesame seeds.

Calcium: 190 mg	Iron: 3.1 mg	Magnesium: 77 mg	Selenium: 7.2 mcg	Zinc: 1.9 mg

Calories: 329 | Protein: 15 g | Carbohydrate: 42 g | Fiber: 10 g | Fat: 10 g | Sodium: 555 mg

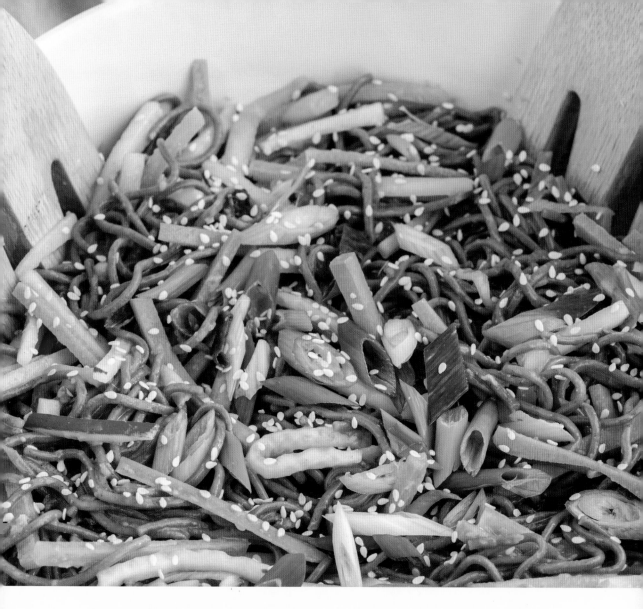

CHEF'S NOTES

Substitutions

Use zucchini noodles (lightly sautéed or raw) in place of buckwheat noodles.

Use another whole-grain or legume noodle of choice in place of buckwheat noodles.

Substitute kale or other leafy greens for the spinach.

Substitute any veggies you have on hand for the carrots, radishes, and cucumbers (for example, jicama, broccoli, or beets).

Storage

Store the noodles in an airtight container in the refrigerator for up to 2 days and the dressing in a separate airtight container in the refrigerator for 5 to 7 days.

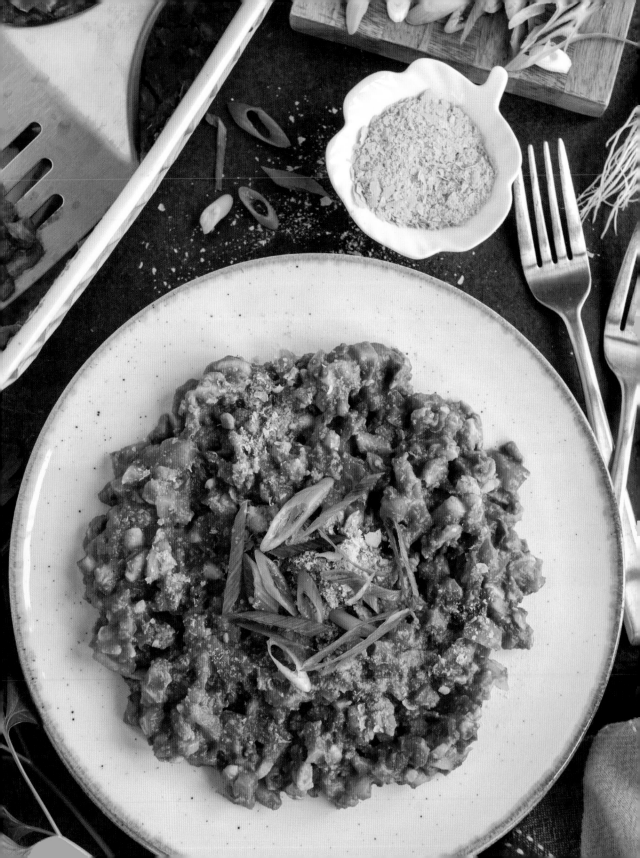

ONE-POT MEALS

A TASTE OF AFRICA FONIO PILAF

If you haven't guessed by its name, the star of this one-pot meal is fonio, an ancient grain from Africa that has a fluffy texture and slightly nutty flavor. It's brimming with nutrients such as iron, magnesium, zinc, B vitamins, and protein. Together with savory vegetables, cooling mint, crunchy pistachios, and healing spices, this is a nourishing, all-in-one meal that is simple to prepare and a delight to enjoy.

Serves: 4   **Prep time:** 15 minutes   **Cooking time:** 5 minutes

1 cup diced yellow onion

1 cup seeded and diced tomatoes

½ cup diced bell pepper

¼ cup tomato paste

2 teaspoons ground cumin

1 teaspoon ground coriander

¼ teaspoon ground cinnamon

½ teaspoon ground turmeric

1 teaspoon sweet paprika (see Chef's Notes)

⅛ teaspoon allspice

2 pinches cayenne pepper, optional (see Chef's Notes)

2 cups low-sodium vegetable broth

1 cup dry fonio, rinsed

1½ cups home-cooked or 1 15-ounce can chickpeas, drained

1 cup chopped spinach

¼ cup chopped cilantro or parsley

1 to 2 teaspoons minced mint, optional

2 to 4 tablespoons chopped pistachios, optional

4 lemon wedges

1. In a medium pot over medium-high heat, sauté the onion, tomatoes, and bell peppers, cooking for 2 minutes or until the onions start to soften.

2. Stir in the tomato paste, cumin, coriander, cinnamon, turmeric, paprika, allspice, and cayenne pepper.

3. Add the vegetable broth and bring the mixture to a boil. Add the fonio, stir to combine all ingredients, and reduce the heat to simmer for 1 minute. Remove the pilaf from the heat, cover, and allow it to sit for 4 minutes.

4. Remove the lid and stir in the chickpeas, spinach, cilantro, and mint until the spinach is wilted.

5. Divide between plates or bowls, garnish with pistachio, and serve with lemon wedges.

| Calcium: 72 mg | Iron: 2.7 mg | Magnesium: 49 mg | Selenium: 3.6 mcg | Zinc: 0.9 mg |

Calories: 333 | Protein: 9 g | Carbohydrate: 58 g | Fiber: 8 g | Fat: 4 g | Sodium: 210 mg

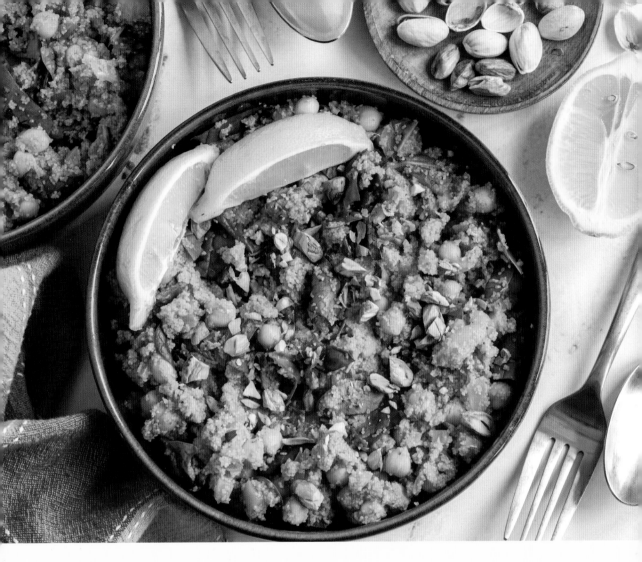

CHEF'S NOTES

Substitutions

Substitute white or purple onion or shallots for yellow onion.

Instead of paprika and cayenne, use 1 tablespoon of harissa powder or paste.

If you like a smoky flavor, substitute smoked paprika for sweet paprika.

Substitute bulgur, cracked freekeh, or quinoa for the fonio. For bulgur, use a 2:1 water-to-grain ratio (similar to fonio) and allow it to sit for 10 to 15 minutes. For cracked freekeh, use a 2.5:1 water-to-grain ratio and simmer for 20 minutes. For quinoa, use a 2:1 water-to-grain ratio and simmer for 15 to 20 minutes.

Instead of chickpeas, use another cooked white bean of choice.

Storage

Store leftovers in an airtight container in the refrigerator for up to 5 days or freeze for up to 1 month.

ALL-IN-ONE MEXICALI QUINOA

Quinoa, corn, black beans, tomatoes, jalapeños, and lime create a fiesta of flavors in this All-In-One Mexicali Quinoa. Plus, this simple dish has plenty of protein, fiber, and wholesome veggies for a meal that the entire family will enjoy!

Serves: 4   **Prep time:** 10 minutes   **Cooking time:** 25 minutes

3 cloves garlic, minced

2 jalapeños, seeded and minced

¾ cup diced tomatoes

¾ cup frozen and thawed or fresh corn

¾ cup home-cooked or 8 ounces canned black beans, drained

1 teaspoon chili powder

1 teaspoon ground cumin

1 teaspoon onion powder

½ teaspoon ground coriander

¼ teaspoon salt, optional

¾ cup dry quinoa, rinsed

1½ cups low-sodium vegetable broth

1 tablespoon lime zest

2 tablespoons lime juice

¼ cup chopped cilantro, optional

1. In a medium pot over medium-high heat, cook the garlic and jalapeños, stirring until fragrant, about one minute.

2. Add the tomatoes, corn, and beans. Stir for another minute.

3. Stir in the chili powder, cumin, onion powder, ground coriander, and salt. Add the quinoa and vegetable broth. Bring the mixture to a boil, reduce the heat to low, cover, and simmer for 20 minutes or until the quinoa is tender.

4. Remove from the heat and let sit, covered, for 10 minutes.

5. Stir in the lime zest, lime juice, and cilantro.

CHEF'S NOTES

Substitutions

Substitute red beans, white beans, or pinto beans for the black beans.

Substitute lemon juice for the lime juice.

Substitute brown rice, black rice, wild rice, or your favorite whole grain of choice for the quinoa. Note that you may need to increase the amount of vegetable broth and the cooking time depending on the grain you choose.

Storage

Store leftovers in an airtight container in the refrigerator for up to 5 days or freeze for up to 3 months.

Calcium: 54 mg	Iron: 2.9 mg	Magnesium: 93 mg	Selenium: 4.1 mcg	Zinc: 3.1 mg

Calories: 204 | Protein: 8.5 g | Carbohydrate: 30 g | Fiber: 7 g | Fat: 2.5 g | Sodium: 359 mg

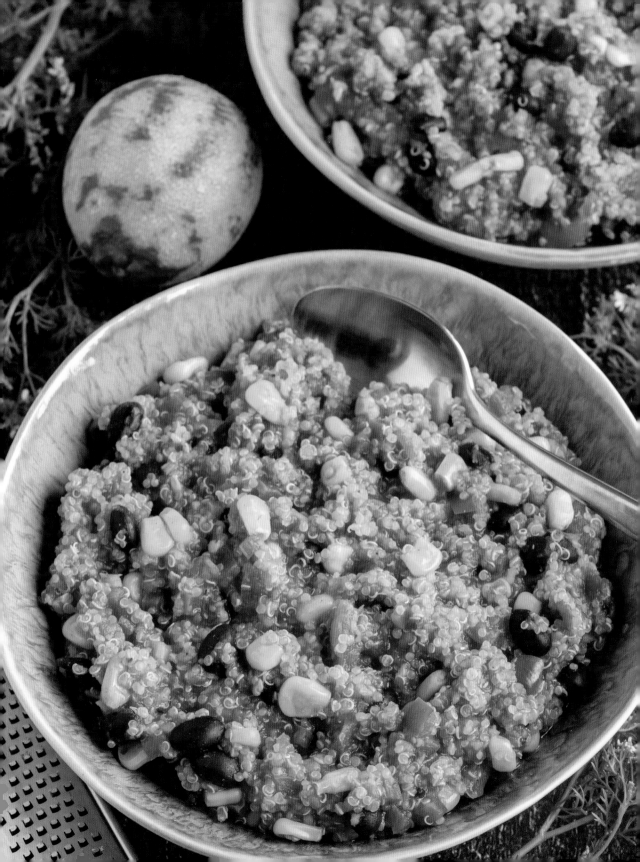

POT-TO-PLATE TEMPEH SAUSAGE PASTA

Technically, this recipe requires two pots if you are preparing the pasta and the tempeh at the same time, but the results come together quickly and easily to make one delicious plant-tastic meal. Tempeh is a hearty plant protein that takes on the flavor of savory herbs and spices to transform into meaty "sausage" crumbles. Chickpea, soy, or hemp-based tempeh varieties all work well. The result is a healthy and delicious plant-based dish that gets even better with the addition of red tomato sauce and fiber-rich pasta.

Serves: 4   **Prep time:** 15 minutes   **Cooking time:** 15 minutes

8 ounces dry whole-grain or legume pasta

16 ounces red pasta sauce of your choice

2 cups chopped spinach

2 tablespoons minced parsley

Vegan Walnut Parmesan (page 114) to taste, optional

Tempeh Sausage

2 teaspoons fennel seeds

8 ounces tempeh, crumbled

½ teaspoon garlic powder

1½ teaspoons dried oregano

1 teaspoon smoked paprika

½ teaspoon onion powder

1 teaspoon minced sage

½ teaspoon crushed red pepper flakes, optional

2 tablespoons coconut aminos or reduced-sodium tamari

1½ teaspoons vegan Worcestershire sauce

1 tablespoon maple syrup

1. Make your pasta according to the package instructions, drain, and set it aside.

2. Make the Tempeh Sausage: Heat a large pan over medium heat. Add the fennel seeds and cook until fragrant, about 1 to 2 minutes. Add the tempeh along with 1 cup of water. Increase the heat to medium-high and cook until the water is absorbed, stirring occasionally, about 3 to 5 minutes.

3. Meanwhile, in a small bowl, combine the garlic powder, oregano, paprika, onion powder, sage, and crushed red pepper flakes. Reduce the heat under the tempeh to medium and add the spice mixture. Cook for 1 minute, until fragrant.

4. In a small bowl, whisk together the coconut aminos, Worcestershire sauce, and maple syrup and add these to the tempeh. Cook for 3 to 5 minutes or until the tempeh is browned. Add 1 to 2 tablespoons of water, if needed, to deglaze the pan.

5. Add the pasta, pasta sauce, spinach, and parsley to the tempeh. Stir to combine and warm through until the spinach is tender.

6. Top with crushed red pepper flakes and Vegan Walnut Parmesan.

Calcium: 59.5 mg	Iron: 3.6 mg	Magnesium: 101 mg	Omega-3s: .2 g	Selenium: 3.4 mcg	Zinc: 0.6 mg

Calories: 323 | Protein: 9.5 g | Carbohydrate: 44 g | Fiber: 7 g | Fat: 9.5 g | Sodium: 615 mg

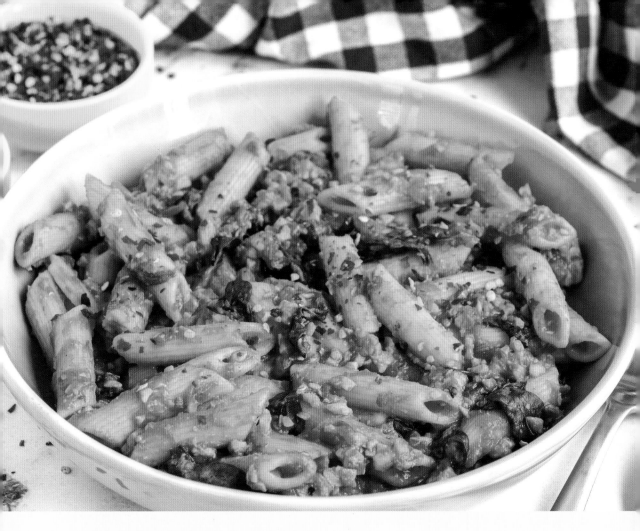

CHEF'S NOTES

Time-Saving Tips

Make the tempeh sausage ahead of time and store it in an airtight container in the refrigerator for up to 3 days.

Prepare the Vegan Walnut Parmesan ahead of time.

Substitutions

Use another leafy green in place of spinach.

Substitute basil for the parsley.

Gluten-Free: Use zucchini or sweet potato noodles in place of whole-grain or legume noodles.

Storage

Store leftovers in an airtight container in the refrigerator for up to 5 days.

WHOLESOME 'N' HEARTY ONE-POT FARRO ROMA

Hearty, fiber-rich farro is a great whole-grain choice to pair with antioxidant-rich squash, protein-packed chickpeas, and a heap of healing herbs and aromatics. When you combine them with lemon zest and a sprinkle of pistachios on top, you've got a one-pot meal that is sure to garner rave reviews and save you time in the kitchen.

Serves: 2   **Prep time:** 15 minutes   **Cooking time:** 25 minutes

1 cup diced onion

2½ cups diced summer squash

8 ounces mushrooms, chopped (approximately 2 cups)

2 large garlic cloves, minced

1 tablespoon sherry vinegar

6 tablespoons tomato paste

1 tablespoon fresh rosemary or thyme, minced

1 teaspoon dried oregano

1 large lemon, zested and juiced (zest divided)

½ teaspoon salt, optional

¼ teaspoon ground black pepper, optional

3 cups low-sodium vegetable broth

1 cup farro, rinsed, soaked, and drained (see page 242)

1½ cups home-cooked or 1 15-ounce can chickpeas, drained

¼ cup chopped pistachios

Crushed red pepper flakes to taste, optional

Vegan Walnut Parmesan (page 114) to taste, optional

1. Heat a large stockpot over medium-high heat. Add the onion, squash, and mushrooms and cook for 2 minutes, stirring occasionally and adding 1 to 2 tablespoons of water as needed to deglaze the pot.

2. Stir in the garlic cloves, vinegar, tomato paste, rosemary, oregano, half of the lemon zest (approximately ½ tablespoon), salt, and pepper, and cook until fragrant, about one minute.

3. Stir in the vegetable broth, farro, and chickpeas. Bring the mixture to a boil and then reduce the heat to simmer. Cover and cook for 20 minutes or until all the liquid has been absorbed, stirring occasionally to prevent the farro from sticking to the bottom of the pot. If there is still a significant amount of liquid in the pot after 20 minutes and the farro is tender (taste test), remove the lid and allow it to keep simmering until most of the liquid has evaporated, about 3 to 5 minutes. The consistency should be similar to a risotto.

4. Remove from the heat and stir in the remaining lemon zest and the lemon juice, to taste. Divide between four plates and sprinkle with pistachios, crushed red pepper flakes, and Vegan Walnut Parmesan.

Calcium: 93 mg	Iron: 2 mg	Magnesium: 126 mg	Selenium: 45 mcg	Zinc: 2.7 mg

Calories: 371 | Protein: 16.5 g | Carbohydrate: 53 g | Fiber: 14 g | Fat: 6.5 g | Sodium: 248 mg

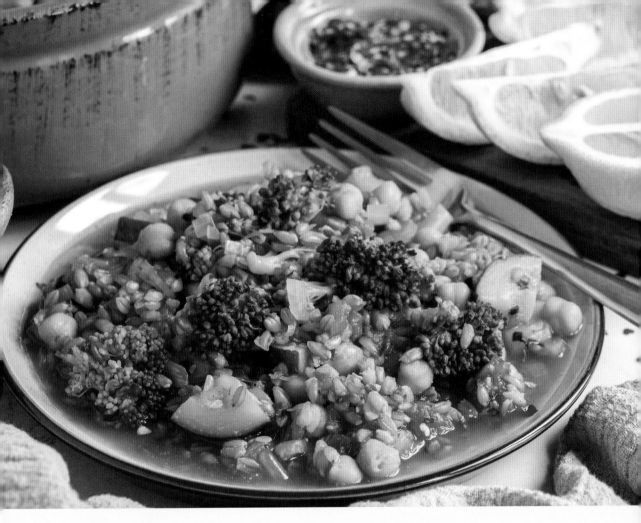

CHEF'S NOTES

Time-Saving Tips

Prepare the Vegan Walnut Parmesan ahead of time or use your favorite store-bought vegan parmesan.

Zest the lemon ahead of time and store the zest in an airtight container in the refrigerator for up to 1 week.

Substitutions

Substitute buckwheat, quinoa, brown rice, millet, or your favorite grain of choice for the farro. (Note that you may need to adjust the amount of vegetable broth and the cooking time depending on the grain you choose. See the Whole Grain Cooking Guide, page 241.) You can also use precooked grains and omit the vegetable broth.

Substitute lentils for the chickpeas.

Substitute diced bell peppers, carrots, or chopped cauliflower in place of summer squash.

Storage

Store in an airtight container in the refrigerator for up to 5 days.

GIVE ME 10 MINUTES TO PREP CHILI

This chili is an ideal go-to when you're in a pinch for time but want something satisfying and bursting with flavor. It's also versatile, and you can use tempeh or any legume of choice as the protein source. Enjoy it on its own, as a filling for tortillas, or scooped up with your favorite chips. It's delicious, easy, and packed with fiber, vitamins, minerals, and phytonutrients.

Serves: 4 **Prep time:** 10 minutes **Cooking time:** 40 minutes

8 ounces tempeh, cut into 4 pieces

1 medium red onion, chopped

1 red bell pepper, chopped

1½ cups home-cooked or 1 15-ounce can fat-free refried black beans

16 ounces homemade or store-bought salsa

1 tablespoon chili powder

1 tablespoon ground cumin

1 teaspoon smoked or sweet paprika

1 teaspoon garlic powder

1 green onion, chopped

1 to 2 tablespoons chopped cilantro, optional

Nutritional yeast to taste, optional

1. Preheat the oven to 350°F.

2. Optional step to boil the tempeh (see Chef's Notes): In a small pan, add the tempeh and enough water to cover it by 1 inch. Bring it to a boil and cook for 10 minutes. Remove from the heat and let the tempeh cool for a few minutes before crumbling it with clean hands, adding it to the bowl you'll use in the next step.

3. In a large bowl, combine the crumbled tempeh, onion, bell pepper, beans, salsa, chili powder, cumin, paprika, and garlic powder.

4. Scoop the mixture into an 8-inch or 9-inch round baking dish. Bake for 35 to 40 minutes or until the center is hot.

5. Remove it from the oven and top with green onions, cilantro, and nutritional yeast (which will also add B12).

Calcium: 160 mg	Iron: 11.5 mg	Magnesium: 125 mg	Omega-3s: .2 g	Selenium: 3.9 mcg	Zinc: 2.1 mg

Calories: 260 | Protein: 19 g | Carbohydrate: 20 g | Fiber: 12 g | Fat: 8 g | Sodium: 1010 mg*

*To reduce the sodium in this recipe, look for low-sodium salsa or use homemade salsa.

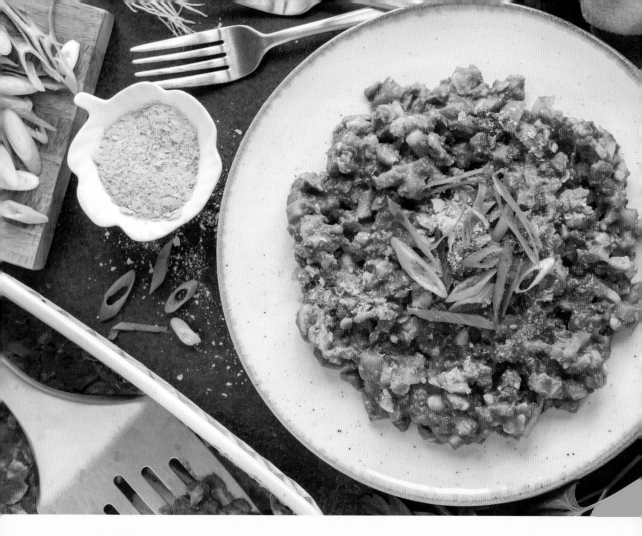

CHEF'S NOTES

Other Tips

Boiling or steaming tempeh for 10 minutes can minimize its bitterness and allow it to absorb more of the flavors that are paired with it. It's not a mandatory step if you don't have time.

Add a dollop of cashew cheese or mix in your favorite leafy greens. You can also sprinkle hemp or chia seeds on top.

If you like more heat, add 1 to 2 diced jalapeños to the chili before cooking.

Substitutions

Substitute white or yellow onion for red onion.

Substitute yellow or orange bell pepper for red bell pepper.

Substitute 1½ cups of black or other beans in place of the tempeh.

Storage

Store in an airtight container in the refrigerator for up to 5 days.

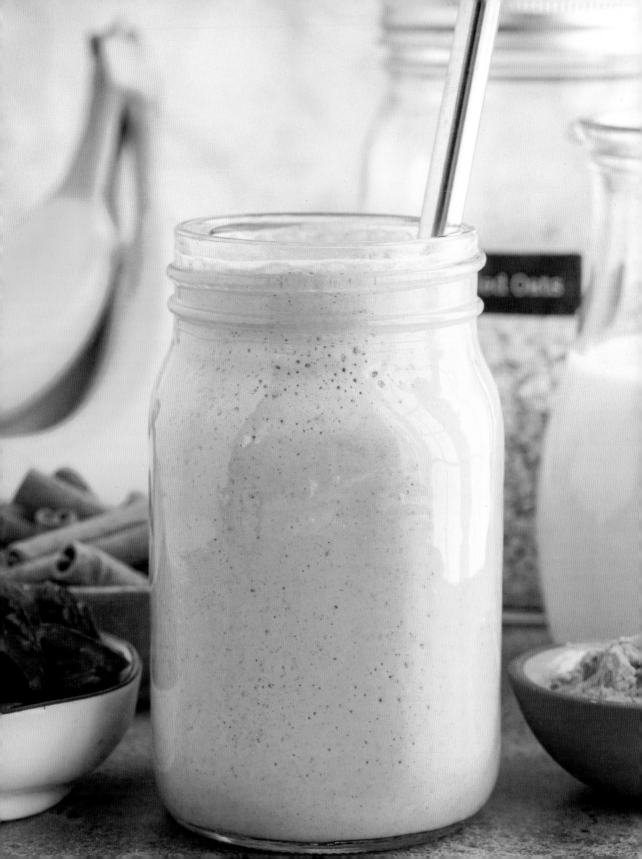

BLENDED MEALS

APPLE PIE FOR BREAKFAST SMOOTHIE

This creamy smoothie is reminiscent of the classic apple pie and ice cream combination we know and love. If you opt to use fortified plant-based milk, it's a good source of vitamins D and B$_{12}$, and it's brimming with fiber, protein, omega-3s, and healing spices.

Serves: 2   **Prep time:** 10 minutes   **Cooking time:** none

1 cup plain, unsweetened plant-based milk
1 cup rolled oats
2 tablespoons flaxseed meal
4 pitted Medjool dates
¼ cup raw walnuts
2 cups roughly chopped apples
½ teaspoon ground cinnamon
2 dashes ground nutmeg
1 tablespoon lemon juice

1. In a blender, blend all ingredients until smooth.
2. Add a handful of ice, if desired, and blend again.
3. Taste and add additional ingredients or plant-based milk to achieve the desired consistency.

CHEF'S NOTES

Substitutions
Substitute chia seeds for the flaxseed meal.
Substitute almonds or pecans for the walnuts.
Substitute pears for the apples.

Storage
Store in an airtight container in the refrigerator for up to 2 days.

Calcium: 311 mg	Iron: 4.5 mg	Magnesium: 311 mg	Omega-3s: 2.3 g	Selenium: 12.5 mcg	Zinc: 2.2 mg	Vitamin B$_{12}$*: 1.25 mcg	Vitamin D*: 100 IU

Calories: 529 | Protein: 14.5 g | Carbohydrate: 72 g | Fiber: 13.5 g | Fat: 17 g | Sodium: 65 mg

*If using fortified plant-based milk.

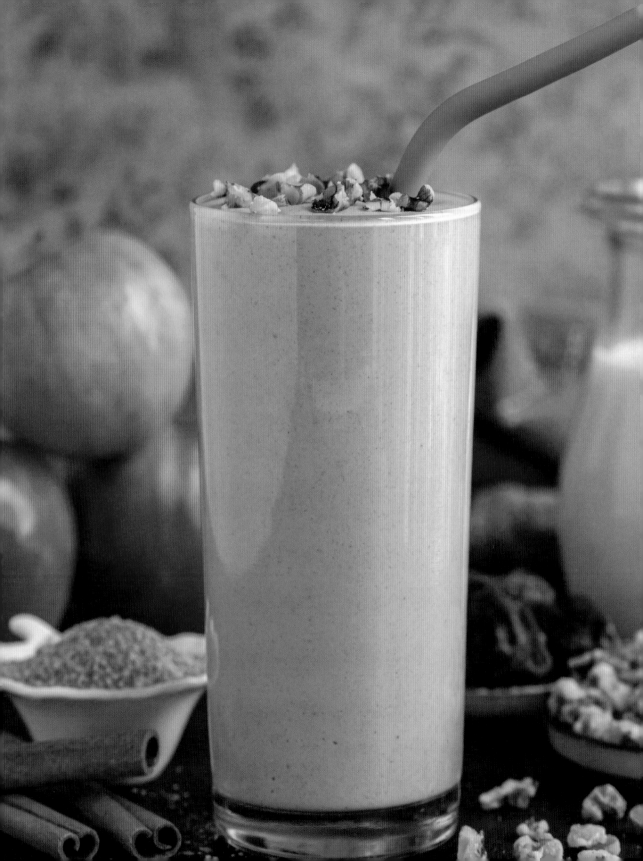

ISLAND TIME KIWI COOLER

With so many tropical fruits packed into this smoothie, it feels like you're on island time with every sip! An ideal balance of tangy and sweet, this bright-green tropical delight is also full of fiber, protein, and healthy omega-3 fats thanks to vitamin C–rich kiwi and pineapple, avocado, hemp seeds, and superfood dark leafy greens. This blended meal is perfect to enjoy any time your mind wants to drift to paradise!

Serves: 2 **Prep time:** 10 minutes **Cooking time:** none

2 whole kiwis, peeled or unpeeled

1 cup cubed fresh or frozen pineapple

1 avocado

1 handful spinach

1 cup plain, unsweetened plant-based milk

2 tablespoons hemp seeds

2 teaspoons lime juice

Shredded unsweetened coconut to taste, optional

1. In a blender, blend all the ingredients except the coconut until smooth.

2. Add a handful of ice, if desired, and blend again.

3. Taste and add additional ingredients of choice.

4. Divide the cooler between glasses and sprinkle with shredded coconut.

CHEF'S NOTES

Substitutions

In place of kiwi, use mandarin oranges or strawberries.

In place of hemp seeds, try flaxseed, chia, or your favorite nut or seed of choice.

Storage

Store in an airtight container in the refrigerator for up to 2 days.

Calcium: 289 mg	Iron: 3.6 mg	Magnesium: 129 mg	Omega-3s: 1 g	Zinc: 1.9 mg	Vitamin B₁₂*: 1.25 mcg	Vitamin D*: 100 IU

Calories: 334 | Protein: 10.5 g | Carbohydrate: 21.5 g | Fiber: 10 g | Fat: 21.5 g | Sodium: 83 mg

*If using fortified plant-based milk.

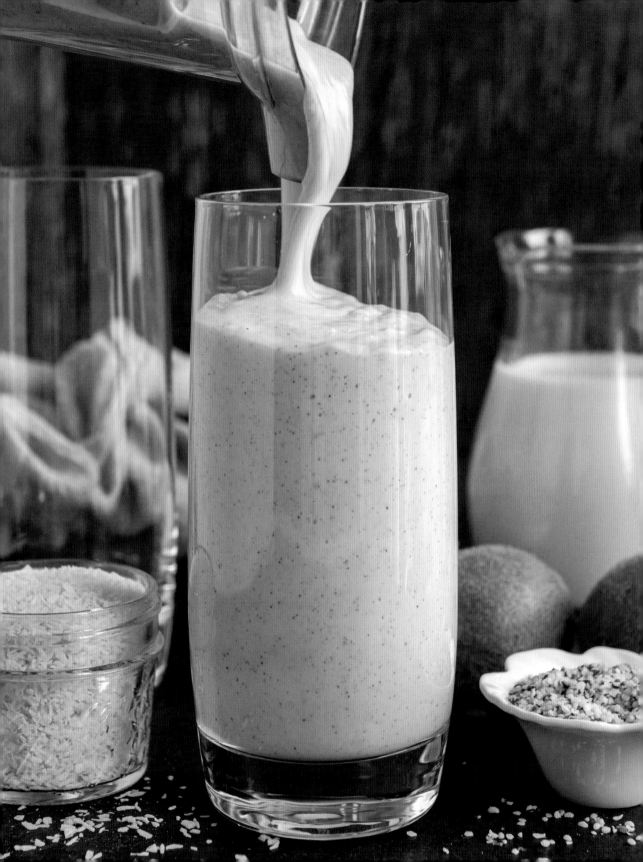

WRAP ME IN COMFORT COLD BREW SMOOTHIE

If you are a coffee lover (and even if you are not, as the espresso is optional), this smoothie is for you! This cold brew–infused recipe is packed with creamy whole coconut, sweet banana, chocolaty cacao nibs, adaptogenic chaga mushrooms, and, of course, antioxidant-rich espresso. Full of notable nutrients and great tasting, it also starts your day off with a gentle energy boost.

Serves: 2 **Prep time:** 10 minutes **Cooking time:** none

½ cup frozen riced cauliflower

1 medium banana

4 pitted Medjool dates

2 tablespoons coconut meat or
 1 tablespoon tahini

2 tablespoons cacao nibs

2 ounces brewed espresso, caffeinated
 or decaffeinated, optional

2 teaspoons chaga powder

1 cup plain, unsweetened
 plant-based milk

1. In a blender, blend all ingredients until smooth.

2. Add a handful of ice, if desired, and blend again.

3. Taste and add additional ingredients of choice.

CHEF'S NOTES

Substitutions

In place of banana, use ¼ cup silken tofu.

Use another mushroom powder in place of chaga.

Storage

Store in an airtight container in the refrigerator for up to 2 days. You may need to add water and blend again as it may thicken when it's stored.

Calcium: 331 mg	Iron: 3.3 mg	Magnesium: 80 mg	Selenium: 5.8 mcg	Zinc: 1 mg	Vitamin B₁₂*: 1.25 mcg	Vitamin D*: 100 IU

Calories: 420 | Protein: 10 g | Carbohydrate: 55 g | Fiber: 11.5 g | Fat: 15 g | Sodium: 60 mg

*If using fortified plant-based milk.

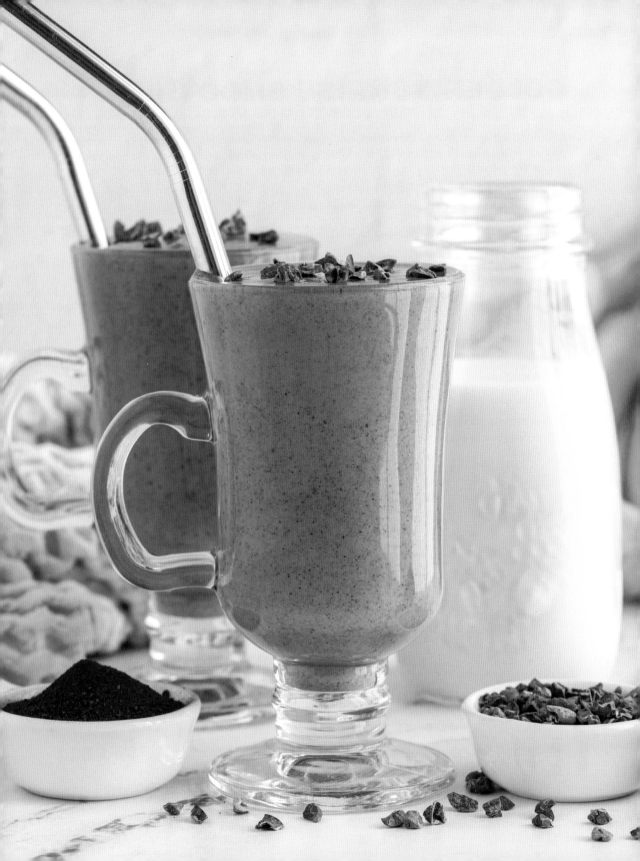

GOLDEN SUNRISE SMOOTHIE

"Early to bed and early to rise makes a man healthy, wealthy, and wise," as the saying goes. Full of anti-inflammatory and antioxidant-rich ingredients, this smoothie has a positive influence on your immune system and overall health thanks to its beneficial fiber, protein, and nourishing spices. With all of these benefits, consuming this slightly sweet and perfectly spiced smoothie is a one-way ticket to real nutrient bliss!

Serves: 2 **Prep time:** 10 minutes **Cooking time:** none

2 fresh or frozen bananas

1½ cups plain, unsweetened plant-based yogurt

1 cup plain, unsweetened plant-based milk

¼ cup rolled oats

2 tablespoons tahini

4 pitted Medjool dates

1 teaspoon ground turmeric

1 teaspoon maca powder, optional

1 teaspoon ground cinnamon

2 pinches ground nutmeg

2 pinches ground black pepper, optional

1. In a blender or food processor, blend all the ingredients until creamy and smooth.

2. Add a handful of ice, if desired, and blend again.

3. Taste and adjust for additional flavors of choice (add more cinnamon for spice, more turmeric for earthiness, or more tahini for nuttiness).

Calcium: 400 mg	Iron: 6.9 mg	Magnesium: 90 mg	Selenium: 9.4 mcg	Zinc: 1.5 mg	Vitamin B₁₂*: 1.25 mcg	Vitamin D*: 100 IU

Calories: 553 | Protein: 23 g | Carbohydrate: 73 g | Fiber: 11.5 g | Fat: 18.5 | Sodium: 175 mg

*If using fortified plant-based milk.

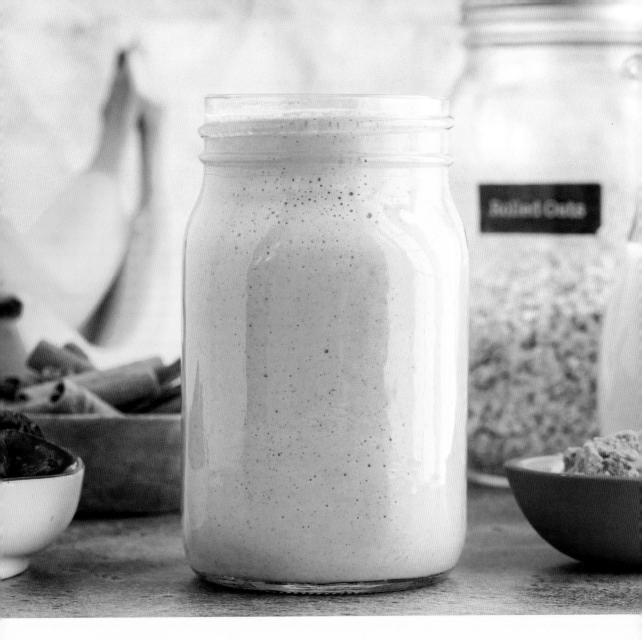

CHEF'S NOTES

Other Tips
You can find maca powder online and, occasionally, in specialty grocery stores or natural food markets.

Storage
Store in an airtight container in the refrigerator for up to 5 days. You may need to add more water and blend again as it may thicken when it's stored.

BEETS 'N' BERRIES SMOOTHIE BOWL

Blueberries and beets may seem like an unlikely pairing, but together they make magical purple bliss! Both contain anthocyanins, making this subtly sweet and highly nourishing smoothie bowl an antioxidant powerhouse. With plenty of fiber, iron, and vitamin C from the beets alone, this unique smoothie bowl is great to enjoy when you are feeling inspired to try something new.

Serves: 2 **Prep time:** 10 minutes **Cooking time:** none

½ cup shredded beet (approximately ½ medium-sized beet)

2 cups frozen blueberries

2 tablespoons lime juice

½ cup plain, unsweetened, plant-based milk

½ cup plain, unsweetened, plant-based yogurt

2 tablespoons hemp seeds

2 tablespoons flaxseed meal

4 Brazil nuts, chopped

2 tablespoons lime zest

1. In a blender or food processor, blend the beet, blueberries, lime juice, and milk until creamy.
2. Transfer to two serving bowls.
3. Divide the yogurt between the two bowls and swirl with a spoon.
4. Divide the remaining ingredients between the two bowls and enjoy!

CHEF'S NOTES

Substitutions

Substitute raspberries, blackberries, strawberries, or cranberries for the blueberries.

In place of Brazil nuts, try walnuts, almonds, hazelnuts, or pumpkin seeds.

Storage

Store in an airtight container in the refrigerator for up to 5 days.

Calcium: 195 mg	Iron: 3.8 mg	Magnesium: 135 mg	Omega-3s: 2.1 g	Selenium: 185 mcg	Zinc: 1.8 mg	Vitamin B$_{12}$*: 65 ug	Vitamin D*: 50 IU

Calories: 375 | Protein: 15 g | Carbohydrate: 32 g | Fiber: 11.5 g | Fat: 19 g | Sodium: 125 mg

*If using fortified plant-based milk.

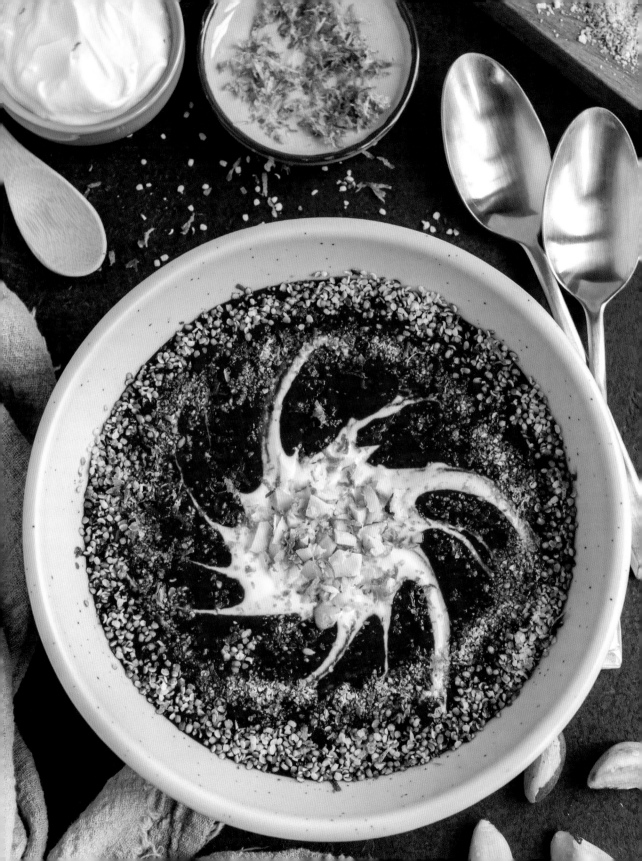

MORNING MOTIVATOR SPICED SHAKE

This delicious shake offers protein and minerals to support a joyful and productive mood, so you'll be ready to tackle whatever the day may bring. Spinach provides a boost of folate, magnesium, and vitamin B_6 (three micronutrients essential for brain power) to make every morning an inspired one.

Serves: 2 **Prep time:** 5 minutes **Cooking time:** none

⅔ cup raw cashews

2 to 4 pitted Medjool dates

¼ cup hemp seeds

1 fresh or frozen banana

2 teaspoons vanilla extract

½ teaspoon ground cinnamon

1 pinch ground nutmeg

2 handfuls spinach

½ teaspoon spirulina, optional

1. In a blender, blend the cashews, 2 dates, hemp seeds, banana, vanilla, cinnamon, nutmeg, spinach, spirulina, and 1½ cups of water until smooth.

2. Taste and add 1 to 2 more dates if you would like more sweetness. Blend again.

3. Add 1 to 2 handfuls of ice, if desired, and blend again.

4. Divide between two drinking glasses and top with a dash of cinnamon, if desired.

CHEF'S NOTES

Substitutions

Use almonds, pecans, or walnuts in place of cashews.

Instead of spinach, use romaine lettuce or another leafy green.

Storage

Store in an airtight container in the refrigerator for up to 3 days. You may need to add more water and blend again as it may thicken when it's stored.

Calcium: 93 mg	Iron: 6 mg	Magnesium: 326 mg	Omega-3s: 2 g	Selenium: 14.5 mcg	Zinc: 4.9 mg
Calories: 510	Protein: 16.5 g	Carbohydrate: 50 g	Fiber: 7 g	Fat: 29 g	Sodium: 37 mg

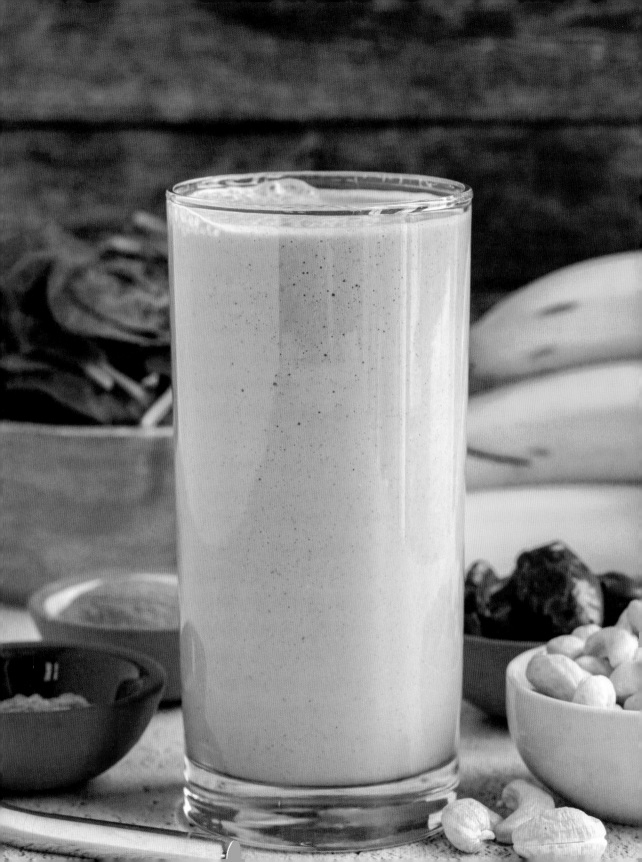

SWEET PUMPKIN SPICE AND EVERYTHING NICE SMOOTHIE BOWL

This may sound like the perfect smoothie bowl for the fall season (and it is!), but it can certainly be enjoyed year-round. Pumpkin is chock-full of beta-carotene, B vitamins, and vitamin C, as well as minerals like iron and calcium. Sprinkle it with buckwheat groats and you'll get protein too!

Serves: 2 **Prep time:** 10 minutes **Cooking time:** none

1 cup homemade or 8 ounces canned pumpkin puree

1 cup plain, unsweetened plant-based milk

2 frozen bananas

2 tablespoons tahini

½ teaspoon ground cinnamon

½ teaspoon ground ginger

2 dashes nutmeg

2 pinches salt, optional

½ cup buckwheat, rinsed, soaked, and drained (see page 241)

¼ cup chopped pecans

2 tablespoons unsweetened or naturally sweetened dried cranberries

½ teaspoon ground cinnamon

1. In a blender or food processor, blend the pumpkin, milk, bananas, tahini, cinnamon, ginger, nutmeg, and salt until smooth.

2. Divide between two bowls.

3. Top with the buckwheat, pecans, cranberries, and cinnamon.

Calcium: 334 mg	Iron: 5.6 mg	Magnesium: 183 mg	Selenium: 11.1 mcg	Zinc: 2.7 mg	Vitamin B₁₂*: 1.25 mcg	Vitamin D*: 100 IU

Calories: 549 | Protein: 15 g | Carbohydrate: 68 g | Fiber: 14 g | Fat: 22 g | Sodium: 89 mg

*If using fortified plant-based milk.

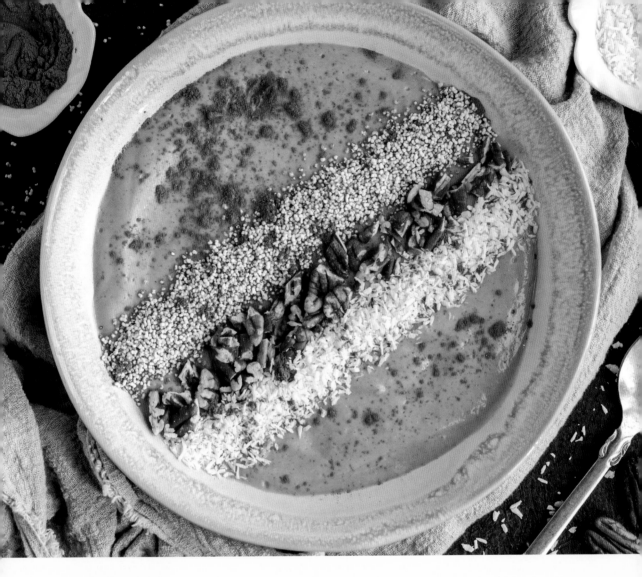

CHEF'S NOTES

Time-Saving Tips

Prepare the base ahead of time and store it in an airtight container in the refrigerator for up to 3 days.

Substitutions

Use raw oats in place of buckwheat.

Add your favorite nut or pumpkin seeds in place of pecans.

In place of tahini, use almond or cashew butter.

Use another dried fruit of choice, like apples or dates, in place of cranberries.

Storage

Store in an airtight container in the refrigerator for up to 3 days.

APPENDIX

How to Cook Beans Guide

This table lists a variety of beans and legumes to add to your diet. Beans are not only a great source of protein and fiber, but they are also concentrated with plenty of the vitamins and minerals your body needs to thrive. Enjoy experimenting with these wholesome varieties—what you can create in the kitchen is endless!

BEANS (1 cup dried)	WATER	SOAK TIME	COOK TIME	COOKED AMOUNT
Adzuki Beans	2½ cups or until completely covered	Hot Soak: 4 hours Quick Soak: 1-2 hours Overnight: 8-12 hours	Stovetop: 35-45 minutes Pressure Cooker: 15-20minutes	3-3½ cups
Black Beans	2½ cups or until completely covered	Hot Soak: 4 hours Quick Soak: 1-2 hours Overnight: 8-12 hours	Stovetop: 50-60 minutes Pressure Cooker: 8-10 minutes	3-3½ cups
Black-Eyed Peas	2½ cups or until completely covered	Hot Soak: 4 hours Quick Soak: 1-2 hours Overnight: 8-12 hours	Stovetop: 45-60 minutes Pressure Cooker: 8-10 minutes	3-3½ cups
Butter Beans/ Lima Beans	2½ cups or until completely covered	Hot Soak: 4 hours Quick Soak: 1-2 hours Overnight: 8-12 hours	Stovetop:45-60 minutes Pressure Cooker: 12-15 minutes	3-3½ cups
Cannellini Beans	2½ cups or until completely covered	Hot Soak: 4 hours Quick Soak: 1-2 hours Overnight: 8-12 hours	Stovetop: 90 minutes-2 hours Pressure Cooker: 20-30 minutes	3-3½ cups
Fava Beans	2½ cups or until completely covered	Hot Soak: 4 hours Quick Soak: 1-2 hours Overnight: 8-12 hours	Stovetop: 50-70 minutes Pressure Cooker: 8-11 minutes	3-3½ cups
Edamame (fresh)	2½ cups or until completely covered	No soaking required	Stovetop: 5-10 minutes Pressure Cooker: 1-2 minutes	1 cup

Garbanzo Beans/ Chickpeas	2½ cups or until completely covered	Hot Soak: 4 hours Quick Soak: 1-2 hours Overnight: 8-12 hours	Stovetop: 90 minutes-3 hours Pressure Cooker: 15-20 minutes	3-3½ cups
Great Northern Beans	2½ cups or until completely covered	Hot Soak: 4 hours Quick Soak: 1-2 hours Overnight: 8-12 hours	Stovetop: 45-60 minutes Pressure Cooker: 12-15 mintues	3-3½ cups
Lentils (Brown)	2½ cups or until completely covered	No soaking required	Stovetop: 30-40 minutes Pressure Cooker: 7-10 minutes	3-3½ cups
Lentils (Green)	2½ cups or until completely covered	No soaking required	Stovetop: 30-40 minutes Pressure Cooker: 7-10 minutes	3-3½ cups
Lentils (Red)	2½ cups or until completely covered	No soaking required	Stovetop: 15-25 minutes Pressure Cooker: 7-8 minutes	3-3½ cups (Note: The red lentils cook down to a paste-like consistency.)
Mung Beans	2½ cups or until completely covered	Hot Soak: 4 hours Quick Soak: 1-2 hours Overnight: 8-12 hours	Stovetop: 50-70 minutes Pressure Cooker: 6-8 minutes	3-3½ cups
Navy Beans	2½ cups or until completely covered	Hot Soak: 4 hours Quick Soak: 1-2 hours Overnight: 8-12 hours	Stovetop: 45-60 minutes Pressure Cooker: 7-10 minutes	3-3½ cups
Pinto Beans	2½ cups or until completely covered	Hot Soak: 4 hours Quick Soak: 1-2 hours Overnight: 8-12 hours	Stovetop: 60-90 minutes Pressure Cooker: 8-10 minutes	3-3½ cups
Red Beans/Small Kidney Beans	2½ cups or until completely covered	Hot Soak: 4 hours Quick Soak: 1-2 hours Overnight: 8-12 hours	Stovetop: 70-90 minutes Pressure Cooker: 12-15 minutes	3-3½ cups
Soybeans	2½ cups or until completely covered	Hot Soak: 4 hours Quick Soak: 1-2 hours Overnight: 8-12 hours	Stovetop: 2½-3 hours Pressure Cooker: 15-20 minutes	3-3½ cups
Split Peas	2½ cups or until completely covered	No soaking required	Stovetop: 35-45 minutes Pressure Cooker: 5-8 minutes	3-3½ cups
Whole Peas	2½ cups or until completely covered	Hot Soak: 4 hours Quick Soak: 1-2 hours Overnight: 8-12 hours	Stovetop: 45-60 minutes Pressure Cooker: 6-10 minutes	3-3½ cups

General Directions

1. Pick through the beans, discarding any discolored or shriveled beans.

2. Rinse the beans well.

3. Soak the beans according to the suggested times and methods above.

4. Place over medium heat; keep water at a gentle simmer to prevent split skins.

5. Beans expand in size as they soak and cook, so it is important to keep an eye on the water-to-bean ratio. Add warm water periodically during the cooking process to keep the beans covered.

6. Stir beans occasionally throughout the cooking process to prevent sticking to the bottom of the pot.

7. Beans take 30 minutes to 2 hours to cook on the stovetop, depending on the variety. You will know the beans are done when they are tender but not mushy.

Cooking Methods

Depending on how you'd like to cook your beans, most bean varieties (after soaking) cook within 30 minutes to 2 hours. Cooking beans using a pressure cooker helps to reduce the time and takes the guesswork out of knowing when the beans are tender—it gets it perfect every time! The pressure and steam also penetrate the tough exterior of beans, making them easier to digest. But, if you don't have one, a pot or slow cooker can work well too.

> **Tip:** Add a bay leaf or a strip of dried kombu (a sea vegetable) when cooking beans. Doing so not only adds flavor, but the kombu can help tenderize the beans and reduce flatulence during digestion. Kombu contains alpha-galactosidase, which helps break down the oligosaccharides in beans that are responsible for their gastrointestinal irritation. You can also add spices, such as fennel, cumin, caraway, ginger, epazote, asafoetida, and turmeric to help make beans more digestible.

Why Pre-Soak Your Beans Before Cooking?

Soaking beans allows the dried beans to absorb water, which begins to dissolve the antinutrients that cause intestinal discomfort and gas. While beans are soaking they are also expanding in size, which results in faster cooking times.

Soaking Methods

Hot Soak: If you are unable to soak your beans overnight, hot soaking is an easy way to help soften the beans and wash away some of the antinutrients before cooking. Simply add 3 to 4 cups of water to a pot and bring to a boil (4 to 5 minutes). Remove the water from the heat, add your beans and cover with a tight-fitting lid. Allow the beans to soak for 4 hours. Then drain the water, add fresh water to the beans, and cook using your preferred method of choice.

Quick Soak: Quick soaking is the fastest method. It will help to soften the beans and remove some antinutrients, but not as effectively as other soaking methods. Lentils are ideal candidates for this method if you're concerned about reducing antinutrient concentrations. Simply add 2 to 3 cups of water to a pot and bring to a boil (4 to 5 minutes). Remove the water from the heat, add your beans and cover with a tight-fitting lid. Allow the beans to soak for 1 to 2 hours. Then drain the water, add fresh water to the beans, and cook using your preferred method.

Overnight Soak: Overnight soaking is the easiest and the most effective method for removing antinutrients. You can soak your beans anywhere from 8 to 24 hours. Place the beans in a large container, add 4 cups of water, and cover the container while the beans soak. If you extend the soaking time past 12 hours, discard the original soaking liquid, rinse, and resoak in fresh water about 2 to 3 times per day. Then drain the water, add fresh water to the beans, and cook using your preferred method.

Batch Cooking

You can cook beans in large batches so you have them ready to go for the week or freeze them for weeks to come. Batch cooking can save you time in the kitchen. Cooked beans keep 3–4 days in the refrigerator and take a minimal amount of time to reheat. Use beans in salads, and grain bowls, as the base for plant burgers, or toss them in your favorite soups or stews. You can also store cooked beans in the freezer for a few months, portioning them in individual containers and using them as you need. After you cook your batched beans, spread them out on a parchment-lined baking sheet so that they cool completely before storing and the beans do not clump together. Freeze the cooled beans, then move them to an airtight container for proper freezer storage.

Whole Grains Cooking Guide

This table lists true grains (oats, wheat varieties, rice varieties, barley, and more) and pseudograins (quinoa, millet, amaranth, buckwheat, teff, wild rice). Pseudograins are seeds with a similar nutrient composition to true grains, so they're often classified as grains. Both true grains and pseudograins are important for overall health. Whole grains are generally chewier (in the best way), more flavorful (nutty and satisfying), and much more nutritious (fiber, protein, B vitamins, and more!) than refined grains. Many of these grains work well for both sweet and savory recipes and can be cooked to various textures, making them versatile, easy to use, and delicious to eat. Use this guide as a resource and for inspiration to try new grains and expand your palate!

GRAIN (1 cup dried grain)	WATER	SOAK TIME	COOK TIME	COOKED AMOUNT
*Amaranth	Stovetop: 1½-2½ cups (depending on the consistency desired. Use more water for a porridge-like consistency.) Pressure Cooker: 1 ½ cups Rice Cooker: 1 cup	3-5 hours	Soaked: 15 minutes Dry: 25-30 minutes Pressure Cooker: 12 minutes with high pressure Rice Cooker: 20 minutes	3½ cups
Barley, hulled	Stovetop: 1 cup (soaked) 3 cups (dry) Pressure Cooker: 1-1½ cups Rice Cooker: 2½ cups	6-12 hours	Soaked: 30-45 minutes Dry: 45-60 minutes Pressure Cooker: 25-30 minutes with high pressure Rice Cooker: 45 minutes	3½ cups
*Buckwheat	Stovetop: ¼-½ cup (soaked) 2 cups (dry) Pressure Cooker: 1 cup Rice Cooker: 1½-2 cups	6-12 hours	Soaked: 3-5 minutes Dry: 20 minutes Pressure Cooker: 5-6 minutes with high pressure Rice cooker: 30-40 minutes minutes	4 cups
Bulgur	Stovetop: 1½-2 cups Pressure Cooker: 1½-2 cups Rice Cooker: 1 cup	Bulgur doesn't need to be soaked since it's precooked.	Dry: 10-12 minutes (may need longer depending on the type of bulgur) Pressure Cooker: 10-12 minutes with low pressure Rice Cooker: 45-50 minutes	3 cups

*Cornmeal (polenta)	Stovetop: 4-5 cups (depending on desired firmness) Pressure Cooker: 4½ cups Slow Cooker: 6 cups	None	Stovetop: 25-35 minutes Pressure Cooker: 4 minutes (instant polenta): 7 minutes with high pressure Slow Cooker: 3-4 hours on high setting; 6-9 hours on low setting	2½ cups
Couscous, whole wheat	Stovetop: 2 cups (hot water) Pressure Cooker: 2 cups (medium-to-large size pearls) Rice Cooker: 1 cup	None	Stovetop: cover and steam for 10 minutes (heat off) Pressure Cooker: 2-3 minutes with high pressure Rice Cooker: 5 minutes on the keep warm setting	3 cups
Farro *Cook farro according to the pasta method.	Stovetop: 3 cups (soaked) 8 cups (dry) Pressure Cooker: 2 cups Rice Cooker: 3 cups	8-12 hours	Soaked: 10 minutes Dry: 30 minutes Pressure Cooker: 10-12 minutes with high pressure Rice Cooker: 30-45 minutes	3 cups
Kamut	Stovetop: 3 cups (soaked) 4 cups (dry) Pressure Cooker: 2½ cups Rice Cooker: 3 cups	8-12 hours	Soaked: 30-45minutes Dry: 45-60 minutes Pressure Cooker: 25 minutes with high pressure Rice Cooker: 40-60 minutes	3 cups
*Millet, hulled	Stovetop: 1½ cups (soaked) 2 cups (dry) Pressure Cooker: 1¾ cups Rice Cooker: 1½ -2 cups	6-12 hours	Soaked: 10-15 minutes Dry: 20 minutes Pressure Cooker: 10 minutes with high pressure Rice Cooker: 20 minutes	4 cups
Oats, steel cut	Stovetop: 2 cups (soaked) 4 cups (dry) Pressure Cooker: 1⅓-1½ cups (porridge-like texture) Rice Cooker: 1½-2 cups	8 hours	Soaked: 12-15 minutes Dry: 15-20 minutes Pressure Cooker: 5 minutes with high pressure Rice Cooker: 30-45 minutes	4 cups
*Quinoa	Stovetop: 1½ cups (soaked) 2 cups (dry) Pressure Cooker: 1¼ cup Rice Cooker: 1½ cup-2 cups	3-4 hours	Soaked: 15-20 minutes Dry: 12-15 minutes Pressure Cooker: 1-2 minutes with high pressure Rice Cooker: 26 minutes	3+ cups

*Rice, brown	Stovetop: 1½–2 cups (soaked) 2½ cups (dry) Pressure Cooker: 1 cup for chewy rice. 1¼ cups; for soft rice Rice Cooker: 1 cup for chewy rice; 1½ cups for soft rice	6-8 hours	Soaked: 15-25 minutes Dry: 45 minutes Pressure Cooker: 20 minutes with high pressure Rice Cooker: 45-60 minutes	3-4 cups
Rye berries	Stovetop: 2½–3 cups water (soaked) 4 cups (dry) Pressure Cooker: 3 cups Rice Cooker: 2 cups	6-8 hours	Soaked: 45-60 minutes Dry: 60 minutes Pressure Cooker: 20-30 with high pressure Rice Cooker: 20-30 minutes	3 cups
*Sorghum	Stovetop: 2½ cups (soaked) 4 cups (dry) Pressure Cooker: 3 cups Rice Cooker: 2¾ cups	6-12 hours	Soaked: 25-40 minutes Dry: 50-60 minutes Pressure Cooker: 30 minutes with high pressure Rice Cooker: 45-60 minutes	3 cups
Spelt berries	Stovetop: 3 cups (soaked) 3 cups (dry) Pressure Cooker: 2½ cups Rice Cooker: 2 cups	6 hours	Soaked: 40-60 minutes Dry: 60-80 minutes Pressure Cooker: 25-30 minutes Rice Cooker: 30-35 minutes	3 cups
*Teff	Stovetop: 1½–2 cups (soaked) 3 cups (dry) Pressure Cooker: 1½–2 cups Rice Cooker: 1 cup–1½ cups	3-4 hours	Soaked: 8-10 minutes Dry: 15-20 minutes Pressure Cooker: 2-3 minutes with high pressure Rice Cooker: 20 minutes	3 cups
Wheat berries	Stovetop: 3 cups (soaked) 4 cups (dry) Pressure Cooker: 3 cups Rice Cooker: 2 cups	8-10 hours	Soaked: 40-60 minutes Dry: 60-90 minutes Pressure Cooker: 25-30 minutes Rice Cooker: 30-35 minutes	3 cups
*Wild Rice	Stovetop: 3 cups (soaked) 4 cups (dry) Pressure Cooker: 3-4 cups Rice Cooker: 2 cups	12-24 hours	Soaked: 30-35 minutes Dry: 40-60 minutes Pressure Cooker: 20-25 minutes with high pressure Rice Cooker: 50 minutes	3 ½ cups

Consider purchasing organic grains whenever possible to minimize exposure to glyphosate.

*Gluten-Free Grains

General Directions

Always rinse and wash your soaked or dry grains before cooking. Cooking most grains is very similar to cooking rice in that just enough water is added until the grain has completely absorbed the water and becomes tender. Place the soaked or dried grains in a pan with fresh water (do not cook grains in the liquid they were soaked in) or vegetable broth, bring it to a boil, then simmer until the liquid is absorbed. Most grains need to be covered while cooking. Pasta is generally cooked in a larger amount of water, with the excess liquid drained after cooking.

Timing Your Grains

Grains can vary in cooking time depending on the age of the grain, length of time the grain was soaked, the type of grain variety, and the pans that are used for cooking. If the grain is not as tender as you'd like when the suggested cooking time is done, you may add more water and continue cooking until the desired consistency is achieved. Or, if the grains have reached your ideal doneness before the liquid has been absorbed, drain off the excess liquid before serving.

Pasta Method

Some grains, like brown rice, farro, wheat berries, and wild rice, can be cooked using the "pasta method," where uncooked whole grains are placed in a large pot of boiling water, boiled until tender, then drained of their excess liquid.

Parboiling Method to Reduce Arsenic Content in Rice

While brown, black, and red rice may be healthier than white rice since they contain more nutrients like fiber, B vitamins, and minerals, they may also be higher in arsenic, a natural element found in soil. The amount of arsenic in rice can vary, depending on the soil in which the rice is grown. The good news is that you can significantly reduce the arsenic content by practicing the parboil method. Here's how: Add fresh water (4 cups for every cup of raw rice) and rice to a pot. Heat on medium-high heat and boil for 5 minutes. Drain the rice, discarding the water. Add fresh water (1¾–2 cups for each cup of parboiled rice) to the rice and simmer, covered, until tender, approximately 25 minutes. and cook the rice with low to medium heat with a lid until the water is absorbed.

Batch Cooking

You can cook whole grains in large batches so you have them ready to go for the week or freeze them for weeks to come. Batch cooking can save you time in the kitchen. Grains keep 3–4 days in the refrigerator and take a minimal amount of time to reheat. Use the grains in salads, grain bowls, or toss them in your favorite soups or stews. You can also store cooked grains in the freezer for a few months, portioning them in individual containers and using them as you need. After you cook your batched grains, spread them out on a parchment-lined baking sheet so that they cool completely before storing and the grains do not clump together. Freeze the cooled grains, then move them to an airtight container for proper freezer storage.

Why Pre-Soak Your Grains Before Cooking?

Many grains can be cooked without soaking. However, grains with a tough outer layer, like whole wheat varieties, can benefit from soaking, which will reduce cooking time and increase digestibility. Soaking grains can also help reduce phytate content, a nutrient that can bind minerals in grains. While phytate can have some health benefits, reducing the phytate content in grains helps to optimize mineral (calcium, iron, zinc) absorption.

If you set out to soak your grains, but do not want to keep up with the length of time suggested, most grains will do well with soaking overnight.

If you are in a pinch, and would like to soak your grains, soaking in hot water reduces soaking time for most grains.

Once your grains have finished soaking, rinse them in a mesh strainer a few times until the water runs clear. Prepare grains in fresh water and your cooking method of choice.

Metric Conversion Chart

STANDARD CUP	FINE POWDER (E.G., FLOUR)	GRAIN (E.G., RICE)	GRANULAR (E.G., SUGAR)	LIQUID SOLIDS (E.G., BUTTER)	LIQUID (E.G., MILK)
1	140 g	150 g	190 g	200 g	240 ml
¾	105 g	113 g	143 g	150 g	180 ml
⅔	93 g	100 g	125 g	133 g	160 ml
½	70 g	75 g	95 g	100 g	120 ml
⅓	47 g	50 g	63 g	67 g	80 ml
¼	35 g	38 g	48 g	50 g	60 ml
⅛	18 g	19 g	24 g	25 g	30 ml

USEFUL EQUIVALENTS FOR COOKING/OVEN TEMPERATURES			
Process	Fahrenheit	Celsius	Gas Mark
Freeze Water	32°F	0°C	
Room Temperature	68°F	20°C	
Boil Water	212°F	100°C	
Bake	325°F	160°C	3
	350°F	180°C	4
	375°F	190°C	5
	400°F	200°C	6
	425°F	220°C	7
	450°F	230°C	8
Broil			Grill

USEFUL EQUIVALENTS FOR LIQUID INGREDIENTS BY VOLUME			
¼ tsp			1 ml
½ tsp			2 ml
1 tsp			5 ml
3 tsp	1 tbsp	½ fl oz	15 ml
	2 tbsp	⅛ cup	1 fl oz	30 ml
	4 tbsp	¼ cup	2 fl oz	60 ml
	5⅓ tbsp	⅓ cup	3 fl oz	80 ml
	8 tbsp	½ cup	4 fl oz	120 ml
	10⅔ tbsp	⅔ cup	5 fl oz	160 ml
	12 tbsp	¾ cup	6 fl oz	180 ml
	16 tbsp	1 cup	8 fl oz	240 ml
	1 pt	2 cups	16 fl oz	480 ml
	1 qt	4 cups	32 fl oz	960 ml

USEFUL EQUIVALENTS FOR DRY INGREDIENTS BY WEIGHT		
(To convert ounces to grams, multiply the number of ounces by 30.)		
1 oz	⅟₁₆ lb	30 g
4 oz	¼ lb	120 g
8 oz	½ lb	240 g
12 oz	¾ lb	360 g
16 oz	1 lb	480 g

USEFUL EQUIVALENTS FOR LENGTH				
(To convert inches to centimeters, multiply the number of inches by 2.5.)				
1 in			2.5 cm	
6 in	½ ft		15 cm	
12 in	1 ft		30 cm	
36 in	3 ft	1 yd	90 cm	
40 in			100 cm	1 m

ENDNOTES

Introduction

1. "Chronic Illnesses: UN Stands Up to Stop 41 Million Avoidable Deaths per Year," UN News, September 27, 2018, https://news.un.org/en/story/2018/09/1021132.

2. "New Study Finds Poor Diet Kills More People Globally Than Tobacco and High Blood Pressure," IMHE, April 3, 2019, https://www.healthdata.org/news-release/new-study-finds-poor-diet-kills-more-people-globally-tobacco-and-high-blood-pressure.

3. "Preventing Heart Disease," Harvard T.H. Chan School of Public Health, August 2022, https://www.hsph.harvard.edu/nutritionsource/disease-prevention/cardiovascular-disease/preventing-cvd/.

4. "Simple Steps to Preventing Diabetes," Harvard T.H. Chan School of Public Health, https://www.hsph.harvard.edu/nutritionsource/disease-prevention/diabetes-prevention/preventing-diabetes-full-story/.

5. "What Do We Know About Diet and Prevention of Alzheimer's Disease?" National Institute on Aging, November 20, 2023, https://www.nia.nih.gov/health/what-do-we-know-about-diet-and-prevention-alzheimers-disease.

6. Lars T. Fadnes et al., "Estimating Impact of Food Choices on Life Expectancy: A Modeling Study," *PLOS Medicine*, February 8, 2022, https://journals.plos.org/plosmedicine/article?id=10.1371/journal.pmed.1003889.

7. Ocean Robbins, "The Blue Zones: Longevity Secrets from Centenarians," Food Revolution Network, September 2, 2022, https://foodrevolution.org/blog/blue-zones-live-to-100/.

8. Ocean Robbins, "Understanding Fat: What Types of Fat Are Good vs Bad for You?" Food Revolution Network, October 19, 2022, https://foodrevolution.org/blog/good-fat-vs-bad-fat-types/.

9. Maki Yazawa, "Mind, Blown: There Are Only *Two* Plant-Based Foods That Contain Saturated Fat, According to RDs," *Well + Good*, January 26, 2023, https://www.wellandgood.com/plant-based-saturated-fat/.

10. United States Department of Agriculture, Agricultural Research Service, "Usual Nutrient Intake from Food and Beverages, by Gender and Age," January 2021, https://www.ars.usda.gov/ARSUserFiles/80400530/pdf/usual/Usual_Intake_gender_WWEIA_2015_2018.pdf.

11. World Health Organization, "The Top 10 Causes of Death," December 9, 2020, https://www.who .int/news-room/fact-sheets/detail/the-top-10-causes-of-death.

12. "Diabetes: Tackle Diabetes With a Plant-Based Diet," Physicians Committee for Responsible Medicine, https://www.pcrm.org/health-topics/diabetes.

13. Ocean Robbins, "IGF-1: The Growth Hormone That Can Fuel Cancer," Food Revolution Network, October 29, 2021, https://foodrevolution.org/blog/what-is-igf-1/.

14. Claire Brown, "Study: The World's Largest Meat and Dairy Companies Combine To Emit More Greenhouse Gases Than Most People Would Have Imagined," Food Revolution Network, August 10, 2018, https://foodrevolution.org/blog/meat-dairy-greenhouse-gases/.

15. Ocean Robbins, "What You Eat Can Impact Climate Change! See 9 Foods That Harm the Planet and 11 Foods That Can Help Save It," August 31, 2021, https://foodrevolution.org/blog/ food-and-climate-change/.

16. Juli Hennings and Harry Lynch, "EarthDate: Depleting the Ogallala Aquifer," Bureau of Economic Geology, https://www.earthdate.org/files/000/002/714/EarthDate_278_C.pdf.

17. Ocean Robbins, "Is Eating Fish Good For You? The Truth About the Health and Environmental Impacts of Eating Fish," Food Revolution Network, November 15, 2019, https://foodrevolution .org/blog/health-and-environmental-impacts-of-eating-fish/.

18. J. Poore and T. Nemecek, "Reducing Food's Environmental Impacts Through Producers and Consumers," *Science* 360, no. 6392 (June 1, 2018): 987–92, https://josephpoore.com/ Science%20360%206392%20987%20-%20Accepted%20Manuscript.pdf.

19. Ocean Robbins, "What's Causing the Global Food Crisis? (And How Plant-Based Diets Can Help!)," Food Revolution Network, November 18, 2022, https://foodrevolution.org/blog/ global-food-crisis-causes-solutions/.

20. Tamika Sims, "Free-Range Chickens and Cage-Free Eggs: The S(coop) on Poultry Labels," *Food Insight*, September 20, 2022, https://foodinsight.org/the-scoop-on-poultry-labels/.

21. Robert H. Schmerling, "What's in Your Supplements?" *Harvard Health Blog*, February 15, 2019, https://www.health.harvard.edu/blog/whats-in-your-supplements-2019021515946.

22. M. J. Stampfer et al., "Vitamin E Consumption and the Risk of Coronary Disease in Women," *New England Journal of Medicine* 328, no. 20 (May 20, 1993): 1444–49, https://pubmed.ncbi.nlm .nih.gov/8479463/.

23. T. C. Campbell and Howard Jacobson, *Whole: Rethinking the Science of Nutrition* (BenBella Books, 2013).

24. Edgar R. Miller III, "Meta-Analysis: High-Dosage Vitamin E Supplementation May Increase All-Cause Mortality," *Annals of Internal Medicine* 142, no. 1 (January 4, 2005):37–46, https://pubmed .ncbi.nlm.nih.gov/15537682/.

25. Goran Bjelakovic, "Mortality in Randomized Trials of Antioxidant Supplements for Primary and Secondary Prevention: Systematic Review and Meta-Analysis," *Journal of the American Medical Association* 297, no. 8 (Feb 28, 2007): 842–57, https://pubmed.ncbi.nlm.nih.gov/17327526/.

26. Alpha-Tocopherol, Beta Carotene Cancer Prevention Study Group, "The Effect of Vitamin E and Beta Carotene on the Incidence of Lung Cancer and Other Cancers in Male Smokers," *New England Journal of Medicine* 330, no. 15 (April 14, 1994): 1029–35, https://pubmed.ncbi.nlm.nih.gov/8127329/.

27. Donald R. Davis, Melvin D. Epp, and Hugh D. Riordan, "Changes in USDA Food Composition Data for 43 Garden Crops, 1950 to 1999," *Journal of the American College of Nutrition* 23, no. 6 (December 2004): 669–82, https://pubmed.ncbi.nlm.nih.gov/15637215/.

Chapter 1

1. James M. Smoliga, Z. Taggart Wilber, and Brooks Taylor Robinson, "Premature Death in Bodybuilders: What Do We Know?" *Sports Medicine* 53, no. 5 (May 2023): 933–48, https://pubmed.ncbi.nlm.nih.gov/36715876/.

2. Campbell and Jacobson, *Whole: Rethinking the Science of Nutrition*.

3. Jillian Kubala and Mikayla Morell, "8 Protein Deficiency Symptoms: Here Are 8 Signs You Might Need More Protein," *Health*, September 5, 2023, https://www.health.com/protein-deficiency-7565059.

4. Dorota Scibior and Hanna Czeczot, "Arginine—Metabolism and Functions in the Human Organism" [article in Polish], *Postepy Higieny i Medycyny Doświadczalnej* (online) 58 (2004): 321–32, https://pubmed.ncbi.nlm.nih.gov/15459550/.

5. National Institutes of Health, Office of Dietary Supplements, Nutrient Recommendations and Databases, https://ods.od.nih.gov/HealthInformation/nutrientrecommendations.aspx.

6. National Research Council, *Recommended Dietary Allowances*, 10th edition (National Academies Press, 1989), https://www.ncbi.nlm.nih.gov/books/NBK234926/.

7. Katie Dodd, "Nutrition Needs for Older Adults: Protein," National Resource Center on Nutrition and Aging, February 14, 2020, https://acl.gov/sites/default/files/nutrition/Nutrition-Needs_Protein_FINAL-2.18.20_508.pdf.

8. Ocean Robbins, "Plant-Based Protein: The Best Sources & How Much You Actually Need," Food Revolution Network, October 26, 2018, https://foodrevolution.org/blog/plant-based-protein/.

9. A.C. Ross, C.L. Taylor, and A.L. Yaktine, "Summary Tables," Dietary Reference Intakes for Calcium and Vitamin D., 2011 https://www.ncbi.nlm.nih.gov/books/NBK56068/table/summarytables.t4/?report=objectonly; https://jissn.biomedcentral.com/articles/10.1186/s12970-017-0177-8.

10. Ocean Robbins, "Plant-Based Lysine: Do You Need Meat to Get Enough Lysine?" Food Revolution Network, June 30, 2023, https://foodrevolution.org/blog/plant-based-lysine-foods/.

11. Michael Greger, "The Protein-Combining Myth," NutritionFacts.Org, Vol. 30 (April 25, 2016), https://nutritionfacts.org/video/the-protein-combining-myth.

12. Gabriela Lucciana Martini et al., "Similar Body Composition, Muscle Size, and Strength Adaptations to Resistance Training in Lacto-Ovo-Vegetarians and Non-Vegetarians," *Applied Physiology, Nutrition, and Metabolism* 48, no. 6 (June 2023), https://doi.org/10.1139/apnm-2022-0258, https://cdnsciencepub.com/doi/10.1139/apnm-2022-0258.

13. Astrid Kolderup Hervik and Birger Svihus, "The Role of Fiber in Energy Balance," *Journal of Nutrition and Metabolism* (January 21, 2019), https://www.hindawi.com/journals/jnme/2019/4983657.

14. Eric Bartholomae and Carol S. Johnston, "Nitrogen Balance at the Recommended Dietary Allowance for Protein in Minimally Active Male Vegans," *Nutrients* 15, no. 14 (July 16, 2023): 3159, https://www.mdpi.com/2072-6643/15/14/3159.

15. Marion Tharrey et al., "Patterns of Plant and Animal Protein Intake Are Strongly Associated with Cardiovascular Mortality: the Adventist Health Study-2 Cohort," *International Journal of Epidemiology* 47, no. 5 (October 1, 2018): 1603–12, https://pubmed.ncbi.nlm.nih.gov/29618018/.

16. Meghan B. Azad et al., "Nonnutritive Sweeteners and Cardiometabolic Health: A Systematic Review and Meta-Analysis of Randomized Controlled Trials and Prospective Cohort Studies," *Canadian Medical Association Journal* 189, no. 28 (July 17, 2017): E929–39, https://www.cmaj.ca/content/189/28/E929.

17. Clean Label Project, "Protein Powder: Our Point of View" (June 12, 2018), https://cleanlabelproject.org/protein-powder-white-paper/.

Chapter 2

1. Yang Yang et al., "Association Between Dietary Fiber and Lower Risk of All-Cause Mortality: A Meta-Analysis of Cohort Studies," *American Journal of Epidemiology* 181, no. 2 (January 15, 2015): 83–91, https://pubmed.ncbi.nlm.nih.gov/25552267/.

2. Yu Peng et al., "Association of Abnormal Bowel Health with Major Chronic Diseases and Risk of Mortality," *Annals of Epidemiology* 75 (November 2022): 39–46, https://www.sciencedirect.com/science/article/pii/S1047279722002265.

3. Ocean Robbins, "What Is Your Poop Telling You? A Guide to Healthy Bowel Habits," Food Revolution Network, May 11, 2022, https://foodrevolution.org/blog/healthy-poop-guide/.

4. Ocean Robbins, "How to Balance Hormones Naturally with Diet & Lifestyle," Food Revolution Network, December 25, 2020, https://foodrevolution.org/blog/balance-hormones-naturally/.

5. Robbins, "How to Balance Hormones Naturally with Diet & Lifestyle."

6. Ocean Robbins, "The Importance of Fiber in Gut Health and Hormonal Balance," Food Revolution Network, March 24, 2023. https://foodrevolution.org/blog/fiber-gut-health-hormones/.

7. Joel Fuhrman, "How to Eat to Reverse and Prevent Diabetes (5 Foods to Eat and 6 to Avoid)," Food Revolution Network, April 6, 2018, https://foodrevolution.org/blog/how-to-eat-to-prevent-diabetes/.

8. Jill Weisenberger, "Fiber: Fiber's Link With Satiety and Weight Control," *Today's Dietitian* 17, no. 2 (February 2015): 14, https://www.todaysdietitian.com/newarchives/021115p14.shtml.

9. Diane E. Threapleton et al., "Dietary Fibre Intake and Risk of Cardiovascular Disease: Systematic review and Meta-Analysis," *British Medical Journal* 347 (December 19, 2013), http://www.bmj.com/content/347/bmj.f6879.

10. World Health Organization, "Diet, Nutrition and the Prevention of Chronic Diseases," WHO Technical Report Series 916 (2003), https://www.who.int/publications/i/item/924120916X.

11. U.S. Department of Agriculture, AskUSDA, "How Much (Dietary) Fiber Should I Eat?" (November 14, 2023), https://ask.usda.gov/s/article/How-much-dietary-fiber-should-I-eat.

12. Skye Gould, "6 Charts That Show How Much More Americans Eat Than They Used To," *Business Insider* (May 10, 2017), https://www.businessinsider.com/daily-calories-americans-eat-increase-2016-07.

13. USDA, Agricultural Research Service, "Usual Nutrient Intake from Food and Beverages, by Gender and Age." https://www.ars.usda.gov/ARSUserFiles/80400530/pdf/usual/Usual_Intake_gender_WWEIA_2015_2018.pdf.

14. James Gallagher, "The Lifesaving Food 90% Aren't Eating Enough Of," BBC (January 10, 2019), https://www.bbc.com/news/health-46827426.

15. "Fiber: Fill Up on 40 Grams of Fiber a Day," Physicians Committee for Responsible Medicine, https://www.pcrm.org/good-nutrition/nutrition-information/fiber.

16. Michaeleen Doucleff, "Is the Secret to a Healthier Microbiome Hidden in the Hadza Diet?" NPR (August 24, 2017), https://www.npr.org/sections/goatsandsoda/2017/08/24/545631521/is-the-secret-to-a-healthier-microbiome-hidden-in-the-hadza-diet.

17. Larisa Gearhart-Serna, "Health Benefits of Dietary Fibers Vary," National Institutes of Health (May 24, 2022), https://www.nih.gov/news-events/nih-research-matters/health-benefits-dietary-fibers-vary.

18. Daniel McDonald et al., "American Gut: An Open Platform for Citizen Science Microbiome Research," *ASM Journals* 3, no. 3 (May 15, 2018), https://journals.asm.org/doi/10.1128/msystems.00031-18.

Chapter 3

1. Ocean Robbins, "Omega-3s: Why Are They Important—And What Are the Best Sources for Your Health?" Food Revolution Network (June 25, 2021), https://foodrevolution.org/blog/omega-3s-vegan/.

2. A. P. Jain, K. K. Aggarwal, and P-Y Zhang, "Omega-3 Fatty Acids and Cardiovascular Disease," *European Review for Medical and Pharmacological Science* 19, no. 3 (2015): 441–45, https://pubmed.ncbi.nlm.nih.gov/25720716/.

3. Ashish Chaddha and Kim A. Eagle, "Omega-3 Fatty Acids and Heart Health," *Circulation* 132, no. 22 (Dec 1, 2015), https://www.ahajournals.org/doi/full/10.1161/CIRCULATIONAHA.114.015176.

4. Juliana Rombaldi Bernardi et al., "Fetal and Neonatal Levels of Omega-3: Effects on Neurodevelopment, Nutrition, and Growth," *Scientific World Journal* 2012 (October 17, 2012), https://doi.org/10.1100/2012/202473.

5. Simon C. Dyall, "Long-Chain Omega-3 Fatty Acids and the Brain: A Review of the Independent and Shared Effects of EPA, DPA and DHA," *Frontiers in Aging Neuroscience* 7, no. 52 (April 21, 2015), https://www.ncbi.nlm.nih.gov/pmc/articles/PMC4404917/.

6. T. A. Ajith, "A Recent Update on the Effects of Omega-3 Fatty Acids in Alzheimer's Disease," *Current Clinical Pharmacology* 13, no. 4 (20118): 252–60, https://pubmed.ncbi.nlm.nih.gov/30084334/.

7. Artemis P. Simopoulos, "Omega-3 Fatty Acids in Inflammation and Autoimmune Diseases," *Journal of the American College of Nutrition* 21, no. 6 (December 2002), https://pubmed.ncbi.nlm.nih.gov/12480795/.

8. Raquel D. S. Freitas and Maria M. Campos, "Protective Effects of Omega-3 Fatty Acids in Cancer-Related Complications," *Nutrients* 11, no. 5 (May 2019): 945, https://www.ncbi.nlm.nih.gov/pmc/articles/PMC6566772/.

9. Eric A. Gurzell et al., "DHA-Enriched Fish Oil Targets B Cell Lipid Microdomains and Enhances Ex Vivo and In Vivo B Cell Function," *Journal of Leukocyte Biology* 93, no. 4 (April 2013): 463–70, https://jlb.onlinelibrary.wiley.com/doi/10.1189/jlb.0812394.

10. Bénédicte M. J. Merle et al., "Circulating Omega-3 Fatty Acids and Neovascular Age-Related Macular Degeneration," *Investigative Ophthalmology and Visual Science* 55, no. 3 (March 2014) 2010–19, https://iovs.arvojournals.org/article.aspx?articleid=2190485.

11. Linus Pauling Institute, Micronutrient Information Center, "Essential Fatty Acids," Oregon State University (June 2019), https://lpi.oregonstate.edu/mic/other-nutrients/essential-fatty-acids.

12. Heart Health, "Why Not Flaxseed Oil?" Harvard Medical School, July 29, 2019, https://www.health.harvard.edu/heart-health/why-not-flaxseed-oil.

13. Linus Pauling Institute, "Essential Fatty Acids," Oregon State University.

14. H. Gerster, "Can Adults Adequately Convert Alpha-Linolenic Acid (18:3n-3) to Eicosapentaenoic Acid (20:5n-3) and Docosahexaenoic Acid (22:6n-3)?" *International Journal of Vitamin and Nutrition Research* 68, no. 3 (1998): 159–73, https://pubmed.ncbi.nlm.nih.gov/9637947/.

15. James J. DiNicolantonio and James H. O'Keefe, "Importance of Maintaining a Low Omega–6/Omega–3 Ratio for Reducing Inflammation, *British Medical Journal* 5, no. 2 (November 15, 2018), https://openheart.bmj.com/content/5/2/e000946.

16. A. P. Simopoulos, "The Importance of the Ratio of Omega-6/Omega-3 Essential Fatty Acids," *Biomedicine and Pharmacotherapy* 56, no. 8 (October 2002): 365–79, https://pubmed.ncbi.nlm.nih.gov/12442909/.

17. National Institutes of Health, Office of Dietary Supplements, "Omega-3 Fatty Acids: Fact Sheet for Health Professionals" (February 15, 2023), https://ods.od.nih.gov/factsheets/Omega3FattyAcids-HealthProfessional/.

18. "Fish Oil Market—Global Industry Assessment & Forecast," *Vantage Market Research* (April 2022), https://www.vantagemarketresearch.com/industry-report/fish-oil-market-1434.

19. Michael J. Orlich, "Vegetarian Dietary Patterns and Mortality in Adventist Health Study," *JAMA Internal Medicine* 173, no. 13 (July 8, 2013): 1230–38, https://www.ncbi.nlm.nih.gov/pmc/articles/PMC4191896/.

20. Tiffany Duong, "Here Are Three Sustainable Seafood Brands to Know for World Oceans Day," *EcoWatch* (June 4, 2021), https://www.ecowatch.com/sustainable-seafood-2653237380.html.

21. Ocean Robbins, "Is Eating Fish Good For You?" Food Revolution Network (November 15, 2019), https://foodrevolution.org/blog/health-and-environmental-impacts-of-eating-fish/

22. Robert H. Schmerling, "Could Eating Fish Increase Your Risk of Cancer?" Harvard Health Publishing, July 26, 2022, https://www.health.harvard.edu/blog/could-eating-fish-increase-your-risk-of-cancer-202207262789.

23. Şevket Metin Kara, Volkan Gul, and Mustafa Kiralan, "Fatty Acid Composition of Hempseed Oils from Different Locations in Turkey," *Spanish Journal of Agricultural Research* 8, no. 2 (June 2010), https://www.researchgate.net/publication/44293885_Fatty_acid_composition_of_hempseed_oils_from_different_locatins_in_Turkey.

24. Amelia R. Sherry, "Spotlight on Stearidonic Acid—Learn More About This Alternative Omega-3 Fatty Acid," *Today's Dietitian* 16, no. 7 (July 2014): 18, https://www.todaysdietitian.com/newarchives/070114p18.shtml.

25. Food Data Central, "Seaweed, Wakame, Raw," USDA Agricultural Research Service (April 2018), https://fdc.nal.usda.gov/fdc-app.html#/food-details/170496/nutrients.

26. Kathy Fackelmann, "Tests Find Many Popular Omega 3 Supplements Are Rancid," George Washington University School of Medicine & Health Sciences (September 28, 2023), https://smhs.gwu.edu/news/tests-find-many-popular-omega-3-supplements-are-rancid.

Chapter 4

1. Jan Trofast, "Berzelius' Discovery of Selenium," *Chemistry International* (September–October 2011): 16–19, https://www.degruyter.com/document/doi/10.1515/ci.2011.33.5.16/pdf.

2. "Selenocysteine," Science Direct, https://www.sciencedirect.com/topics/biochemistry-genetics-and-molecular-biology/selenocysteine.

3. Nicole, "How to Consume Enough Selenium on a Vegan Diet," *Lettuce Veg Out* (October 31, 2023), https://lettucevegout.com/vegan-nutrition/selenium/.

4. P. Goyens et al., "Selenium Deficiency as a Possible Factor in the Pathogenesis of Myxoedematous Endemic Cretinism," *Acta Endocrinology* (Copenhagen) 114, no. 4 (April 1987): 497–502, https://pubmed.ncbi.nlm.nih.gov/3577581/.

5. Josef Köhrle, "Selenium, Iodine and Iron—Essential Trace Elements for Thyroid Hormone Synthesis and Metabolism," *International Journal of Molecular Sciences* 24, no. 4 (February 8, 2023): 3393, https://www.mdpi.com/1422-0067/24/4/3393.

6. Rannapaula Lawrynhuk Urbano Ferreira et al., "Selenium in Human Health and Gut Microflora: Bioavailability of Selenocompounds and Relationship with Diseases," *Frontiers in Nutrition* 8 (June 4, 2021), https://www.frontiersin.org/articles/10.3389/fnut.2021.685317/full.

7. National Institutes of Health, Office of Dietary Supplements, "Selenium: Fact Sheet for Health Professionals" (March 26, 2021), https://ods.od.nih.gov/factsheets/Selenium-HealthProfessional/.

8. Nicole, "How to Consume Enough Selenium on a Vegan Diet."

9. NIH, Office of Dietary Supplements, "Selenium: Fact Sheet for Health Professionals," https://ods.od.nih.gov/factsheets/Selenium-HealthProfessional/.

10. Nicole, "How to Consume Enough Selenium on a Vegan Diet."

Chapter 5

1. Maria Maares and Hajo Haase, "A Guide to Human Zinc Absorption: General Overview and Recent Advances of In Vitro Intestinal Models," *Nutrients* 12, no. 3 (March 2020): 762, https://www.ncbi.nlm.nih.gov/pmc/articles/PMC7146416/.

2. Claudia Andreini et al., "Counting the Zinc-Proteins Encoded in the Human Genome," *Journal of Proteome Research* 5, no. 1 (January 2006): 196–201, https://pubmed.ncbi.nlm.nih.gov/16396512/.

3. Ananda S. Prasad, "Lessons Learned from Experimental Human Model of Zinc Deficiency," *Journal of Immunology Research* 2020 (January 9, 2020), hhttps://doi.org/10.1155/2020/9207279.

4. Roya Kelishadi, Hassan Alikhassy, and Masoud Amiri, "Zinc and Copper Status in Children with High Family Risk of Premature Cardiovascular Disease," *Annals of Saudi Medicine* 22, no. 5–6 (September–November 2002): 291–94, https://pubmed.ncbi.nlm.nih.gov/17146244/.

5. Marcin P. Joachimiak, "Zinc Against COVID-19? Symptom Surveillance and Deficiency Risk Groups," *PLoS Neglected Tropical Diseases* 15, no. 1 (January 4, 2021), https://www.ncbi.nlm.nih.gov/pmc/articles/PMC7781367/.

6. Peter Jaret, "Is Zinc Good for Vision?" *WebMD* (September 21, 2023), https://www.webmd.com/eye-health/zinc-vision.

7. Jack Norris, "Zinc," *Vegan Health* (October 2021), https://veganhealth.org/zinc/.

8. Lönnerdal Bo, "Dietary Factors Influencing Zinc Absorption," *Journal of Nutrition* 130, no. 5 (May 2000): 1378S–83S, https://www.sciencedirect.com/science/article/pii/S0022316622140927.

9. Bo, "Dietary Factors Influencing Zinc Absorption."

10. D. R. Bennett et al., "Zinc Toxicity Following Massive Coin Ingestion," *American Journal of Forensic Medicine and Pathology* 18, no. 2 (June 1997):148–53, https://pubmed.ncbi.nlm.nih.gov/9185931/.

11. G. J. Fosmire, "Zinc Toxicity," *American Journal of Clinical Nutrition* 51, no. 2 (February 1990): 225–27, https://pubmed.ncbi.nlm.nih.gov/2407097/.

12. Ulrika M. Agnew and Todd L. Slesinger, *Zinc Toxicity* (StatPearls, 2024), https://www.ncbi.nlm.nih.gov/books/NBK554548/.

13. Nicole Galan, "What Happens When a Person Takes Too Much Zinc?"*Medical News Today* (October 23, 2019), https://www.medicalnewstoday.com articles/326760#recommended-guidelines.

Chapter 6

1. "How Many Cells Are in Your Body?" *National Geographic* (January 13, 2016), https://www.nationalgeographic.com/science/article/how-many-cells-are-in-your-body.

2. Karolin Roemhild et al., "Iron Metabolism: Pathophysiology and Pharmacology," *Trends in Pharmacological Sciences* 42, no. 8 (August 1, 2021): 640–56, https://www.ncbi.nlm.nih.gov/pmc/articles/PMC7611894/.

3. R. Kongkachuichai, P. Napatthalung, and R. Charoensiri, "Heme and Nonheme Iron Content of Animal Products Commonly Consumed in Thailand," *Journal of Food Composition and Analysis* 15, no. 4 (August 2002): 389–98, https://www.sciencedirect.com/science/article/abs/pii/S088915750291080X.

4. "Do Your Products Contain Genetically Modified Ingredients?" https://faq.impossiblefoods.com/hc/en-us/articles/360023038894-Do-your-products-contain-genetically-modified-ingredients-.

5. Ocean Robbins, "The Truth About Iron + Why Plant-Based Foods Are the Best Way to Get the Iron You Need," Food Revolution Network (January 23, 2019), https://foodrevolution.org/blog/iron-rich-foods/.

6. Jamie Eske, "How Does Oxidative Stress Affect the Body?" *Medical News Today* (April 3, 2019), https://www.medicalnewstoday.com/articles/324863.

7. Sandro Altamura and Martina U. Muckenthaler, "Iron Toxicity in Diseases of Aging: Alzheimer's Disease, Parkinson's Disease and Atherosclerosis," *Journal of Alzheimer's Disease* 16, no. 4 (2009): 879–95, https://pubmed.ncbi.nlm.nih.gov/19387120/.

8. British Nutrition Foundation, "Iron as a Pro-Oxidant" in *Iron: Nutritional and Physiological Significance* (Springer, 1995), 33–41, https://link.springer.com/chapter/10.1007/978-94-011-0585-9_6.

9. Joanna Kaluza, Alicja Wolk, and Susanna C. Larsson, "Heme Iron Intake and Risk of Stroke: A Prospective Study of Men, *Stroke* 44, no. 2 (February 2013): 334–39, https://pubmed.ncbi.nlm.nih.gov/23306319/.

10. Wei Yang et al., "Is Heme Iron Intake Associated with Risk of Coronary Heart Disease? A Meta-Analysis of Prospective Studies," *European Journal of Nutrition* 53, no. 2 (2014): 395–400, https://pubmed.ncbi.nlm.nih.gov/23708150/.

11. Wei Bao et al., "Dietary Iron Intake, Body Iron Stores, and the Risk of Type 2 Diabetes: A Systematic Review and Meta-Analysis," *BMC Medicine* 10, no. 1 (October 10, 2012): 119, https://pubmed.ncbi.nlm.nih.gov/23046549/.

12. Nadia M. Bastide, Fabrice H.F. Pierre, and Denis E. Corpet, "Heme Iron from Meat and Risk of Colorectal Cancer: A Meta-Analysis and a Review of the Mechanisms Involved," *Cancer Prevention Research* (Philadelphia) 4, no. 2 (February 2011): 177–84, https://aacrjournals.org/cancerpreventionresearch/article/4/2/177/49367/Heme-Iron-from-Meat-and-Risk-of-Colorectal-Cancer.

13. Gwyneth K. Davey et al., "EPIC-Oxford: Lifestyle Characteristics and Nutrient Intakes in a Cohort of 33,883 Meat-Eaters and 31,546 Non Meat-Eaters in the UK," *Public Health Nutrition* 6, no. 3 (May 2003): 259–69, https://pubmed.ncbi.nlm.nih.gov/12740075/.

14. Lisa M. Haider et al., "The Effect of Vegetarian Diets on Iron Status in Adults: A Systematic Review and Meta-Analysis," *Critical Reviews in Food Science and Nutrition* 58, no. 8 (May 24, 2018): 1359–74, https://pubmed.ncbi.nlm.nih.gov/27880062/.

15. National Institutes of Health, Office of Dietary Supplements, "Iron: Fact Sheet for Health Professionals" (January 15, 2023), https://ods.od.nih.gov/factsheets/Iron-HealthProfessional/#h2.

16. Mayo Clinic Staff, "Anemia" (May 11, 2023), https://www.mayoclinic.org/diseases-conditions/anemia/symptoms-causes/syc-20351360.

17. Ocean Robbins, "What Are Antinutrients? And Do You Need to Avoid Them?" Food Revolution Network, June 17, 2022, https://foodrevolution.org/blog/what-are-antinutrients/.

18. Michael Greger, "Does Coffee Inhibit Iron Absorption? What Are the Effects of Having Too Much Iron?" NutritionFacts.org, March 8, 2023, https://nutritionfacts.org/video/does-coffee-inhibit-iron-absorption-what-are-the-effects-of-having-too-much-iron/.

19. Meredith James, "Vegan Sources of Vitamin A: The Plant Eater's Guide," Tofubud, https://tofubud.com/blogs/tips/vegan-sources-of-vitamin-a.

20. P. D. Prinsen Geerligs, B. J. Brabin, A. A. Omari, "Food Prepared in Iron Cooking Pots as an Intervention for Reducing Iron Deficiency Anaemia in Developing Countries: A Systematic Review," *Journal of Human Nutrition and Dietetics* 16, no. 4 (August 2003): 275–81, https://pubmed.ncbi.nlm.nih.gov/12859709/.

21. Ocean Robbins, "Amazing Alliums—Why These Disease-Fighting Veggies Are Worth Eating Every Day!" Food Revolution Network, January 25, 2019, https://foodrevolution.org/blog/allium-vegetables/.

22. Centers for Disease Control and Prevention, Genomics & Precision Health, "Hereditary Hemochromatosis," May 20, 2022, https://www.cdc.gov/genomics/disease/hemochromatosis.htm.

Chapter 7

1. National Institutes of Health, Office of Dietary Supplements, "Magnesium: Fact Sheet for Health Professionals," June 2, 2022, https://ods.od.nih.gov/factsheets/Magnesium-HealthProfessional.

2. James J. DiNicolantonio, James H. O'Keefe, and William Wilson, "Subclinical Magnesium Deficiency: A Principal Driver of Cardiovascular Disease and a Public Health Crisis," *Open Heart* 5, no. 1 (January 13, 2018): e000668, https://www.ncbi.nlm.nih.gov/pmc/articles/PMC5786912/.

3. Andrea Rosanoff, Connie M. Weaver, and Robert K. Rude, "Suboptimal Magnesium Status in the United States: Are the Health Consequences Underestimated?" *Nutrition Reviews* 70, no. 3 (March 2012):153–64, https://pubmed.ncbi.nlm.nih.gov/22364157/.

4. DiNicolantonio, O'Keefe, and Wilson, "Subclinical Magnesium Deficiency."

5. NIH, Office of Dietary Supplements, "Magnesium: Fact Sheet for Health Professionals."

6. Linus Pauling Institute, Micronutrient Information Center, "Magnesium," Oregon State University (February 2019), https://lpi.oregonstate.edu/mic/minerals/magnesium.

7. Faheemuddin Ahmed and Abdul Mohammed, "Magnesium: The Forgotten Electrolyte—A Review on Hypomagnesemia," *Medical Sciences* (Basel) 7, no. 4 (April 2019): 56, https://www.ncbi.nlm.nih.gov/pmc/articles/PMC6524065/.

8. Jiang Wu et al., "Circulating Magnesium Levels and Incidence of Coronary Heart Diseases, Hypertension, and Type 2 Diabetes Mellitus: A Meta-Analysis of Prospective Cohort Studies," *Nutrition Journal* 16, no. 1 (September 19, 2017): 60, https://www.ncbi.nlm.nih.gov/pmc/articles/PMC5606028/.

9. S. Miller et al., "Effects of Magnesium on Atrial Fibrillation after Cardiac Surgery: A Meta-Analysis," *Heart* 91, no. 5 (May 2005): 618–23, https://www.ncbi.nlm.nih.gov/pmc/articles/PMC1768903/.

10. Xin Fang et al., "Dose-Response Relationship between Dietary Magnesium Intake and Risk of Type 2 Diabetes Mellitus: A Systematic Review and Meta-Regression Analysis of Prospective Cohort Studies," *Nutrients* 8, no. 11 (November 2016): 739, https://www.ncbi.nlm.nih.gov/pmc/articles/PMC5133122/.

11. Ailsa A. Welch, Jane Skinner, and Mary Hickson, "Dietary Magnesium May Be Protective for Aging of Bone and Skeletal Muscle in Middle and Younger Older Age Men and Women: Cross-Sectional Findings from the UK Biobank Cohort," *Nutrients* 9, no. 11 (November 2017): 1189, https://www.ncbi.nlm.nih.gov/pmc/articles/PMC5707661/.

12. Behnood Abbasi et al., "The Effect of Magnesium Supplementation on Primary Insomnia in Elderly: A Double-Blind Placebo-Controlled Clinical Trial," *Journal of Research in Medical Sciences* 17, no. 12 (December 2012): 1161–69, https://pubmed.ncbi.nlm.nih.gov/23853635/.

13. Robert Vink and Mihai Nechifor, eds., *Magnesium in the Central Nervous System* (University of Adelaide Press, 2011), https://www.ncbi.nlm.nih.gov/books/NBK507271/.

14. Vink and Nechifor, eds., *Magnesium in the Central Nervous System.*

15. Emily K. Tarleton et al., "Role of Magnesium Supplementation in the Treatment of Depression: A Randomized Clinical Trial," *PLoS One* 12, no. 6 (June 2017): e0180067, https://www.ncbi.nlm.nih.gov/pmc/articles/PMC5487054/.

16. National Institutes of Health, Office of Dietary Supplements, "Magnesium: Fact Sheet for Consumers," https://ods.od.nih.gov/factsheets/Magnesium-Consumer/.

17. D. Siegenberg et al., "Ascorbic Acid Prevents the Dose-Dependent Inhibitory Effects of Polyphenols and Phytates on Nonheme-Iron Absorption," *American Journal of Clinical Nutrition* 52, no. 2 (February 1991): 537–41, https://pubmed.ncbi.nlm.nih.gov/1989423/.

18. Rena Goldman, "Ten Foods High in Magnesium," *Medical News Today*, November 8, 2023, https://www.medicalnewstoday.com/articles/318595.

19. Franziska Spritzler, "10 Magnesium-Rich Foods That Are Super Healthy," *Healthline*, January 24, 2024, https://www.healthline.com/nutrition/10-foods-high-in-magnesium.

20. NIH, Office of Dietary Supplements, "Magnesium: Fact Sheet for Health Professionals."

Chapter 8

1. T. K. Kenyon, "Science and Celebrity: Humphry Davy's Rising Star," Science History Institute, December 23, 2008, https://sciencehistory.org/stories/magazine/science-and-celebrity-humphry-davys-rising-star/.

2. Martha, "How Much Money Has the Dairy Industry Spend on Advertising?" IGSID.org, November 9, 2021, https://www.icsid.org/business/how-much-money-has-the-dairy-industry-spend-on-advertising/.

3. National Institutes of Health, Office of Dietary Supplements, "Calcium: Fact Sheet for Consumers," September 14, 2023, https://ods.od.nih.gov/factsheets/Calcium-Consumer/.

4. Andrew R. Marks, "Calcium and the Heart: A Question of Life and Death," *Journal of Clinical Investigation* 111, no. 5 (March 1, 2003): 597–600, https://www.ncbi.nlm.nih.gov/pmc/articles/PMC151912/.

5. NIH, Office of Dietary Supplements, "Calcium: Fact Sheet for Consumers."

6. NIH, Office of Dietary Supplements, "Calcium: Fact Sheet for Health Professionals," January 3, 2034, https://ods.od.nih.gov/factsheets/Calcium-HealthProfessional/.

7. Judith C. Thalheimer, "Questions on Calcium and Vitamin D Recommendations," *Today's Geriatric Medicine* 9, no. 4 (July/August 2016): 30, http://www.todaysgeriatricmedicine.com/archive/JA16p30.shtml.

8. "Dairy Lobbying," OpenSecrets.org, https://www.opensecrets.org/industries/lobbying.php?ind=A04++.

9. Markham Heid, "Experts Say Lobbying Skewed the U.S. Dietary Guidelines," *Time*, January 8, 2016, https://time.com/4130043/lobbying-politics-dietary-guidelines/.

10. Harvard Medical Publishing, "How Much Calcium Do You Really Need?" February 2, 2022, https://www.health.harvard.edu/staying-healthy/how-much-calcium-do-you-really-need.

11. Roland L. Weinsier and Carlos L. Krumdieck, "Dairy Foods and Bone Health: Examination of the Evidence," *American Journal of Clinical Nutrition* 72, no. 3 (September 2000): 681–89, https://www.sciencedirect.com/science/article/pii/S0002916523067588.

12. James Colquhoun, "The Truth About Calcium and Osteoporosis," *Food Matters*, November 24, 2009, https://www.foodmatters.com/article/the-truth-about-calcium-and-osteoporosis.

13. Emily Yoffe, "Got Osteoporosis? Maybe All That Milk You've Been Drinking Is to Blame," *Slate*, August 3, 1999, https://slate.com/news-and-politics/1999/08/got-osteoporosis.html.

14. Dagfinn Aune et al., "Dairy Products, Calcium, and Prostate Cancer Risk: A Systematic Review and Meta-Analysis of Cohort Studies," *American Journal of Clinical Nutrition* 101, no. 1 (January 2015): 87–117, https://www.ncbi.nlm.nih.gov/pubmed/25527754.

15. J. Ji, J. Sundquist, and K. Sundquist, "Lactose Intolerance and Risk of Lung, Breast and Ovarian Cancers: Aetiological Clues from a Population-Based Study in Sweden," *British Journal of Cancer* 112, no. 1 (January 6, 2015): 149–52, https://www.ncbi.nlm.nih.gov/pubmed/25314053.

16. "Dairy," NutritionFacts.org, https://nutritionfacts.org/topics/dairy/.

17. Helen Thompson, "An Evolutionary Whodunit: How Did Humans Develop Lactose Tolerance?" NPR, December 28, 2012, https://www.npr.org/sections/thesalt/2012/12/27/168144785/an-evolutionary-whodunit-how-did-humans-develop-lactose-tolerance.

18. Ocean Robbins, "The Surprising Truth About Antibiotics, Factory Farms, and Food Recalls," Food Revolution Network, November 29, 2023, https://foodrevolution.org/blog/antibiotic-resistance-factory-farms/.

19. Birgit Teucher et al., "Sodium and Bone Health: Impact of Moderately High and Low Salt Intakes on Calcium Metabolism in Postmenopausal Women," *Journal of Bone and Mineral Research* 23, no. 9 (September 2008): 1477–85, https://pubmed.ncbi.nlm.nih.gov/18410231/.

20. E. A. Krall, B. Dawson-Hughes, "Smoking Increases Bone Loss and Decreases Intestinal Calcium Absorption," *Journal of Bone and Mineral Research* 14, no. 2 (February 1999): 215–20, https://pubmed.ncbi.nlm.nih.gov/9933475/.

21. C. M. Weaver and K. L. Plawecki, "Dietary Calcium: Adequacy of a Vegetarian Diet," *American Journal of Clinical Nutrition* 59 (5 Supplement, May 1994): 1238S–241S, https://pubmed.ncbi.nlm.nih.gov/8172128/.

22. R. P. Heaney and C. M. Weaver, "Calcium Absorption from Kale," *American Journal of Clinical Nutrition* 51, no. 4 (April 1990): 656–57, https://pubmed.ncbi.nlm.nih.gov/2321572/.

23. Catherine Burt Driver, "Osteoporosis and Calcium," *eMedicine Health*, https://www.emedicinehealth.com/osteoporosis_and_calcium/article_em.htm.

24. A. Zittermann et al., "Evidence for an Acute Rise of Intestinal Calcium Absorption in Response to Aerobic Exercise," *European Journal of Nutrition* 41, no. 5 (October 2002):189–96, https://pubmed.ncbi.nlm.nih.gov/12395212/.

25. Jack Norris, "Calcium," Vegan Health, https://veganhealth.org/calcium-part-2.

26. Charles Patrick Davis, "Kidney Stones: Symptoms, Causes, and Treatment," MedicineNet (7/1/2021), https://www.medicinenet.com/kidney_stone_pictures_slideshow/article.htm.

27. Mark J. Bolland et al., "Vascular Events in Healthy Older Women Receiving Calcium Supplementation: Randomised Controlled Trial," *British Journal of Medicine* 336 (February 2, 2008): 262–26, https://pubmed.ncbi.nlm.nih.gov/18198394/.

28. National Institutes of Health, Office of Dietary Supplements, "Calcium: Fact Sheet for Consumers," September 14, 2023, https://ods.od.nih.gov/factsheets/Calcium-Consumer/.

Chapter 9

1. "Dichlorine, Dibromine, and Diiodine," LibreTexts, https://chem.libretexts.org/Bookshelves/ Inorganic_Chemistry/Map%3A_Inorganic_Chemistry_(Housecroft)/17%3A_The_Group_17 _Elements/17.04%3A_The_Elements/17.4B%3A_Dichlorine_Dibromine_and_Diiodine.

2. National Institutes of Health, National Institute of Diabetes and Digestive and Kidney Diseases, "Hypothyroidism (Underactive Thyroid)" (March 2021), https://www.niddk.nih.gov/ health-information/endocrine-diseases/hypothyroidism.

3. "Goiter," American Thyroid Association, https://www.thyroid.org/goiter/.

4. National Institutes of Health, National Institute of Diabetes and Digestive and Kidney Diseases, "Hyperthyroidism (Overactive Thyroid)" (August 2021), https://www.niddk.nih.gov/ health-information/endocrine-diseases/hyperthyroidism.

5. National Institutes of Health, Office of Dietary Supplements, "Iodine: Fact Sheet for Consumers" (July 2, 2022), https://ods.od.nih.gov/factsheets/Iodine-Consumer/.

6. NIH, Office of Dietary Supplements, "Iodine: Fact Sheet for Consumers."

7. Global Health Now, "Iodized Salt," Johns Hopkins Bloomberg School of Public Health, https:// globalhealthnow.org/object/iodized-salt.

8. Ocean Robbins, "Are Sea Vegetables Good for You and the Planet?—And Are Some Better Than Others?" Food Revolution Network, October 20, 2021, https://foodrevolution.org/blog/ are-sea-vegetables-good-for-you/.

9. Theodore T. Zava and David T. Zava, "Assessment of Japanese Iodine Intake Based on Seaweed Consumption in Japan: A Literature-Based Analysis," *Thyroid Research* 4 (October 5, 2011): 14, https://www.ncbi.nlm.nih.gov/pmc/articles/PMC3204293/.

10. National Institutes of Health, Office of Dietary Supplements, "Vitamin K: Fact Sheet for Health Professionals" (March 29, 2021), https://ods.od.nih.gov/factsheets/VitaminK-HealthProfessional/.

11. Ocean Robbins, "Vitamin K: Benefits, How to Get It, and How Much You Need," Food Revolution Network, February 17, 2021, https://foodrevolution.org/blog/vitamin-k-benefits/.

12. Linus Pauling Institute, Micronutrient Information Center, "Vitamin K," Oregon State University (July 2022), https://lpi.oregonstate.edu/mic/vitamins/vitamin-K.

13. Sarah Cockayne et al., "Vitamin K and the Prevention of Fractures: Systematic Review and Meta-Analysis of Randomized Controlled Trials," *Archives of Internal Medicine* 166, no. 12 (June 26, 2006): 1256–61, https://pubmed.ncbi.nlm.nih.gov/16801507/.

14. A. Zittermann, "Effects of Vitamin K on Calcium and Bone Metabolism," *Current Opinion in Clinical Nutrition and Metabolic Care* 4, no. 6 (November 2001): 483–87, https://pubmed.ncbi.nlm .nih.gov/11706280/.

15. M. Kyla Shea and Rachel M. Holden, "Vitamin K Status and Vascular Calcification: Evidence from Observational and Clinical Studies," *Advances in Nutrition* 3, no. 2 (March 1, 2012): 158–65, https://pubmed.ncbi.nlm.nih.gov/22516723/.

16. Guylaine Ferland, "Vitamin K and the Nervous System: An Overview of Its Actions," *Advances in Nutrition* 3, no. 2 (March 1, 2012): 204–12, https://pubmed.ncbi.nlm.nih.gov/22516728/.

17. Guylaine Ferland, "Vitamin K, an Emerging Nutrient in Brain Function," *Biofactors 38,* no. 2 (March–April 2012): 151–57, https://pubmed.ncbi.nlm.nih.gov/22419547/.

18. Mitsuru Ishizuka et al., "Effect of Menatetrenone, a Vitamin K2 Analog, on Recurrence of Hepatocellular Carcinoma after Surgical Resection: A Prospective Randomized Controlled Trial," *Anticancer Research* 32, no. 12 (December 2012): 5415–20, https://pubmed.ncbi.nlm.nih.gov/23225445/.

19. Maurice Halder et al., "Vitamin K: Double Bonds beyond Coagulation Insights into Differences between Vitamin K1 and K2 in Health and Disease," *International Journal of Molecular Sciences* 20, no. 4 (February 2019): 896, https://www.ncbi.nlm.nih.gov/pmc/articles/PMC6413124/.

20. Robin J. Marles, Amy L. Roe, and Hellen A. Oketch-Rabah, "US Pharmacopeial Convention Safety Evaluation of Menaquinone-7, a Form of Vitamin K," *Nutrition Reviews* 75, no. 1 (July 1, 2017): 553–78, https://pubmed.ncbi.nlm.nih.gov/28838081/.

21. Halder et al., "Vitamin K: Double Bonds beyond Coagulation."

22. *WebMD* Editorial Contributors, "Top Foods High in Vitamin K2," *WebMD*, November 16, 2022, https://www.webmd.com/diet/foods-high-in-vitamin-k2.

23. L. J. Schurgers and C. Vermeer, "Determination of Phylloquinone and Menaquinones in Food. Effect of Food Matrix on Circulating Vitamin K Concentrations," *Haemostasis* 30, no. 6 (November–December 2000): 298–307, https://pubmed.ncbi.nlm.nih.gov/11356998/.

24. Linus Pauling Institute, Micronutrient Information Center, "Vitamin B12," Oregon State University (November 2023), https://lpi.oregonstate.edu/mic/vitamins/vitamin-B12.

25. Paul Ganguly and Sreyoshi Fatima Alam, "Role of Homocysteine in the Development of Cardiovascular Disease," *Nutrition Journal* 14, no. 6 (published online January 10, 2015), https://www.ncbi.nlm.nih.gov/pmc/articles/PMC4326479/.

26. A. David Smith et al., "Homocysteine and Dementia: An International Consensus Statement," *Journal of Alzheimer's Disease* 62, no. 2 (February 20, 2018): 561–70, https://www.ncbi.nlm.nih.gov/pmc/articles/PMC5836397/.

27. T. A. Ajith, "Homocysteine in Ocular Diseases," *Clinica Chimica Acta* 450 (October 23, 2015): 316–21, https://pubmed.ncbi.nlm.nih.gov/26343924/.

28. Sameh M. Senousy et al., "Association between Biomarkers of Vitamin B12 Status and the Risk of Neural Tube Defects," *Journal of Obstetrics and Gynaecology Research* 44, no. 10 (October 2018): 1902–8, https://pubmed.ncbi.nlm.nih.gov/30043514/.

29. Jarosław Krzywański et al., "Vitamin B12 Status and Optimal Range for Hemoglobin Formation in Elite Athletes," *Nutrients* 12, no. 4 (April 9, 2020): 1038, https://pubmed.ncbi.nlm.nih.gov/32283824/.

30. "Are You Vitamin B$_{12}$ Deficient?" *Agricultural Research* (August 2000), https://agresearchmag.ars.usda.gov/ar/archive/2000/aug/vita0800.pdf.

31. "B12 and the AHDB," *Surge*, https://www.surgeactivism.org/b12ahdb.

32. Fumio Watanabe et al., "Vitamin B$_{12}$-Containing Plant Food Sources for Vegetarians," *Nutrients* 6, no. 5 (May 2014): 1861–73, https://www.ncbi.nlm.nih.gov/pmc/articles/PMC4042564/.

33. Watanabe et al., "Vitamin B$_{12}$-Containing Plant Food Sources for Vegetarians."

34. Palni Kundra et al., "Healthy Adult Gut Microbiota Sustains Its Own Vitamin B12 Requirement in an *in Vitro* Hatch Fermentation Model," *Frontiers in Nutrition* 9 (December 2022), Sec. Nutrition and Microbes, https://www.frontiersin.org/articles/10.3389/fnut.2022.1070155/full.

35. Jean-Louis Guéant, Rosa-Maria Guéant-Rodriguez, and David H. Alpers, "Chapter Nine—Vitamin B12 Absorption and Malabsorption," *Vitamins and Hormones* 119 (2022), 241–74, https://doi.org/10.1016/bs.vh.2022.01.016.

36. Pankaj Vashi et al., "Methylmalonic Acid and Homocysteine as Indicators of Vitamin B-12 Deficiency in Cancer," *PLoS One* 11, no. 1 (January 25, 2016): e0147843, https://www.ncbi.nlm.nih.gov/pmc/articles/PMC4725715/.

37. K. Okuda et al., "Intestinal Absorption and Concurrent Chemical Changes of Methylcobalamin," *Journal of Laboratory and Clinical Medicine* 81, no. 4 (April 1973): 557–67, https://pubmed.ncbi.nlm.nih.gov/4696188/.

38. You and Your Hormones, "Vitamin D," Society for Endocrinology, November 2021, https://www.yourhormones.info/hormones/vitamin-d/.

39. National Institutes of Health, Office of Dietary Supplements, "Vitamin D: Fact Sheet for Health Professionals" (September 18, 2023), https://ods.od.nih.gov/factsheets/VitaminD-HealthProfessional/.

40. Pacharee Manoy et al., "Vitamin D Supplementation Improves Quality of Life and Physical Performance in Osteoarthritis Patients," *Nutrients* 9, no. 8 (August 2017): 799, https://www.ncbi.nlm.nih.gov/pmc/articles/PMC5579593/.

41. NIH, Office of Dietary Supplements, "Vitamin D: Fact Sheet for Health Professionals."

42. Jianmin Han et al., "25-Hydroxyvitamin D and Total Cancer Incidence and Mortality: A Meta-Analysis of Prospective Cohort Studies," *Nutrients* 11, no. 10 (September 26, 2019): 2295, https://pubmed.ncbi.nlm.nih.gov/31561503/.

43. Andraž Dovnik and Nina Fokter Dovnik, "Vitamin D and Ovarian Cancer: Systematic Review of the Literature with a Focus on Molecular Mechanisms," *Cells* 9, no. 2 (February 2020): 335, https://www.ncbi.nlm.nih.gov/pmc/articles/PMC7072673/.

44. Runhua Zhang et al., "Serum 25-Hydroxyvitamin D and the Risk of Cardiovascular Disease: Dose-Response Meta-Analysis of Prospective Studies," *American Journal of Clinical Nutrition* 105, no. 4 (April 2017): 810–19, https://pubmed.ncbi.nlm.nih.gov/28251933/.

45. Kassandra L. Munger et al., "25-Hydroxyvitamin D Deficiency and Risk of MS among Women in the Finnish Maternity Cohort," *Neurology* 89, no. 15 (October 10, 2017): 1578–83, https://pubmed.ncbi.nlm.nih.gov/28904091/.

46. Chen-Yen Yang et al., "The Implication of Vitamin D and Autoimmunity: a Comprehensive Review," *Clinical Reviews in Allergy and Immunology* 45, no. 2 (October 2013): 217–26, https://www.ncbi.nlm.nih.gov/pmc/articles/PMC6047889/.

47. Xinyi Li et al., "The Effect of Vitamin D Supplementation on Glycemic Control in Type 2 Diabetes Patients: A Systematic Review and Meta-Analysis," *Nutrients* 10, no. 3 (March 19, 2018): 375, https://pubmed.ncbi.nlm.nih.gov/29562681/.

48. Shamaila Rafiq and Per Bendix Jeppesen, "Is Hypovitaminosis D Related to Incidence of Type 2 Diabetes and High Fasting Glucose Level in Healthy Subjects: A Systematic Review and Meta-Analysis of Observational Studies," *Nutrients* 10, no. 1 (January 10, 2018): 59, https://pubmed.ncbi.nlm.nih.gov/29320437/.

49. Petre Cristian Ilie, Simina Stefanescu, and Lee Smith, "The Role of Vitamin D in the Prevention of Coronavirus Disease 2019 Infection and Mortality," *Aging Clinical and Experimental Research* 32, no. 7 (May 6, 2020): 1195–98, https://www.ncbi.nlm.nih.gov/pmc/articles/PMC7202265/.

50. Marta Entrenas Castillo et al., "Effect of Calcifediol Treatment and Best Available Therapy versus Best Available Therapy on Intensive Care Unit Admission and Mortality among Patients Hospitalized for COVID-19: A Pilot Randomized Clinical Study," *Journal of Steroid Biochemistry and Molecular Biology* 203 (October 2020): 105751,https://www.sciencedirect.com/science/article/pii/S0960076020302764?via%3Dihub#bibl0005.

51. Beata M. Gruber-Bzura, "Vitamin D and Influenza—Prevention or Therapy?" *International Journal of Molecular Sciences* 19, no. 8 (August 2018): 2419, https://www.ncbi.nlm.nih.gov/pmc/articles/PMC6121423/.

52. Rita Moretti, Maria Elisa Morelli, and Paola Caruso, "Vitamin D in Neurological Diseases: A Rationale for a Pathogenic Impact," *International Journal of Molecular Sciences* 19, no. 8 (August 2018): 2245, https://www.ncbi.nlm.nih.gov/pmc/articles/PMC6121649/.

53. Sue Penckofer et al., "Vitamin D Supplementation Improves Mood in Women with Type 2 Diabetes," *Journal of Diabetes Research* 2017 (September 7, 2017): 8232863, https://www.ncbi.nlm.nih.gov/pmc/articles/PMC5610883/.

54. Megan Brooks, "Endocrine Society Issues Practice Guideline on Vitamin D," *Medscape*, June 7, 2011, https://www.medscape.com/viewarticle/744128.

55. Glenn Cardwell et al., "A Review of Mushrooms as a Potential Source of Dietary Vitamin D," *Nutrients* 10, no. 10 (October 2018): 1498, https://www.ncbi.nlm.nih.gov/pmc/articles/PMC6213178/#:~:text=Whole%20oyster%20mushrooms%20have%20been,46%2C51%2C52%5D.

56. Omeed Sizar et al, *Vitamin D Deficiency* (Statpearls Publishing, 2024), https://www.ncbi.nlm.nih.gov/books/NBK532266/.

57. "Micellization," Science Direct, https://www.sciencedirect.com/topics/chemistry/micellization.

58. Ching-Yun Hsu et al., "Use of Lipid Nanocarriers to Improve Oral Delivery of Vitamins," *Nutrients* 11, no. 1 (January 2019): 68, https://pubmed.ncbi.nlm.nih.gov/30609658/.

59. H. M. Trang et al., "Evidence That Vitamin D3 Increases Serum 25-Hydroxyvitamin D More Efficiently Than Does Vitamin D2," *American Journal of Clinical Nutrition* 68, no. 4 (October 1998): 854–58, https://pubmed.ncbi.nlm.nih.gov/9771862/.

60. NIH, Office of Dietary Supplements, "Vitamin D: Fact Sheet for Health Professionals."

INDEX

A

African fonio pilaf, 210–11

age, protein and, 9

aioli, plant-based, 98

air fryers/air frying, 84, 85

Air-Fryer Crunchy Chickpea and Cauliflower Tacos, 190–91

ALA. *See* omega-3 fatty acids

All-In-One Mexicali Quinoa, 212–13

almonds

    about: calcium and, 62; fiber and, 21; magnesium and, 56; protein and, 11

    Creamy Almond Meets Crunchy Slaw, 116–17

    other recipes with, 102–03, 106–07, 158–59, 172–73

amino acids, 5, 6, 7, 10. *See also* protein

Apple Pie for Breakfast Smoothie, 222–23

apricots, iron and, 48

asparagus

    Asparagus and Black Bean Tasty Tostadas, 188–89

    Living and Thriving Zucchini Noodles with Raw Marinara Sauce, 202–03

    Sip and Shine Asparagus Soup, 140–41

    Tortilla Pizza with, 162–63

avocados

    about: fiber and, 21; oil-free sautéing and, 86

    Delightfully Creamy Avocado Salad with Maple Tahini Dressing, 108–09

    Island Time Kiwi Cooler, 224–25

    other recipes with, 130–31, 170–71, 178–79, 192–93

    other salads/bowls with, 96–97, 106–07, 150–51, 152–53, 154–55

    other wraps/sandwiches with, 100–01, 172–73, 180–81, 184–85, 186–87, 190–91

    Smashed Avocado Chickpea Salad Wrap, 174–75

    Turn Up the Beet Burger with Smashed Avocado and Pickled Onions, 166–67

B

bananas

    Banana Bliss Chocolate Chip Millet Muffins, 94–95

    Golden Sunrise Smoothie, 228–29

Banh Mi Oh My Vietnamese-Inspired Tacos, 184–85

basil, in Kale Walnut Basil Pesto, 170–71

beans and other legumes. *See also* black beans; chickpeas; lentils

    about: canned, 81; cooking, 81; reducing gassiness from, 86–7; soaking, 81; zinc and, 39

    All-In-One Mexicali Quinoa, 212–13

    Asparagus and Black Bean Tasty Tostadas, 188–89

    Clean Out the Pantry Everyday Tacos, 186–87

    Creamy Dreamy Mushrooms, Greens, and Beans Soup, 136–37

    Give Me 10 Minutes to Prep Chili, 218–19

    other recipes with, 120–21, 146–47, 166–67

    other soup recipes with, 128–29, 130–31

    Super Greens and Beans Detox Salad, 112–13

    Turn Up the Beet Burger with Smashed Avocado and Pickled Onions, 166–67

    Under the Italian Sun-Dried Tomato, Cannellini, and Spinach Salad, 110–11

    Warm and Smoky White Bean and Spinach Flautas, 192–93

beets

    Beets 'n' Berries Smoothie Bowl, 230–31

    Turn Up the Beet Burger with Smashed Avocado and Pickled Onions, 166–67

berries

    about: raspberries and fiber, 21

    Beets 'n' Berries Smoothie Bowl, 230–31

    Berrylicious Poppy Seed Pancakes, 92–93

Tangy Blueberry Dressing, 144
black beans
    about: calcium and, 62; cooking, 255, 256–58;
        fiber and, 17, 19, 21; magnesium and, 57;
        protein and, 11
    All-In-One Mexicali Quinoa, 212–13
    Asparagus and Black Bean Tasty Tostadas, 188–89
    Clean Out the Pantry Everyday Tacos, 186–87
    Crunchy Southwest Salad with Zingy Lime
        Dressing, 120–21
    Give Me 10 Minutes to Prep Chili, 218–19
blended meals, 221–35
    Apple Pie for Breakfast Smoothie, 222–23
    Beets 'n' Berries Smoothie Bowl, 230–31
    Golden Sunrise Smoothie, 228–29
    Island Time Kiwi Cooler, 224–25
    Morning Motivator Spiced Shake, 232–33
    Sweet Pumpkin Spice and Everything Nice
        Smoothie Bowl, 234–35
    Wrap Me in Comfort Cold Brew Smoothie,
        226–27
blender, 83
bok choy, 132–33, 154–55
A Bowl of Goodness Tortilla Soup, 130–31
bowls, 143–59. *See also* salads
    Beets 'n' Berries Smoothie Bowl, 230–31
    Bountiful Bulgur Bowl with Savory Orange
        Vinaigrette, 148–49
    Deconstructed Sushi Bowl, 152–53
    Fantastically Fermented Natto Black Rice Bowl,
        154–55
    Purple Paradise Power Bowl, 144–45
    Sweet on You Chili Broccoli and Tofu Bowl,
        156–57
    Sweet Potato Lentil Bowl with Silky Green Tahini
        Sauce, 158–59
    Sweet Pumpkin Spice and Everything Nice
        Smoothie Bowl, 234–35
    The Ultimate Loaded Mashed Potato Bowl,
        146–47
    Zesty Fiesta Mushroom Chorizo Taco Bowl,
        150–51
breads and such. *See also* sandwiches and wraps
    Banana Bliss Chocolate Chip Millet Muffins,
        94–95
    Meet Me in the Mediterranean Tortilla Pizza with
        Tofu Ricotta, 162–63

breakfasts, 89–103
    Banana Bliss Chocolate Chip Millet Muffins,
        94–95
    Berrylicious Poppy Seed Pancakes, 92–93
    Morning Zen Buckwheat Muesli, 102–03
    Rise 'n' Shine Breakfast Hash, 98–99
    Simply Savory Polenta and Greens Breakfast Bowl,
        96–97
    Three-Grain Peaches and Cream Breakfast Bowl,
        90–91
    Wrapped in Wellness Tofu Scramble, 100–101
breastfeeding, protein and, 8–9
Bright and Lively Citrus Salad, 106–107
broccoli
    about: calcium and, 62; sprouts, recipes with,
        178–79, 180–81
    Sweet on You Chili Broccoli and Tofu Bowl,
        156–57
    Veggielicious Mac 'n' Cheese with, 196
buckwheat
    about: cooking, 81, 259, 262–63
    Berrylicious Poppy Seed Pancakes, 92–93
    Morning Zen Buckwheat Muesli, 102–103
    salad with, 108–109
    Simple and Savory Buckwheat Soup, 128–29
    Sweet Pumpkin Spice and Everything Nice
        Smoothie Bowl, 234–35
    Three-Grain Peaches and Cream Breakfast Bowl,
        90–91
    Zesty Ginger Soba Noodle Salad, 206–207
bulgur
    about: cooking, 91, 259, 262–63
    Bountiful Bulgur Bowl with Savory Orange
        Vinaigrette, 148–49
    Super Greens and Beans Detox Salad, 112–13
    Yummy Tabbouleh Salad, 124–25
burgers. *See* sandwiches and wraps
Buttery Vegan Corn Chowder, 138–39

C

cabbage
    Creamy Almond Meets Crunchy Slaw, 116–17
    Deconstructed Sushi Bowl, 152–53
    Lettuce Go to the Farmers Market Salad, 118–19
    Pea-Nuts About You Thai Millet Salad, 122–23
    Pile 'Em High Pad Thai Tofu Burgers, 176–77

Purple Paradise Power Bowl, 144–45
Sweet 'n' Smoky BBQ Tempeh Collard Wrap, 172–73
calcium, 59–63
    about: overview/summary of, 59–61, 63
    amount needed, 61
    benefits and functions, 59–61, 63
    dairy and, 61
    forms and sources of, 59
    magnesium and, 55–56
plant-based sources, 62–63 (*See also specific sources*)
    supplements, 63
cashews
    about: as creamy sauce base, 86; iron and, 48; magnesium and, 56; selenium and, 33; soaking, 87
    Cashew Sour Cream, 100–101
    Clean Out the Pantry Everyday Tacos, 186–87
    5-Minute Cheesy Sauce, 146–47
    Morning Motivator Spiced Shake, 232–33
    other recipes with, 136–37, 156–57, 198–99, 232–33
cauliflower
    about: magnesium and, 56; vitamin K and, 68
    Air Fryer Crunchy Chickpea and Cauliflower Tacos, 190–91
    Nourish and Thrive Immune Support Soup, 134–35
    Veggielicious Mac 'n' Cheese, 196–97
    Wrap Me in Comfort Cold Brew Smoothie, 226–27
    YUM-ami Cacio e Pepe, 198–99
cheese
    Meet Me in the Mediterranean Tortilla Pizza with Tofu Ricotta, 162–63
    Vegan Walnut Parmesan, 114–15
    Veggielicious Mac 'n' Cheese, 196–97
chia seeds
    about: calcium and, 62; chia and flax "eggs," 85; fiber and, 21; magnesium and, 56; omega-3s and, 28, 29
    recipes with, 94–95, 102–103
chickpeas
    about: cooking, 256–58; fiber and, 21; iron and, 48; protein and, 11
    Air-Fryer Crunchy Chickpea and Cauliflower Tacos, 190–91

Bountiful Bulgur Bowl with Savory Orange Vinaigrette, 148–49
Creamy Dreamy Mushrooms, Greens, and Beans Soup, 136–37
Moroccan Baked Chickpeas, 148–49
Nourish and Thrive Immune Support Soup, 134–35
other recipes with, 216–17
Purple Paradise Power Bowl, 144–45
salad recipe with, 118–19
Smashed Avocado Chickpea Salad Wrap, 174–75
A Taste of Africa Fonio Pilaf, 210–11
Wholesome 'n' Hearty One-Pot Farro Roma, 216–17
chili, 10 minutes to prep, 218–19
chocolate
    about: magnesium and, 57
    Banana Bliss Chocolate Chip Millet Muffins, 94–95
citrus
    about: brightening up dishes with, 86
    Bright and Lively Citrus Salad, 106–107
    Savory Orange Vinaigrette, 148–49
    Zingy Lime Dressing, 120
Clean Out the Pantry Everyday Tacos, 186–87
coffee, in Wrap Me in Comfort Cold Brew Smoothie, 226–27
collard greens
    about: calcium and, 62
    other recipes with, 128–29, 174–75
    Sweet 'n' Smoky BBQ Tempeh Collard Wrap, 172–73
corn and polenta. *See also* tacos and tostadas
    Bountiful Bulgur Bowl with Savory Orange Vinaigrette, 148–49
    A Bowl of Goodness Tortilla Soup, 130–31
    Buttery Vegan Corn Chowder, 138–39
    Simply Savory Polenta and Greens Breakfast Bowl, 96–97
couscous, 13, 34, 242, 244–45
Creamy Almond Meets Crunchy Slaw, 116–17
Creamy and Cozy Veggie Ramen, 132–33
Creamy Dreamy Mushrooms, Greens, and Beans Soup, 136–37
Creamy Ginger Dressing, 112
cutting boards, 82

D

dairy, calcium and, 61
date paste, 86
Deconstructed Sushi Bowl, 152–53
detox salad, 112–13
DHA. *See* omega-3 fatty acids
diet, plant-rich
    benefits of, xiii–xiv
    depleted soil and, xviii–xix
    environmental impact, xv
    ethical considerations, xv
    fiber and, xv
    practicality of, xv
    quality of life, longevity and, xiii–xv
dressings. *See* sauces and dressings
Dukkah Seasoning, 158–59

E

edamame
    about: cooking, 237; iron and, 48; protein and, 11
    recipes with, 116–17, 132–33, 152–53, 200–201
environment, plant-rich diet and, xv
EPA. *See* omega-3 fatty acids
equipment, kitchen, 82–4
espresso, in Wrap Me in Comfort Cold Brew
    Smoothie, 226–27
essential amino acid requirements, 10
ethics, plant-rich diet and, xv

F

Fantastically Fermented Natto Black Rice Bowl,
    154–55
farro, 216–17, 242, 244
fiber, 15–21
    about: overview/summary of, 15–16, 21; plant-rich
        diet and, xv
    amount needed, 18–19
    benefits of, 15–18
    how to get enough, 20–21
    Island Time Kiwi Cooler, 224–25
    plant-based sources, 21 (*See also specific sources*)
    prebiotic-rich foods and, 19–20
    soluble and insoluble, 19
    types of, 19–20
    volume of, camping anecdote and, 15–16

flautas, smoky white bean and spinach, 192–93
fonio pilaf, a taste of Africa, 230–31
food processor, 83
frozen fruits and veggies, 80–1
    fruit. *See also specific fruit*
    about: chopping, 85; organic, 86; time-saving tips
        (precut, canned, frozen), 80–1, 85
    Apple Pie for Breakfast Smoothie, 222–23

G

Garden of Goodness Sandwich, 180–81
gassiness, reducing from beans, 86–7
ginger
    Creamy Ginger Dressing, 112
    Ginger Dressing, 206–207
Golden Sunrise Smoothie, 228–29
    grains. *See also* breads and such; buckwheat; bulgur;
        pasta; quinoa; rice, brown; rice and wild rice
    about: cooking by grain type, 259–63; precooked,
        81; soaking, 87, 245; whole grains, 87
    Banana Bliss Chocolate Chip Millet Muffins, 94–5
    Delightfully Creamy Avocado Salad with Maple
        Tahini Dressing, 108–109
    Morning Zen Buckwheat Muesli, 102–103
    A Taste of Africa Fonio Pilaf, 210–11
    Wholesome 'n' Hearty One-Pot Farro Roma,
        216–17
Green Tahini Sauce, 158–59
greens. *See also* collard greens; kale; salads; spinach
    about: iron and, 48
    Creamy Dreamy Mushrooms, Greens, and Beans
        Soup, 136–37
    other recipes with, 128–29, 164–65
sandwiches with (*See* sandwiches and wraps)
    Simply Savory Polenta and Greens Breakfast Bowl,
        96–97
gyro, tempeh, 164–65

H

hash, breakfast, 98–9
hemp seeds
    about: omega-3s and, 28, 29; protein and, 11; zinc
        and, 39
    recipes with, 102–103, 106–107, 124–25, 224–25,
        232–33

I

immune support soup, 134–35
ingredients. *See also specific ingredients*
  money-saving tips, 84–5
  prepping ahead of time, 82
  time-saving tips, 80–4
iodine, 65–68
iron, 43–49
  about: overview/summary of, 43, 49
  absorption of, 45, 47, 48
  "antinutrients," 47, 48
  avoiding excessive, 48
  benefits and functions, 43–45
  excessive, 43, 45–46, 48
  getting enough, 47–48
  as "Goldilocks" nutrient, 43
  types of (heme and nonheme), 45, 46, 47, 48
Island Time Kiwi Cooler, 224–25
It's Slice to Meet You Plant-Powered Pesto Pizza,
  170–71

J

jackfruit, tortilla soup with, 130–31

K

kala namak, 85
kale
  about: calcium and, 62
  Kale Salad, 190–91
  Kale Walnut Basil Pesto, 170–71
  other recipes with, 98–99, 134–35, 136–37,
    144–45, 146–47
  other salads/bowls with, 112–13, 118–19, 120–21
kitchen equipment, time-saving, 82–4
kiwi cooler, 224–25
knives, 82

L

lactation, protein and, 8–9
  lemon/lime. *See* citrus
lentils
  about: calcium and, 63; cooking, 81, 238–39; fiber
    and, 21; iron and, 48; protein and, 11; selenium
    and, 33; zinc and, 39
  Rise 'n' Shine Breakfast Hash, 98–99

Super Greens and Beans Detox Salad, 112–13
Sweet Potato Lentil Bowl with Silky Green Tahini
  Sauce, 158–59
Zesty Fiesta Mushroom Chorizo Taco Bowl,
  150–51
Lettuce Go to the Farmers Market Salad, 118–19
lima beans, 21, 237, 239–40

M

magnesium, 51–57
  about: overview/summary of, 51–53, 57
  amount needed, 55–56
  "antinutrients," 55
  benefits and functions, 53, 54–55
  calcium/zinc supplements and, 55–56
  deficiency, symptoms/causes, 53, 57
  food sources of, 56–57 (*See also specific sources*)
  getting enough from food, 51–53
  importance of, 51
  loss of, causes of, 57
  phytic acid and, 55
  supplements, 57
mandoline, 83
maple syrup, 86
marinara sauce, raw, 202–203
mayo, spicy, 168
Meet Me in the Mediterranean Tortilla Pizza with
  Tofu Ricotta, 162–63
metric conversion chart, 246
Miso Peanut Dressing, 118
Miso Zen Spicy Noodle Bowl, 200–201
money-saving tips, 84–5
Morning Motivator Spiced Shake, 232–33
Morning Zen Buckwheat Muesli, 102–103
muesli, 102–103
multifunction cookers, 83–4
mushrooms
  about: selenium and, 33; zinc and, 39
  Banh Mi Oh My Vietnamese-Inspired Tacos,
    184–5
  Creamy Dreamy Mushrooms, Greens, and Beans
    Soup, 136–37
  Miso Zen Spicy Noodle Bowl, 200–201
  other recipes with, 106–107, 98–9, 128–29,
    132–33, 156–57, 198–99, 216–17
  Presto Pesto Pasta, 204–205

Zesty Fiesta Mushroom Chorizo Taco Bowl, 150–51

N

noodles/pasta
Creamy and Cozy Veggie Ramen, 132–33
Living and Thriving Zucchini Noodles with Raw Marinara Sauce, 202–203
Miso Zen Spicy Noodle Bowl, 200–201
Perfectly Balanced 15-Minute Pasta Salad, 114–15
Pot-to-Plate Tempeh Sausage Pasta, 214–15
Presto Pesto Pasta, 204–205
Veggielicious Mac 'n' Cheese, 196–97
YUM-ami Cacio e Pepe, 198–99
Zesty Ginger Soba Noodle Salad, 206–207
Nourish and Thrive Immune Support Soup, 134–35
nutrients. *See also specific nutrients*
about: overview of, xvi; this book and, xix
depleted soil and, xxviii–xix
plant-based diet and, xix
nuts and seeds. *See also* almonds; cashews; chia seeds; hemp seeds; peanuts and peanut butter; tahini sauces
about: chia and flax "eggs," 85; nut-free options, 86; protein and, 11, 12, 13; sesame seeds and calcium, 62
Berrylicious Poppy Seed Pancakes, 92–3
Creamy Almond Meets Crunchy Slaw, 116–17
Sweet and Savory Pecan Topping, 90
Vegan Walnut Parmesan, 114–15

O

oats
about: fiber and, 21
Apple Pie for Breakfast Smoothie, 228–29
Morning Zen Buckwheat Muesli, 102–103
other recipes with, 92–3, 166–67
oil-free sautéing, 86
omega-3 fatty acids, 23–29
about: overview/summary of, 23–24, 29
ALA (alpha-linoleic acid), 23, 25–26, 28
amount needed, 26
descriptions, functions, and effects, 25–26
DHA (docosahexaenoic acid), 23, 25–26, 27, 28–29

EPA (eicosapentaenoic acid), 23, 25–26, 27, 28–29
fish, fish oil and, 26–28, 29
importance and benefits/functions, 23–24
plant-based sources, 28–29
types of, 23
one-pot, one-pan meals, 209–19
about: overview of, 82
All-In-One Mexicali Quinoa, 212–13
Give Me 10 Minutes to Prep Chili, 218–19
Pot-to-Plate Tempeh Sausage Pasta, 214–15
A Taste of Africa Fonio Pilaf, 210–11
onions, pickled red, 166
organic food, 86

P

pancakes, poppy seed, 92–3
pasta. *See* noodles/pasta
peaches and cream breakfast bowl, three-grain, 90–1
peanuts and peanut butter
about: magnesium and, 56; protein and, 11
Miso Peanut Dressing, 118
Pea-Nuts About You Thai Millet Salad, 122–23
peas
about: cooking, 238, 239–40; fiber and, 21; zinc and, 39
recipes with, 122–23, 204–205
Perfectly Balanced 15-Minute Pasta Salad, 114–15
physical activity, protein and, 7–8
phytic acid, 55
Pickled Red Onions, 166
Pico de Gallo, 188–9
pizza
It's Slice to Meet You Plant-Powered Pesto Pizza, 170–71
Meet Me in the Mediterranean Tortilla Pizza with Tofu Ricotta, 162–63
polenta, 96–97, 242, 244–45
potatoes. *See also* sweet potatoes
about: magnesium and, 57
The Ultimate Loaded Mashed Potato Bowl, 146–47
Pot-to-Plate Tempeh Sausage Pasta, 214–15
powders, protein, 12–13
practicality of diet, xvi

pregnancy, lactation, 18–19

pregnancy, protein and, 8–9

prepping ahead of time, 82

protein, 3–13

about: plant-based diet overview/summary and, 5–6, 13

age and, 9

amino acids and, 5, 6, 7, 10

animal vs. plant, 10–2

author's father and, 3–5

deficiency, symptoms, 6

defined, 5, 6

diets high in, 11–12

essential amino acid requirements, 10

excessive, 11–12

muscle strength and, 3–5

physical activity and, 7–8

plant-based, 10–11, 13

powders, about, 12–13

pregnancy, lactation and, 8–9

quality of, 10–11

requirements, 6–10, 13

sources of plant, 11 (*See also specific sources*)

stress and, 8, 9

weight and, 7

pumpkin

about: seeds, and magnesium/zinc, 39, 56

Sweet Pumpkin Spice and Everything Nice Smoothie Bowl, 234–35

Q

quinoa

about: cooking, 81, 242, 244–45; magnesium and, 56; protein and, 11; zinc and, 39

All-In-One Mexicali Quinoa, 212–13

other recipes with, 90–91, 106–107, 110–11

R

Raw Marinara Sauce, 202–203

recipes. *See also specific main ingredients; specific recipes*

about: overview of, 80

global recommendations, 85–7

money-saving tips, 84–5

time-saving tips, 80–4

rice, brown

about: magnesium and, 57; selenium and, 33

Creamy and Cozy Veggie Ramen, 132–33

Deconstructed Sushi Bowl, 152–53

Fantastically Fermented Natto Black Rice Bowl, 154–55

Rolled Up with Love Vegetable Temaki Hand Roll, 178–79

Sweet on You Chili Broccoli and Tofu Bowl, 156–57

Zesty Fiesta Mushroom Chorizo Taco Bowl, 150–51

rice and wild rice

about: cooking, 243, 244–45; zinc and, 39

Fantastically Fermented Natto Black Rice Bowl, 154–55

Rise 'n' Shine Breakfast Hash, 98–99

Rolled Up with Love Vegetable Temaki Hand Roll, 178–79

S

salad dressings. *See* sauces and dressings

salads, 105–25. *See also* bowls

Bright and Lively Citrus Salad, 106–107

Creamy Almond Meets Crunchy Slaw, 116–17

Crunchy Southwest Salad with Zingy Lime Dressing, 120–21

Delightfully Creamy Avocado Salad with Maple Tahini Dressing, 108–109

dressings (*See* sauces and dressings; *specific salads*)

Kale Salad, 190

Lettuce Go to the Farmers Market Salad, 118–19

Pea-Nuts About You Thai Millet Salad, 122–23

Perfectly Balanced 15-Minute Pasta Salad, 114–15

Smashed Avocado Chickpea Salad Wrap, 174–75

Super Greens and Beans Detox Salad, 112–13

Under the Italian Sun-Dried Tomato, Cannellini, and Spinach Salad, 110–11

Yummy Tabbouleh Salad, 124–25

salt, kala namak, 85

salt, tips for using, 87

sandwiches and wraps. *See also* pizza; tacos and tostadas

Garden of Goodness Sandwich, 180–81

Pile 'Em High Pad Thai Tofu Burgers, 176–77

Rolled Up with Love Vegetable Temaki Hand Roll, 178–79

Seoul-ful TLT with Pickled Veggies and Spicy Mayo, 168–69

Smashed Avocado Chickpea Salad Wrap, 174–75

Smothered in Tzatziki Tempeh Gyro, 164–65

Sweet 'n' Smoky BBQ Tempeh Collard Wrap, 172–73

Turn Up the Beet Burger with Smashed Avocado and Pickled Onions, 166–67

Wrapped in Wellness Tofu Scramble, 100–101

sauces and dressings
  about: making ahead, 85
  BBQ Sauce, 172–73
  Cashew Sour Cream, 100–101
  Creamy Ginger Dressing, 112
  5-Minute Cheesy Sauce, 146–47
  Ginger Dressing, 206–207
  Green Tahini Sauce, 158–59
  Kale Walnut Basil Pesto, 170–71
  Miso Peanut Dressing, 118
  Pico de Gallo, 188–89
  Plant-Based Aioli, 98
  Raw Marinara Sauce, 202–203
  Savory Orange Vinaigrette, 148–49
  Spicy Mayo, 168
  Sweet and Savory Pecan Topping, 90
  Tahini Sauce, 100–101
  Tangy Blueberry Dressing, 144
  Turmeric Tahini Sauce, 180–81
  Tzatziki Sauce, 164
  Vegan Walnut Parmesan, 114–15
  Zingy Lime Dressing, 120

sausage, tempeh, 214–15

sautéing, oil-free, 86

seeds. See chia seeds; nuts and seeds; tahini sauces

selenium, 31–35
  about: overview/summary of, 31, 35
  amount needed, 33, 34–35
  benefits and functions, 31–33
  excessive, selenosis and, 34–35

sources of, 33–34 (See also specific sources)
  supplements, 35

selenosis, 34–35

Seoul-ful TLT with Pickled Veggies and Spicy Mayo, 168–69

silicone spatulas, 84

Simple and Savory Buckwheat Soup, 128–29

Simply Savory Polenta and Greens Breakfast Bowl, 96–7

Sip and Shine Asparagus Soup, 140–41

slaws. See salads

Smashed Avocado Chickpea Salad Wrap, 174–75

smoothies. See blended meals

Smothered in Tzatziki Tempeh Gyro, 164–65

soil, depleted, xviii–xix

soups and stews, 127–40
  A Bowl of Goodness Tortilla Soup, 130–31
  Buttery Vegan Corn Chowder, 138–39
  Creamy and Cozy Veggie Ramen, 132–33
  Creamy Dreamy Mushrooms, Greens, and Beans Soup, 136–37
  Nourish and Thrive Immune Support Soup, 134–35
  Simple and Savory Buckwheat Soup, 128–29
  Sip and Shine Asparagus Soup, 140–41

sour cream, cashew, 100–101

spinach. See also greens
  about: magnesium and, 56; selenium and, 33
  Bright and Lively Citrus Salad, 106–107
  other recipes with, 100–101, 210–11; bowl, 148–49, 158–59; coolers/shakes, 224–25, 232–33; pasta, 198–99, 214–15; salad, 206–207; sandwiches and wraps, 164–65, 180–81
  Warm and Smoky White Bean and Spinach Flautas, 192–93
  Under the Italian Sun-Dried Tomato, Cannellini, and Spinach Salad, 110–11
  YUM-ami Cacio e Pepe, 198–99

squash
  Veggielicious Mac 'n' Cheese, 196–97
  Wholesome 'n' Hearty One-Pot Farro Roma, 216–17

storage containers, 84

stress, protein and, 8, 9

supplements. See also specific nutrients
  about: coming up short, xviii–xix; effectiveness compared to whole foods, xviii–xix; key ingredients warranting, 65; notable nutrients and, xvi–xix; quality and consistency issues, xvi–xviii
  calcium, 63

iodine, 65–68
magnesium, 57
omega-3 fatty acids, 29
protein powders, 12–13
selenium, 35
vitamin B$_{12}$, 70–73
vitamin D, 74–76
vitamin K, 68–70
zinc, 40–41
sushi bowl, deconstructed, 152–53
Sweet 'n' Smoky BBQ Tempeh Collard Wrap, 172–73
Sweet on You Chili Broccoli and Tofu Bowl, 156–57
sweet potatoes
    other recipes with, 144–45
    Purple Paradise Power Bowl, 138–39
    Rise N' Shine Breakfast Hash, 98–99
    Sweet Potato Lentil Bowl with Silky Green Tahini Sauce, 158–59
Sweet Pumpkin Spice and Everything Nice Smoothie Bowl, 234–35
sweetener, whole-food, 87

T

tabbouleh salad, 124–25
tacos and tostadas, 183–83
    Air Fryer Crunchy Chickpea and Cauliflower Tacos, 190–91
    Asparagus and Black Bean Tasty Tostadas, 188–89
    Banh Mi Oh My Vietnamese-Inspired Tacos, 184–85
    Clean Out the Pantry Everyday Tacos, 186–87
    Warm and Smoky White Bean and Spinach Flautas, 192–93
    Zesty Fiesta Mushroom Chorizo Taco Bowl, 150–51
tahini sauces
    Green Tahini Sauce, 158–59
    Tahini Sauce, 100–101
    Turmeric Tahini Sauce, 180–81
A Taste of Africa Fonio Pilaf, 210–11
tempeh. *See also* tofu
    about: iron and, 48; protein and, 11; time-saving tips, 81–2
    Give Me 10 Minutes to Prep Chili, 218–19

Pot-to-Plate Tempeh Sausage Pasta, 214–15
    Smothered in Tzatziki Tempeh Gyro, 164–65
    Sweet 'n' Smoky BBQ Tempeh Collard Wrap, 172–73
time-saving tips, 80–84. *See also specific recipes*
tofu. *See also* tempeh
    about: calcium and, 62; iron and, 48; pressing, 81, 87; protein and, 11; selenium and, 33, 34; time-saving tips, 81; zinc and, 39
    Meet Me in the Mediterranean Tortilla Pizza with Tofu Ricotta, 162–63
    other recipes with, 140–41, 172–73
    Pile 'Em High Pad Thai Tofu Burgers, 176–77
    Rise 'n' Shine Breakfast Hash, 98–9
    Rolled Up with Love Vegetable Temaki Hand Roll, 178–79
    Seoul-ful TLT with Pickled Veggies and Spicy Mayo, 168–69
    Sweet on You Chili Broccoli and Tofu Bowl, 156–57
    Wrapped in Wellness Tofu Scramble, 100–101
tortillas. *See also* tacos and tostadas
    A Bowl of Goodness Tortilla Soup, 130–31
    Crunchy Tortilla Strips, 120–21
    Meet Me in the Mediterranean Tortilla Pizza with Tofu Ricotta, 162–63
Turmeric Tahini Sauce, 180–81
Turn Up the Beet Burger with Smashed Avocado and Pickled Onions, 166–67
Tzatziki Sauce, 164

U

Under the Italian Sun-Dried Tomato, Cannellini, and Spinach Salad, 110–11

V

vegetables. *See also specific vegetables*
    about: chopping, 85; organic, 86; time-saving tips (precut, canned, frozen), 80–81, 85
    Creamy and Cozy Veggie Ramen, 132–33
    Rolled Up with Love Vegetable Temaki Hand Roll, 178–79
    Seoul-ful TLT with Pickled Veggies and Spicy Mayo, 168–69
    Veggielicious Mac 'n' Cheese, 196–97

vitamin B$_{12}$, 70–73
vitamin D, 74–77
vitamin K, 68–70

W

weight, protein and, 7
Wholesome 'n' Hearty One-Pot Farro Roma, 216–17
Wrap Me in Comfort Cold Brew Smoothie, 226–27
Wrapped in Wellness Tofu Scramble, 100–101

Y

yogurt
Golden Sunrise Smoothie, 228–29
Three-Grain Peaches and Cream Breakfast Bowl, 90–1

Tzatziki Sauce, 164
YUM-ami Cacio e Pepe, 198–99
Yummy Tabbouleh Salad, 124–25

Z

zinc, 37–41
about: overview/summary of, 37, 41
amount needed, 39
"antinutrients," 39
benefits and functions, 41
excessive, 41
getting enough from food, 39–40
plant-based sources, 39 *(See also specific sources)*
supplements, 40–41
Zingy Lime Dressing, 120

ACKNOWLEDGMENTS

We extend our heartfelt gratitude to our cherished partners, Phoenix Robbins and Ricky Russert, whose unwavering support, honest feedback, and enduring love sustain us through late-night research endeavors and wild culinary experiments. To our beloved family members and friends, your nurturing presence enriches our lives, and we are eternally grateful to each and every one of you.

Thank you to Howard Jacobson, who played a massive and essential role in the creation of this book. Howie—your eloquence, humor, and wisdom are extraordinary. Working with you is a profound honor and a true joy.

We are greatly thankful for the love, life, and work of Deo and John Robbins (Ocean's mom and dad), who have deeply touched both of us (in very different yet utterly profound ways), and led the way to Food Revolution Network.

Special thanks to Bobbie and John Dandrea, recipe and taste testers, and Nichole's mom and dad.

We'd like to extend a special thank-you to our official and wonderful recipe testers, Gabrielle Merritt, Tracey Taylor, Patricia Walker, and Adrienne Davis, who put their plant-based culinary caps on with enthusiasm, professionalism, openness, and vigor. Your thoughtful feedback and suggestions for the recipes played a sizable role in shaping this book. Working with all of you has been a joy and a privilege of the highest magnitude.

Profound gratitude to AnnMarie Roth—your steadfast guidance shepherded this project at every turn. Roselynne Mackay, your awe-inspiring creativity brought a unique dimension to our work. Angela MacNeil, your photographic brilliance breathed life into our recipes. Liana Minassian, your framework provided the foundation for this book. Esther Ender, your meticulous proofreading and flexibility ensured the book's accuracy and coherence.

We owe immense thanks to the entire team at Food Revolution Network for your invaluable support, making this book possible.

To Reid Tracy, Patty Gift, Lisa Cheng, Monica O'Connor, and the entire editorial and design teams at Hay House—your belief in us and inspiration brought this project to life. Working alongside you all has been a true pleasure.

Lastly, dear reader, we extend our gratitude to you for your conscientiousness about what you eat and its impact on your health and the environment. Together, one delectable bite at a time, we are crafting healthier lives and a more sustainable future for life on this planet. Thank you for joining us on this delicious journey.

ABOUT THE AUTHORS

OCEAN ROBBINS is a father and a husband; a gardener and a dancer; a TEDx speaker and best-selling author; and is co-founder and CEO of the million-member Food Revolution Network. Born in a log cabin and raised on food his family grew in their garden, his work is rooted in a health-conscious family legacy. Ocean's journey from founding the nonprofit YES! at age 16 to leading a global food revolution movement embodies his commitment to healthy people and a healthy planet.

Ocean's best-selling books, *31-Day Food Revolution* and *Real Superfoods*, offer practical guidance on adopting diets that benefit both human and planetary wellness. His influential TEDx talk, "Eating Your Way To Happiness," has reached over a million viewers, and he's organized and hosted online courses and Summits that have reached more than two million people. Recognized with several prestigious awards, including a National Jefferson Award for Outstanding Public Service and the Freedom's Flame Award, along with a former adjunct professorship at Chapman University, Ocean is on a mission to transform our food system, drive down the chronic disease epidemic, and mobilize people worldwide to be part of the solution.

www.foodrevolution.org

NICHOLE DANDREA-RUSSERT, MS, RDN, is Food Revolution Network's Lead Dietitian and Recipe Developer. Her focus is on plant-based eating for the body and the mind, and for the health of the planet. She is the author of *The Fiber Effect: Stop Counting Calories and Start Counting Fiber for Better Health, The Vegan Athlete's Nutrition Handbook: The Essential Guide for Plant-Based Performance,* and co-author, with Ocean Robbins, of *Real Superfoods*. She's a nutrition spokesperson for The Weather Channel's AMHQ and Pattrn, and has been featured in *Eating Well, Women's Health, Yoga Journal, Forbes Health,* and *Business Insider.* She lives in Atlanta with her husband and rescue pup, Mariposa.

www.purelyplanted.com

Hay House Titles of Related Interest

YOU CAN HEAL YOUR LIFE, the movie,
starring Louise Hay & Friends
(available as an online streaming video)
www.hayhouse.com/louise-movie

THE SHIFT, the movie,
starring Dr. Wayne W. Dyer
(available as an online streaming video)
www.hayhouse.com/the-shift-movie

***

*BEAT CANCER KITCHEN: Deliciously Simple Plant-Based
Anticancer Recipes*, by Chris Wark

*FOOD BABE KITCHEN: More than 100 Delicious, Real Food Recipes
to Change Your Body and Your Life*, by Vani Hari

*THE FOOD MATTERS COOKBOOK: A Simple Gluten-Free Guide
to Transforming Your Health One Meal at a Time*,
by James Colquhoun & Laurentine ten Bosch

*GROW A NEW BODY COOKBOOK: Upgrade Your Brain and Heal
Your Gut with 90+ Plant-Based Recipes*, by Alberto Villoldo, Ph.D.

All of the above are available at your local bookstore,
or may be ordered by contacting Hay House.

***

We hope you enjoyed this Hay House book. If you'd like to receive our online catalog featuring additional information on Hay House books and products, or if you'd like to find out more about the Hay Foundation, please contact:

Hay House LLC, P.O. Box 5100, Carlsbad, CA 92018-5100
(760) 431-7695 or (800) 654-5126
www.hayhouse.com® • www.hayfoundation.org

———

Published in Australia by:
Hay House Australia Publishing Pty Ltd
18/36 Ralph St., Alexandria NSW 2015
Phone: +61 (02) 9669 4299
www.hayhouse.com.au

Published in the United Kingdom by:
Hay House UK Ltd
The Sixth Floor, Watson House,
54 Baker Street, London W1U 7BU
Phone: +44 (0) 203 927 7290
www.hayhouse.co.uk

Published in India by:
Hay House Publishers (India) Pvt Ltd
Muskaan Complex, Plot No. 3,
B-2, Vasant Kunj, New Delhi 110 070
Phone: +91 11 41761620
www.hayhouse.co.in

———

Let Your Soul Grow

Experience life-changing transformation—one video at a time—with guidance from the world's leading experts.

www.healyourlifeplus.com

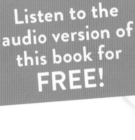